Measuring coverage of essei
and newborn care interventions: A

Edited by

Agbessi Amouzou (Department of International Health, Johns Hopkins
Bloomberg School of Public Health, Baltimore, Maryland, USA)
Liliana Carvajal-Aguirre, **Shane M Khan**, **Vrinda Mehra** (Data and Analytics,
Division of Data, Research and Policy, UNICEF, New York, New York, USA)
Kavita Singh (MEASURE Evaluation/Carolina Population Center, Department of Maternal
and Child Health, UNC-Chapel Hill, Chapel Hill, North Carolina, USA)
Lara ME Vaz (Department of Global Health, Save the Children, Washington DC, USA)

Published in the United Kingdom by Inishmore Laser Scientific Publishing Ltd

Inishmore Laser Scientific Publishing Ltd
Caledonian Exchange, 19a Canning Street, Edinburgh
United Kingdom, EH3 8HE

Printed in Croatia by LaserPlus, Ltd

ISBN-13: 978-1-9999564-1-7

Front cover photocredit: logo produced by United Nations Children's Fund, Data
& Analytics, Division of Data, Research and Policy, New York, NY, USA

Measuring coverage of essential maternal and newborn care interventions: An unfinished agenda

Edited by

Agbessi Amouzou (Department of International Health, Johns Hopkins
Bloomberg School of Public Health, Baltimore, Maryland, USA)
Liliana Carvajal-Aguirre, **Shane M Khan**, **Vrinda Mehra** (Data and Analytics,
Division of Data, Research and Policy, UNICEF, New York, New York, USA)
Kavita Singh (MEASURE Evaluation/Carolina Population Center, Department of Maternal
and Child Health, UNC-Chapel Hill, Chapel Hill, North Carolina, USA)
Lara ME Vaz (Department of Global Health, Save the Children, Washington DC, USA)

2019

Contents

PREFACE

About this collection

Newborn deaths now comprise nearly half of all deaths in children under the age of five years, and improvements in maternal mortality worldwide has been slower than expected. The global community has reached consensus on a recommended package of essential interventions for saving mothers and newborn lives that include interventions delivered to mothers and newborns, and on a set of associated indicators to enable assessment of progress with their scale-up. The Every Newborn Action Plan (ENAP), launched in 2014, includes a monitoring framework and an approach to increase the availability of high quality data on these indicators. The Sustainable Development Goal Framework also includes explicit targets on maternal and neonatal mortality – a reflection of the growing recognition of maternal and newborn survival as core to overall development. These global calls to action have spurred efforts to collect more data on maternal and newborn health. Large population-based household survey programs such as the USAID supported Demographic Health Surveys (DHS) and the UNICEF supported Multiple Indicator Cluster Surveys (MICS), for example, have added new questions and modules to generate better data on newborns. More information on the intrapartum and postnatal periods is also now being collected through health facility surveys and routine health information system.

This book represents a collective effort of experts from academic, non-governmental institutions, large household survey programs, and United Nations agencies to examine how well these new data meet global and national monitoring needs, and any associations they show between the uptake of essential maternal and newborn interventions and health outcomes for the mother and baby. The papers included in the supplement describe the coverage, availability and quality of maternal and newborn interventions, identify data gaps on maternal and newborn health, and compare the methodology used in the MICS and DHS for the measurement of newborn indicators.

Funding for this supplement was provided by the Bill & Melinda Gates Foundation through grants to UNICEF and Countdown to 2015 and Countdown to 2030, by the United States Agency for International Development(USAID) through MEASURE Evaluation (cooperative agreement AID–OAA–

L–14–00004. The views expressed are not necessarily those of USAID or the United States government. Funding for specific papers is noted in the funding section of each paper.

This collection was edited in a collaboration effort by researchers from various institutions: Agbessi Amouzou form the Department of International Health, Johns Hopkins Bloomberg School of Public Health, Baltimore, Maryland, USA. Liliana Carvajal-Aguirre, Shane M Khan and Vrinda Mehra from Data and Analytics, Division of Data, Research and Policy, UNICEF HQ. Kavita Singh from Evaluation/Carolina Population Center, Department of Maternal and Child Health, UNC-Chapel Hill, Chapel Hill, North Carolina, USA and Lara ME Vaz from Department of Global Health, Save the Children, Washington DC, USA.

Acknowledgement

We are grateful to all authors, reviewers and institutions including Johns Hopkins University – Institute for International Programs, the London School of Hygiene and Tropical Medicine, Save the Children-Saving Newborn Lives, MEASURE Evaluation/University of North Carolina Chapel Hill, The Demographic and Health Surveys (DHS) Program, United Nations Children's Fund, USAID, World Health Organization, and others, for their valuable contributions to this collection. We are thankful to Jennifer Harris Requejo from UNICEF for her support in finalizing and publishing this collection

SECTION 1

Commentaries and overview

Why improving the measurement and monitoring of essential maternal and newborn health interventions matters

Jennifer Harris Requejo[1], Shams El Arifeen[2]

[1] United Nations Children's Fund, Data and Analytics, Division of Data, Research and Policy, New York, NY, USA
[2] International Centre for Diarrhoeal Disease Research, Dhaka, Bangladesh

The goal of ending preventable maternal and newborn mortality is achievable. Many maternal and newborn deaths can be averted through family planning services, and the timely provision of high quality care throughout pregnancy, childbirth, and the postnatal period. Yet, progress in increasing universal access to these life-saving interventions has been uneven and slower than we hoped. There are still approximately 2.5 million newborn deaths and 300,000 maternal deaths per year, most occurring in countries with the highest resource constraints and weakest health care infrastructures [1,2].

The positive news is that these stark numbers have not gone unnoticed, and great strides have been made in identifying essential packages of care for saving the lives of mothers and their newborn babies. Global consensus has also been reached on a core set of indicators for assessing progress in scaling-up these essential packages. Targets for reducing maternal and newborn mortality are in the Sustainable Development Goal (SDG) Framework, and many of these core indicators are embedded within other global accountability frameworks such as the Global Strategy for Women's, Children's and Adolescents' Health (2016-2030), Countdown to 2030, Every Newborn Action Plan, and Ending Preventable Maternal Mortality.

But, why does it matter if maternal and newborn health related indicators feature prominently in global accountability frameworks? The simple answer is the maxim we know so well: What gets measured gets done. And this translates into all of us doing our part to make it possible for every woman to have a healthy pregnancy and positive birth outcome for herself and her newborn baby.

The inclusion of maternal and newborn health indicators in global accountability frameworks has spurred a surge of data collection efforts in recent years

– new questions and modules have been added, for example, to large-scale population-based surveys such as the UNICEF supported Multiple Indicator Cluster Surveys (MICS) and the USAID supported Demographic and Health Surveys (DHS), and to health facility assessments such as MEASURE's Service Provision Assessment, and WHO's Service Availability and Readiness Assessment. There are also ongoing efforts to provide guidance to countries, through a set of modules (DHIS2 modules) produced under the umbrella of the Health Data Collaborative, on a standard set of indicators to collect through their routine health information systems.

All these data collection efforts have greatly increased the availability of data on essential maternal and newborn health interventions. The aim of this supplement is to take stock of where we are now: Are these efforts enough to meet global and national monitoring needs for maternal and newborn health? What else needs to be done to improve the measurement of maternal and newborn health indicators so that we all can be held to account for achieving the ambitious SDG targets? This supplement is organized into three sections. The first provides an overview of the data landscape for essential maternal and newborn health interventions. The second section includes papers that focus on the policy and programmatic implications of accurately measuring and regularly monitoring key maternal and newborn health indicators. These studies demonstrate what can be learned from analyses of available data about progress in individual and in groups of countries. They highlight where improvements are being made, where more work is needed, and context specific opportunities for increasing both the supply of and demand for essential maternal and newborn care. The set of papers in the third section highlights methodological work completed or underway on improving the measurement of maternal and newborn interventions and how this work helps address existing data gaps (e.g., in data capture approaches, and in defining indicators).

Several actionable messages emerge from the collection. These include a recommendation to increase data collection approaches that capture information about effective coverage and the quality of care, essential data for determining the impact interventions have on health outcomes. The study by Carvajal-Aguirre et al., for example, revealed large gaps in 20 countries in sub-Saharan Africa on the content of health services, indicating the urgent need for these countries to improve health service readiness to deliver all recommended maternal and newborn interventions. One such approach proposed to address these gaps is to improve the interoperability of household and health facility surveys, and to develop robust methods for linking different survey modalities [4]. Improving the quality of data captured through country health information systems would also enable more real time assessments of service provision, equipping program managers with the information they need to better determine where resources should be allocated and where course correction is needed.

Although the escalation in data availability on maternal and newborn health interventions is a laudable achievement, studies in this collection show that further work is needed on harmonizing data collection efforts to improve comparability across them. The study by Amouzou et al., for example, found that the MICS and DHS use different questions and methodologies for capturing information on postnatal care which reduces comparability across the two survey programs and the ability to develop time trends [5]. Other authors point out that data is still lacking on newborn practices which must be remedied (e.g., through innovative approaches that will help overcome existing challenges in collecting this information), and they present the limitations of using early initiation of breastfeeding as a proxy measure for essential newborn care [6]. The individual country papers show how data helps reveal context specific issues and the need to tailor intervention delivery strategies accordingly.

This supplement is timely given the ambitious global development agenda and the growing awareness of maternal and newborn survival as essential to its achievement. It shows the power of data to: 1) inform us about how well we are doing in improving coverage of essential maternal and newborn interventions within and across countries, and 2) why investments in the measurement agenda are critical for increasing our ability to know what we need to know about the success of policies and programs in saving maternal and newborn lives.

References

1 UN-interagency Group for Child Mortality Estimation. 2018. Levels & Trends in Child Mortality: Report 2018. New York: United Nations Children's Fund; 2018.

2 World Health Organization, UNICEF, UNFPA, World Bank Group and the United Nations Population Division. Trends in Maternal Mortality: 1990 to 2015. Geneva: World Health Organization.

3 Carvajal-Aguirre L, Amouzou A, Mehra V, Ziqi M, Zaka N, Newby H. Gap between contact and content in maternal and newborn care: An analysis of data from 20 countries in sub–Saharan Africa. J Glob Health. 2017;7:020501

4 Carvajal-Aguirre L, Mehra V, Amouzou A, Khan SM, Vaz L, Guenther T, et al. Does health facility service environment matter for the receipt of essential newborn care? Linking health facility and household survey data in Malawi. J Glob Health. 2017;7:020508.

5 Amouzou A, Mehra V, Carvajal-Aguirre L, Khan SM, Sitrin D, Vaz LM. Measuring postnatal care contacts for mothers and newborns: An analysis of data from the MICS and DHS surveys. J Glob Health. 2017;7: 020502.

6 Sitrin D, Perin J, Vaz LM, Carvajal-Aguirre L, Khan SM, Fishel J, et al. Evidence from household surveys for measuring coverage of newborn care practices. J Glob Health. 2017;7:020503.

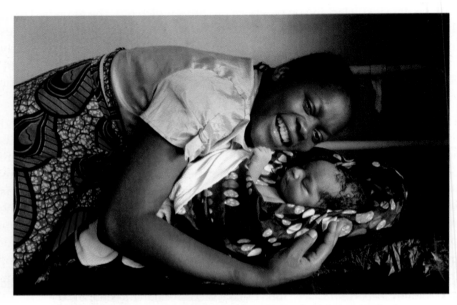

Photo: (c) UNICEF/UN018538/Chikondi (used with permission).

Measuring coverage of essential maternal and newborn care interventions: An unfinished agenda to define the data matrix for action in maternal and newborn health

Allisyn Moran[1], Tanya Marchant[2]

---

[1] Department of Maternal, Newborn, Child and Adolescent Health, World Health Organization, Geneva, Switzerland
[2] Department of Disease Control, London School of Hygiene and Tropical Medicine, London, UK

This collection provides crucial evidence on progress made and outstanding challenges on the road to improving maternal and newborn health using national household data (Demographic and Health Surveys; Multiple Indicator Cluster Surveys) and facility data (Service Provision Assessment) on multi-country coverage of maternal and newborn care seeking and care provision. Of the 11 manuscripts in this collection, six point to the need for more high quality, respectful care provided by health professionals working in enabling environments. Here we consider which data are fit for this improvement purpose.

THE MATERNAL AND NEWBORN MEASUREMENT DYAD

The Sustainable Development Goals have aided the alignment of global strategies across reproductive, maternal, newborn, child and adolescent health. Central to this is recognition that in-service provision as well as measurement it is essential to keep the mother and baby together as a dyad, especially around the time of birth when the majority of maternal and newborn deaths occur. Despite the considerable progress by household and facility surveys to illuminate evidence on the content of care, robust data on quality life-saving care at birth remains scarce in many settings [1-3], and there continues to be a need for global guidance on best measurement methods.

DATA FIT FOR THE PROGRAMMATIC CONTEXT

As practised by disease-specific initiatives such as UNAIDS [4], improving programmes for mothers and newborns requires a combination of data sources. Core indicators from national survey platforms are an essential part of the data matrix, but timely data from delivery rooms that can prospectively inform the decisions of health system actors at multiple levels are also needed. Inevitably this means that well-functioning health management information systems plus civil registration and vital statistics platforms are essential, especially when supported by innovations to summarise and visualize these data. Additional platforms may also be needed to provide more granular quality assessments, for example sentinel surveillance in communities and special studies in facilities.

When optimized, these data sources in combination have powerful potential to advance the quality of maternal and newborn care. But defining a complex data matrix alone cannot remove the barrier that poor quality of care poses to maternal and newborn survival: careful guidance is needed to help actors prioritize and organize evidence for action. Considerable work has already been carried out to understand data needs and method limitations [5]. Work is under way to develop guidance on indicators and data collection tools for measurement of maternal and newborn programmes including suggestions for maximizing use of all data sources; however, as research is conducted, the guidance will need to be updated and refined to reflect new recommendations. To further accelerate progress now the maternal and newborn health community must work to make sense of when and how each data source can be made to work together.

References

1 Moxon SG, Ruysen H, Kerber KJ, Amouzou A, Fourniers S, Grove J, et al. Count every newborn; a measurement improvement roadmap for coverage data. BMC Pregnancy Childbirth. 2015;15 Suppl 2:S8. Medline:26391444 doi:10.1186/1471-2393-15-S2-S8

2 Marchant T, Bryce J, Victora C, Moran AC, Claeson M, Requejo J, et al. Improved measurement for mothers, newborns and children in the era of the Sustainable Development Goals. J Glob Health. 2016;6:010506. Medline:27418960 doi:10.7189/jogh.06.010506

3 Munos MK, Stanton CK, Bryce J. Core Group for Improving Coverage Measurement for MNCH. Improving coverage measurement for reproductive, maternal, neonatal and child health: gaps and opportunities. J Glob Health. 2017;7:010801. Medline:28607675 doi:10.7189/jogh.07.010801

4 UNAIDS. Global AIDS Monitoring 2017: Indicators for monitoring the 2016 United Nations Political Declaration on HIV and AIDS. Available: http://www.unaids.org/sites/default/files/media_asset/2017-Global-AIDS-Monitoring_en.pdf. Accessed: 23 October 2017.

5 World Health Organization. Mother and Newborn Information for Tracking Outcomes and Results (MONITOR) technical advisory group. Available: http://www.who.int/maternal child adolescent/epidemiology/monitor/en/. Accessed: 23 October 2017.

Measuring coverage of essential maternal and newborn care interventions: An unfinished agenda

Liliana Carvajal–Aguirre[1], Lara ME Vaz[2], Kavita Singh[3,4], Deborah Sitrin[5], Allisyn C Moran[6], Shane M Khan[1], Agbessi Amouzou[7]

[1] Data and Analytics, Division of Data, Research and Policy, UNICEF, New York City, New York, USA

[2] Department of Global Health, Save the Children, Washington DC, USA

[3] MEASURE Evaluation/Carolina Population Center, University of North Carolina at Chapel Hill, Chapel Hill, North Carolina, USA

[4] Department of Maternal and Child Health, Gillings School of Global Public Health, Chapel Hill, North Carolina, USA

[5] Jhpiego, Baltimore, Maryland, USA

[6] Department of Maternal, Newborn, Child and Adolescent Health, World Health Organization, Geneva, Switzerland

[7] Institute for International Health, Department of International Health, Johns Hopkins Bloomberg School of Public Health, Baltimore, Maryland, USA

Over the past few decades, the agenda for newborn health has shifted remarkably, taking newborns from being nearly invisible in the global health agenda of 1990s to being central in discussions today. Despite this change, the decline in neonatal mortality from 1990 to 2016 has been slower than that of post–neonatal under–five mortality: 49% compared with 62% globally [1]. Newborn deaths represent 46% of all under–five deaths–of the 5.6 million under–5 deaths in 2016, nearly 2.7 million deaths occurred in the neonatal period, with a large proportion dying within the first week following birth [1,2]. Preterm birth complications (35%), intrapartum–related events (24%) and sepsis (15%) – most of which are preventable–have been identified as leading causes of neonatal deaths [3]. Although maternal mortality was estimated by the UN inter–agency group to have declined by 44% between 1990 and 2015, the reduction was far below the 75% MDG target. Approximately 303 000 women die each year from complications of pregnancy and childbirth, with 99% of deaths in low– and middle–income countries, making maternal mortality one of the indicators with the largest disparity between rich and poor countries [4]. With the majority of maternal and newborn deaths occurring around the time of birth, quality and equitable maternal and newborn care are essential to improve survival. Several global partnerships and initiatives such as the United Nations Every Woman Every Child movement (EWEC) and Every Newborn Action Plan (ENAP) have called for more focused attention on newborn health in order to end preventable newborn and child deaths [5,6]. The 2030 agenda of Sustainable Development Goals (SDG) and accompanying Global Strategy for Women's Children's and Adolescents' Health (2016–2030) include a specific target for all countries to reduce neonatal mortality to at least as low as 12 per 1000 live births, further reinforcing and strengthening commitment to neonatal survival [7].

Available research and evidence on newborn health clearly highlight impending challenges and strategies to improve newborn survival. The 2013 PLOS Medicine collection on "Measuring Coverage of MNCH" and the 2014 Lancet Every Newborn Series noted gaps in the availability of metrics and data on newborn care. Additionally, the globally agreed upon monitoring frameworks as ENAP, Ending Preventable Maternal Mortality (EPMM), the Global Strategy for Women's, Children's and Health (2016–2030) and Countdown to 2030 – have all identified critical areas where further indicator development and data collection are needed and have begun work to test or validate indicators [8]. There is also increased recognition of the role of data in measuring progress toward the promise of an equitable future in the SDG era. This has resulted in an explicit SDG target to support countries to increase the availability of high–quality, timely and disaggregated data, including data related to newborn health.

To date, large–scale household surveys such as the UNICEF–supported Multiple Indicator Cluster Surveys (MICS) and the USAID–supported Demographic and Health Surveys (DHS) are the primary sources of population–level coverage estimates of newborn health interventions [9,10]. Household surveys have been extremely important for national and sub–national monitoring of key indicators and are invaluable as a public source of data for examining sub–national inequalities and understanding coverage gaps in intervention as well as for research purposes. However, studies have indicated that the validity of coverage measures from household surveys can vary across indicators [11–13]. Household survey programs work constantly on revisiting and refining approaches to data collection. Following the 2013 recommendation of the Newborn Indicators Technical Working Group, some new indicators to measure care in the immediate newborn period have been added by the two household survey programmes. In addition, newborn–care related content is now also included and measured through health facility assessments.

With the increasing focus on the need for data on newborns, and availability of new data, it is time to understand these data and take stock of the findings but also of gaps. In the current context in which newborn survival is central to the global health agenda, there is an urgent need to strengthen the collection of data on newborn care, particularly on aspects related to quality of care and to identify and fill remaining gaps as well as ensure the data are aligned with global and national monitoring needs. Attuned to this context, the series of papers in this collection provide program and policy findings on measurement of maternal and newborn care and outcomes, with implications for future measurement implementation and research. The supplement provides an analysis and description of the associations and patterns of coverage and quality of recommended maternal and newborn care practices and interventions as captured at the population and facility level. It further strengthens evidence of limitation of current coverage indicators and the need for effective coverage measurement that incorporates quality of care provided. Several papers in the supplement highlight the scope of facility level data in assessing readiness to provide newborn care. Finally, the supplement assesses gaps and quality of available data on newborn health and measurement approaches across measurement platforms.

MEASURING PROGRESS AND CHALLENGES IN MATERNAL AND NEWBORN HEALTH

Maternal and Newborn health–related measurement (data and metrics)

Improving measurement of newborn health is at the core of this supplement. Though the quality, frequency and visibility of data for newborn health have improved notably compared to a decade ago [14], gaps in availability and quality of data on newborns remain. To accelerate and monitor progress towards the global target of reducing neonatal mortality, a set of core indicators has been proposed and incorporated in several monitoring frameworks. Some core indicators like, skilled birth attendant and exclusive and early initiation of breastfeeding have been established and reported on for decades through data collected in MICS, DHS and other household surveys. As a result, nearly 75% of the countries have data available for these indicators [8,15]. On the other hand, some indicators used for global reporting, such as "postnatal care for mothers and newborns," have been agreed upon more recently, with essential care indicators such as "thermal care" recommended for data collection in household surveys only in 2013. As highlighted by Sitrin et al in this supplement, only twelve national surveys between 2005 and 2014 included at least one indicator for immediate newborn care in addition to breastfeeding [16]. The supplement includes a series of papers addressing gaps and assessing the quality of many of these core indicators. Main findings are described below (**Table 1**).

Postnatal care (PNC) is an important strategy to improve newborn survival. Some issues related to measurement of postnatal contacts were mentioned in the PLOS One series, "Measuring Coverage of MNCH"; it also described a few changes made to MICS and DHS questionnaires, in an attempt to address issues revealed through formative research on indicator for postnatal care. However, there has not been a systematic assessment comparing the measurement approaches implemented by MICS and DHS, the two largest

Table 1. *Data on maternal and newborn indicators across current global monitoring frameworks and assessed in the current collection*

MATERNAL AND NEW-BORN HEALTH–RELATED INDICATORS	GAPS (AS IDENTIFIED IN THE CURRENT SERIES)	RECOMMENDATION (BASED ON STUDIES IN THE SERIES)
Content of antenatal care	Large gap between contacts and content of antenatal care	Coverage indicators should include elements of content of care to identify true effectiveness of maternal and child health interventions.
Skilled attendant at birth	Skilled attendants even in health facilities may not be equipped to save newborns	Need to supplement and link coverage data with health facility level data and quality of care indicators.
Postnatal care for mothers and babies	Difference in data collection tools eg, questionnaires and the methodology adopted to measure PNC across survey programs has created comparability issues in coverage levels	Need to harmonize data collection tools across survey programs. Need to determine differences in coverage by individual, household, regional characteristics. Individual characteristics should include delivery–related factors.
Essential newborn care with early initiation of breastfeeding as tracer indicator: • immediate and thorough drying; • immediate skin–to–skin contact; •delayed cord clamping; • early initiation of BF	• Early initiation of breastfeeding is not a high performing tracer indicator of essential newborn care, •Coverage of skin to skin and thermal care is low	Need to collect data on newborn care practices other than breastfeeding initiation through standardized questions in household level surveys.
Service readiness for newborn care in facilities	Lack of qualified staff	Improve training and increase capacity of staff across health sectors. Increase availability of essential commodities

sources of population–based MNCH coverage data in low and middle–income countries, which left open the question of how questionnaire differences may affect the comparability and interpretation of PNC coverage across surveys and countries. The study comparing measurement of postnatal care across the two survey programs in this supplement reveals a difference in the way questions on postnatal care for mothers and newborns are framed in MICS and DHS. MICS and DHS surveys have also followed different methodological approaches to compute the global indicator of postnatal contacts for mothers and newborns within two days following delivery, resulting in comparability issues in coverage levels across the two programs. As the evidence shows, this has implications for accurate measurement of coverage of postnatal care [17]. With an increased focus on quality of care provided, content of postnatal care may provide more helpful monitoring information to track reduction of neonatal mortality in the future.

The Every Newborn Action Plan proposed several indicators to track impact, coverage and equity of newborn health–related interventions. It proposed early breastfeeding as a tracer for essential newborn care, due to the data availability and evidence of benefits of breastfeeding. A methodological paper in this series assessed the correlation between early breastfeeding initiation and other newborn care practices [16]. The analysis found that breastfeeding initiation is not a good tracer indicator for newborn care practices and recommends improved methodologies for accurate measurement of these practices.

The quality of newborn health interventions is a significant gap that is not currently being addressed by the globally agreed upon coverage indicators to assess newborn health. It is increasingly recognized that global measures of coverage of maternal and newborn health capture main contacts with the health system but provide little information about the quality of care received. In this supplement, we assessed the gap between contact and content –as a proxy for quality–of maternal and newborn health services in 20 sub–Saharan countries and found that the gap between contact and content is excessively large in all [18].

Newborn health policy and program

Over the past several years, there have been major advances in agenda setting for newborn health, including implementation of several globally endorsed action plans and monitoring frameworks. There has been a notable increase in the number of publications focused on newborn health, and evidence is now available for interventions that address the three main causes of newborn deaths. Recent research indicates that increased coverage and quality of pre-conception, antenatal, intrapartum, and postnatal interventions by 2025 has the potential to avert 71% of neonatal deaths (1.9 million, range 1.6–2.1 million) [19]. A study in this supplement analyzed the recently available data on newborn care practices and found very low coverage of skin -to -skin contact despite its protective effects against neonatal morbidity and mortality [20]. Singh et al. examined the role of individual and health system characteristics on receipt of postnatal care and found coverage to be low in Bangladesh, particularly for newborns of mothers who delivered at home and who did not report a complication. Such analysis result in better identification of the most vulnerable newborns and provide valuable programmatic insights to improve coverage [21].

Quality of newborn health interventions emerged as a key missed opportunity to accelerate newborn survival in three studies that analyze survey data from 20 sub–Saharan countries, Bangladesh and Haiti [22–24]. Two studies using health facility data assessed the service readiness to deliver life-saving newborn interventions and found that health facilities are not yet equipped to save newborns at risk of dying [23,24]. An assessment of health service environment in Malawi revealed that newborns in districts with high service readiness have higher odds of receiving essential newborn care. This study highlights that there is an urgent need to increase the level of service readiness across all facilities and in particular, the quality and training of the staff, so that all newborns – irrespective of the health facility, district or region of delivery–are able to receive all recommended essential interventions.

RECOMMENDATIONS – CALL TO ACTION

Poor quality in newborn care is a major barrier to newborn survival, and we strongly recommend strengthening measurement of elements of content of care to improve the measurement of the coverage of maternal, neonatal and child health care. Recently, the World Health Organization and the Lancet quality improvement commission have proposed standards of care and measures assessing quality of maternal and newborn health care [25,26]. We propose that linking household survey data on coverage of interventions with facility–level data on service availability and readiness could help better measure effective coverage and identify its determinants and barriers.

It is encouraging to note that newborn health measurement is now central to many global initiatives, and new indicators are being added to household surveys and facility assessments. However, to track progress over time and make comparisons between countries, there is an urgent need to harmonize data collection across household surveys and facility assessments. To assess whether newborns are receiving life–saving interventions, the existing standardized questions regarding newborn care practices such as thermal care and skin–to–skin contact need to be consistently added to national household surveys. The DHS now includes an optional newborn module which outlines standardized questions on newborn care, which could be added to DHS surveys.MICS also includes standard questions. However, there is some evidence of poor validity of household survey indicators especially related to timing or sequence of events around the time of birth or questions which are composite of several events such as breastfeeding within one hour of birth, newborn dried and placed on mother's skin. For instance, these studies confirm that many indicators of intrapartum care and associated morbidities have generally low validity and reliability when assessed by women's reports. However, some salient indicators are reported with acceptable accuracy, most notably skilled attendance at birth and cesarean section [12,27]. Other strategies must be developed for those indicators with low validity and reliability and caution must be taken when interpreting results. Newborns also require data that can inform the decisions of more local health system actors. At the district level a manager who wants to optimize the health system can use national survey data to benchmark indicators at the regional level once every three to five years. But to know which inputs and health worker processes are optimized in the district, where actions are needed, and crucially whether outcomes improve as a result, different data platforms are required. The Health Management Information System (HMIS) and a well-functioning civil registration and vital statistics system have the potential to support this need and innovations to summarize and visualize these data so fit for district-level management could play an important role.Currently, UNICEF, WHO, and UNFPA are developing a standardized list of indicators for maternal and newborn health that can be consistently tracked and reported through HMIS and DHIS2.Other projects, such as the Maternal and Child Survival Program and the Quality, Equity and Dignity Network are testing and implementing these indicators, with a focus on using data for decision making at all levels.Data from HMIS will be crucial for monitoring progress toward national and global targets.

References

1 United Nations Inter-agency Group for Child Mortality Estimation (IGME). Levels and Trends in Child Mortality: Report 2017, New York: UNICEF; 2017.

2 UNICEF. Committing to child survival: A promise renewed – Progress report 2015. New York: UNICEF; 2015.

3 WHO and Maternal and Child Epidemiology Estimation Group (MCEE) provisional estimates 2015. Geneva: WHO; 2015.

4 WHO, UNICEF, UNFPA, World Bank, UNPD. Trends in maternal mortality: 1990 to 2015. Geneva: WHO; 2015.

5 WHO. Every Newborn Action Plan Metrics: WHO technical consultation on newborn health indicators. Geneva: WHO; 2015.

6 Commission on Information and Accountability. Keeping promises, measuring results: commission on information and accountability for women's and children's health. Geneva: WHO; 2011.

7 United Nations. Sustainable Development Goals. Available: http://www.un.org/sustainabledevelopment/sustainable-development-goals/. Accessed: 1 October 2017.

8 UNICEF. Is every child counted? Status of data for children in the SDGs. New York: UNICEF; 2016.

9 UNICEF. Statistics and monitoring: Multiple Indicator Cluster Surveys. Available: http://mics.unicef.org/surveys. Accessed: 1 October 2017.

10 The DHS Program. Demographic and Health Surveys. Available: https://dhsprogram.com/. Accessed: 1 October 2017.

11 Blanc AK, Diaz C, McCarthy KJ, Berdichevsky K. Measuring progress in maternal and newborn heatlh care in Mexico: validating indicators of health system contact and quality of care. BMC Pregnancy Childbirth. 2016;16:255. Medline:27577266 doi:10.1186/s12884-016-1047-0

12 Blanc AK, Warren C, McCarthy KJ, Kimani J, Ndwiga C. RamaRao S. Assessing the validity of indicators of the quality of maternal and newborn health care in Kenya. J Glob Health. 2016;6:010405. Medline:27231541 doi:10.7189/jogh.06.010405

13 Bryce J, Arnold F, Blanc A, Hancioglu A, Newby H, Requejo R, et al. Measuring coverage in MNCH: new findings, new strategies, and recommendations for action. PLoS Med. 2013;10:e1001423. Medline:23667340 doi:10.1371/journal.pmed.1001423

14 Darmstadt GL, Kinney MV, Chopra M, Cousens S, Kak L, Paul VK, et al; Lancet Every Newborn Study Group. Who has been caring for the baby? Lancet 2014; 384:174-88. Medline:24853603 doi:10.1016/S0140-6736(14)60458-X

15 Global Databases UNICEF. 2016. Available: https://data.unicef.org/. Accessed: 1 October 2017.

16 Sitrin D, Perin J, Vaz L, Carvajal-Aguirre L, Khan S, Fishel J, Amouzou A. Evidence from household surveys for measuring coverage of newborn care practices. J Glob Health. 2017;7:020503. doi:10.7189/jogh.07.020503

17 Amouzou A, Mehra V, Carvajal-Aguirre L, Sitrin D, Vaz L, Khan S. Measuring postnatal care contacts for mothers and newborns: An analysis of data from the MICS and DHS surveys. J Glob Health. 2017;7:020502. doi:10.7189/jogh.07.020502

18 Carvajal-Aguirre L, Amouzou A, Mehra V, Ziqi M, Zaka N, Newby H. Gap between contact and content in maternal and newborn care: An analysis of data from 20 countries in sub-Saharan Africa. J Glob Health. 2017;7:020501. doi:10.7189/jogh.07.020501

19 Bhutta ZA, Das JK, Bahl R, Lawn JE, Salam RA, Paul VK, et al. Can available interventions end preventable deaths in mothers, newborn babies, and stillbirths, and at what cost? Lancet. 2014;384:347-70. Medline:24853604 doi:10.1016/S0140-6736(14)60792-3

20 Singh K, Khan S, Carvajal-Aguirre L, Brodish P, Amouzou A, Moran A. The importance of skin-to-skin contact for early initiation of breastfeeding in Nigeria and Bangladesh. J Glob Health. 2017;7:020506. doi:10.7189/jogh.07.020506

21 Singh K, Brodish P, Chowdhury ME, Biswas TK, Kim ET, Godwin C et al. Postnatal care for newborns in Bangladesh: The Importance of health-related factors and location. J Glob Health. 2017;7:020508. doi:10.7189/jogh.07.020508

22 Amouzou A, Ziqi M, Carvajal-Aguirre L, Quinley J. Skilled attendant at birth and newborn survival in Sub-Saharan Africa. J Glob Health. 2017;7:020504. doi:10.7189/jogh.07.020504

23 Winter R, Yourkavitch J, Wang W, Mallick L. Assessment of health facility capacity to provide newborn care in Bangladesh, Haiti, Malawi, Senegal, and Tanzania. J Glob Health. 2017;7:020510. doi:10.7189/jogh.07.020510

24 Carvajal-Aguirre L, Mehra V, Amouzou A, Khan S, Vaz L, Guenther T, et al. Does health facility service environment matter for the receipt of essential newborn care? Linking health facility and household survey data in Malawi. J Glob Health. 2017;7:020509. doi:10.7189/jogh.07.020509

25 World Health Organization. Consultation on improving measurement of the quality of maternal, newborn and child care in health facilities. Geneva: WHO; 2014.

26 Kruk ME, Pate M, Mullan Z. Introducing The Lancet Global Health Commission on High-Quality Health Systems in the SDG era. Lancet Glob Health. 2017;5:e480-1. Medline:28302563 doi:10.1016/S2214-109X(17)30101-8

27 Stanton CK, Rawlins B, Drake M, dos Anjos M, Cantor D, Chongo L, et al. Measuring coverage in MNCH: testing the validity of women's self-report of key maternal and newborn health interventions during the peripartum period in Mozambique. PLoS One. 2013;8:e60694. Medline:23667427 doi:10.1371/journal.pone.0060694

SECTION 2

Coverage of maternal and newborn care interventions – policy and programmatic implications

Skilled attendant at birth and newborn survival in Sub–Saharan Africa

Agbessi Amouzou[1], Meng Ziqi[2], Liliana Carvajal-Aguirre[2], John Quinley[2]

[1] Institute for International Programs, Department of International Health, Johns Hopkins Bloomberg School of Public Health, Baltimore, USA

[2] UNICEF, New York, NY, USA

Background Recent studies have shown higher neonatal mortality among births delivered by a skilled attendant at birth (SAB) compared to those who were not in sub–Saharan African countries. Deaths during the neonatal period are concentrated in the first 7 days of life, with about one third of these deaths occurring during the first day of life. We reassessed the relationship between SAB and neonatal mortality by distinguishing deaths on the first day of life from those on days 2–27.

Methods We used data on births in the past five years from recent demographic and health survey (DHS) between 2010 and 2014 in 20 countries in sub–Saharan Africa. The main categorical outcome was 1) newborns who died within the first day of birth (day 0–1), 2) newborns who died between days 2–27, and 3) newborns who survived the neonatal period. We ran generalized linear mixed model with multinomial distribution and random effect for country on pooled data. Additionally, we ran a separate model restricted to births with SAB and assessed the association of receipt of seven antenatal care (ANC) and two immediate postnatal care interventions on risk of death on days 0–1 and days 2–27. These variables were assessed as proxy of quality of antenatal and postnatal care.

Results We found no statistically significant difference in risk of death on first day of life between newborns with SAB compared to those without. However, after the first day of life, newborns delivered with SAB were 16% less likely to die within 2–27 days than those without SAB (OR = 0.84, 95% CI = 0.71–0.99). Among births with skilled attendant, those who were weighed at birth and those who were initiated early on breastfeeding were significantly less likely to die on days 0–1 (respectively OR = 0.42 95% CI = 0.29–0.62 and OR = 0.24, 95% CI 0.18–0.31) or on days 2–27 (OR = 0.60, 95% CI = 0.45–0.81 and OR = 0.59, 95% CI = 47–0.74, respectively). Newborns whose mothers received an additional ANC intervention had no improved survival chances during days 0–1 of life. However, there was significant association on days 2–27 where newborns whose mothers received an additional ANC interventions had higher survival chances (OR = 0.95, 95% CI = 0.93–0.98).

Conclusion Findings demonstrate the vulnerability of newborns immediately after birth, compounded with insufficient quality of care. Improving the quality of care around the time of birth will significantly improve survival and therefore accelerate reduction in neonatal mortality in sub–Saharan African countries. Improved approaches for measuring skilled attendant at birth are also needed.

Global level of mortality among children under–five has been halved since 1990, with a decline from 91 deaths per 1000 live birth to 43 in 2015. A similar decline was also observed in sub–Saharan Africa, the region with the highest burden of mortality [1]. The pace of mortality decline was much slower among neonates, with sub–Sahara Africa recording one of the slowest declines of 38% over the same period, just behind Oceania where level of mortality is much lower. Subsequently, there is an increasing share of newborn deaths among all under–five deaths, reaching over a third in sub–Saharan Africa. The increasing mortality compression to the first days of life has raised calls for greater focus on newborn, with the adoption of the Every Newborn Action Plan (ENAP) in June 2014 and the subsequent publication of a Lancet Newborn Series to galvanize evidence–based programming that would accelerate reduction of newborn death toward ending preventable deaths [2]. The ENAP highlighted the strategic benefit of focusing on quality care around the time of birth by ensuring that all pregnancies have access to skilled quality care necessary for a healthy pregnancy and to protect the life of the newborn, and care for small and sick newborns [3,4]. The WHO has defined skilled attendant at birth as "an accredited health professional — such as a midwife, doctor or nurse — who has been educated and trained to proficiency in the skills needed to manage normal (uncomplicated) pregnancies, childbirth and the immediate postnatal period, and in the identification, management and referral of complications in women and newborns" [5]. This definition is currently being revised to clarify the competencies and extend to the notion of competent qualified maternal and newborn health care professional. [6] However, it does not address the limitation in measurement of skilled attendant at birth. In the absence of comparable data on quality skilled care, so far the world has mostly relied on the indicator of access to skilled attendant at delivery to monitor the likelihood that pregnancies receive some sort of quality of delivery care. Despite its limitation, this indicator has been one of the key coverage monitoring indicator in the Millennium Development Goals and more recently also adopted in the Sustainable Development Goals [7]. Skilled attendant at birth is also monitored as a core indicator in the ENAP and the Ending Preventable Maternal Mortality (EPMM) [8]. However, increasing number of studies calls for going beyond monitoring simple contact with a health system to include content and quality of interventions received [9–11]. Furthermore, assessment of the association between births reported to have been delivered with skilled attendant and chances of survival beyond the neonatal period did not generate expected results, especially in sub–Saharan Africa and Asia. In a recent study that included three countries each of three regions – Asia, sub–Saharan Africa and Latin America, Singh and her colleagues showed that skilled delivery did not appear to improve the survival of the newborn on the first day or week of life in the sub–Saharan African and Asian countries [12]. Possible explanations to this counter–intuitive finding highlight low quality of maternal and newborn services such that, although pregnant women come into contact with the health system to deliver, critical interventions needed to save the newborn in case of complications during delivery or postnatal period are not always available [13,14]. Other explanations include selection bias and uncertainty in the measurement of skilled attendant at birth in household surveys. Most women respondents in these surveys are of low schooling and not able to recall the type of cadre of health worker that provided the delivery care [15]. Regarding the selection bias, it is thought that in resource–constrained settings where access to health facility remains challenging and coverage of health facility use relatively low, women accessing delivery services in health facilities are likely to be those of higher potential risk of obstetric complication. A substantial portion of these women arrive late in health facilities, which may also not be properly equipped to promptly attend to the emergency [16–18].

In this study, we reassessed this relationship in a larger number of sub–Saharan African countries and by distinguishing deaths on the first day of life from days 2–27 using a multinomial mixed model. We conjecture that if the selection effect is real, the positive association between SAB and mortality will be seen only during the first day of life, when newborns are particularly vulnerable. Past this period, a negative association should be observed. Regarding quality of care, we also assessed association between the receipt of a series of seven antenatal care and two immediate postnatal care interventions by women and their newborns and mortality on days 0–1 and days 2–27.

DATA AND METHODS

We used data from recent Demographic and Health Surveys (DHSs), conducted in sub–Saharan Africa between 2010 and 2014, with information on child mortality collected using full birth history from women aged 15–49 and selected antenatal and postnatal interventions. Data were available for 20 countries in sub–Saharan Africa. **Table 1** includes the list of the countries. DHSs

Table 1. *Percentage of births with skilled health personnel and neonatal mortality rate by country*

COUNTRY	SURVEY YEAR	PERCENTAGE OF BIRTHS WITH SKILLED HEALTH PERSONNEL	NEONATAL MORTALITY (FIVE YEAR PRECEDING THE SURVEY)*	NUMBER OF LIVE BIRTHS IN THE FIVE YEARS PRECEDING THE SURVEY	DEFINITION OF SKILLED ATTENDANT AT BIRTH
Benin	2011–2012	80.9	23	5147	Doctor, nurse/midwife
Burkina Faso	2010	65.9	28	5790	Doctor, nurse/midwife, auxiliary midwife
Burundi	2010	60.3	31	3007	Doctor, nurse/midwife
Cameroon	2011	63.6	31	4496	Doctor, nurse/midwife
Comoros	2012	82.2	24	1251	Doctor, nurse/midwife
Congo	2011–2012	92.5	22	3625	Doctor, nurse/midwife, Assistant
Cote D'Ivoire	2011–2012	59.4	38	3041	Doctor, nurse/midwife
Democratic Republic of the Congo	2013	80.1	28	7209	Doctor, nurse/midwife
Gabon	2012	89.3	26	2443	Doctor, nurse/midwife
Guinea	2012	45.3	33	2763	Doctor, nurse/midwife, auxiliary midwife
Liberia	2013	61.1	26	2984	Doctor, nurse/midwife
Mozambique	2011	54.3	30	4543	Doctor, nurse/midwife
Niger	2012	29.3	24	4738	Doctor, nurse/midwife
Nigeria	2013	38.1	37	12272	Doctor, nurse/midwife
Rwanda	2010	69.0	27	3119	Doctor, nurse/midwife
Senegal	2010–2011	65.1	29	4771	Doctor, nurse/midwife
Sierra Leone	2013	59.7	39	4652	Doctor, nurse/midwife
Uganda	2011	57.4	27	2949	Doctor, nurse/midwife
United Republic of Tanzania	2010	48.9	26	3010	Doctor/assistant medical officer, nurse/midwife, clinical officer, assistant clinical officer
Zimbabwe	2010–2011	66.2	31	2358	Doctor, nurse/midwife
MEDIAN		62.3			
Correlation between SAB and NMR		−0.42 (*P* < 0.0619)			

*From STATCompiler, StatCompiler.com, accessed on February 2, 2017.

are USAID–funded nationally representative household surveys carried out about every five years in low– and middle–income countries [19]. The survey program started in the mid–1980s and has been a major source of demographic, reproductive and health data in these countries. Data are collected using typically a two–stage cluster sampling (with some variation in some countries), with first stage represented by population census enumeration areas, and the second stage by households. All women of reproductive age (15–49 years) in each sampled household are interviewed. Data are collected on several modules, including a full birth history module that captures information on every live birth a woman respondent ever had and the survival status of these births. For children who died, information is collected on age at death. The breakdown of the age at death depends on the age range. For deaths under one month, age at death is collected in days, starting from day 0 (as day of birth). For deaths over 1 month of age but under two–years, age at death is collected in months, and for deaths over two years, age at death is collected in years. This information is used to estimate mortality among children under–five (neonatal, post–neonatal, infant, under–five mortality). Another module includes information on health care provided during pregnancy, delivery and the postpartum period for all live births in the five years preceding the survey. This module captures data on antenatal care, assistance at delivery and postnatal care. A limited number of interventions delivered during these stages is also collected from women's recall. The module allows computation of births who had a skilled attendant at birth. Skilled birth attendant is captured generally as doctor, nurse, and midwife but there are slight variations across countries with addition of special cadres considered skilled (**Table 1**). Linking this module to the full birth history module allows an analysis of the association between receipt of skilled delivery and neonatal mortality. We based the analysis on children born in the past five years preceding each survey. For the twenty countries with available data, these range from 1251 to 12 272 births for a total of 84 168 births.

Variables

The main outcome is death during the neonatal period. We created three categories: 1) newborns who died on days 0–1, 2) newborns who died between days 2 and 27, and 3) children under–five who survived the neonatal period. We initially also separated out deaths on days 2–7 but results of preliminary analysis were similar to those of deaths on days 8–27. We therefore grouped them together.

In addition to a binary variable on whether a birth was assisted by a skilled attendant at birth or not, we considered an additional main independent variable related to interventions received by the mother during antenatal care to capture quality of ANC. These interventions include urine test, blood test, blood pressure measured, iron supplementation, tetanus protection at birth, counselled on pregnancy complications, tested for HIV and received results. We created a categorical variable of number of interventions received by summing the indicator variable representing each intervention. We use this composite indicator as a proxy for quality of care received by the women during their pregnancy. For postnatal interventions, we considered two immediate postnatal interventions: whether the newborn was weighed at birth and whether the newborn was initiated early on breastfeeding. The latter was captured by asking the mother whether the newborn was breastfed within one hour following birth. We could not consider other available postnatal indicators in the analysis due to possible selection bias that would be introduced, given newborns who died immediately during the first days of life would not have the same exposure time to the chance of receiving these interventions.

We considered as control variables, socio–economic and demographic variables with known effects on mortality. These included residence (urban, rural), wealth quintile (poorest, poorer, middle, richer, richest), marital status (single, married, other), parity (1, 2–4, 5 or more), mother's age at birth (15–19, 20–29, 30–39, 40–49 years), and mother's education level (no schooling, primary, secondary or higher).

Analysis

We first described the coverage of skilled attendant at birth in the twenty countries. For each country, we computed and compared neonatal mortality rate separately for births with a skilled birth attendant and those without. We computed these rates on the three years preceding each survey using a life table approach [20]. To compare the rates, we computed 95% confidence intervals using Jackknife approach [21]. We then pooled all country data and fit a generalized linear mixed model with multinomial distribution and random effect for country. We used the third category of the outcome variables (children under–five who survived the neonatal period) as the reference category. We estimated two models. First, we fit a model of mortality outcome on skilled attendance at birth, adjusting for the control variables described above. Second, we fit a model of mortality outcome on number of ANC interventions received, and the immediate postnatal variables controlling for socio–demographic variables. The latter model included data from 18 countries and was restricted to only births delivered with skilled health personnel to assess the effect of quality of care on newborn death. The mortality computation analyses were carried out in STATA version 13 while the regression models were implemented in SAS.

RESULTS

Table 1 and **Figure 1** show levels of coverage of skilled attendant at birth (SAB) by country. Coverage ranged from 29% in Niger to 93% in Congo with a median of 62%. Table 1 also shows the five–year neonatal mortality rate by country, ranging from 22 deaths per 1000 live births in Congo to 39 deaths per 1000 live births in Sierra Leone. There is a marginally significant inverse relationship between SAB and neonatal mortality: ($r = -0.42$, $P < 0.0619$). While Congo shows the highest coverage of SAB and lowest neonatal mortality, the country with lowest coverage of SAB (Niger) does not have the highest neonatal mortality. **Figure 2** presents the neonatal mortality rate by SAB along with the 95% confidence intervals. The general picture across countries suggests no significant survival advantage during the neonatal period among births with SAB and those without. Based on the confidence intervals, there is no statistically significant difference in neonatal mortality rate among births with SAB compared to those without, except in Burkina Faso where births with SAB have significantly lower neonatal mortality than those without.

Table 2 presents results from the multinomial mixed model regression. Births who survived beyond the neonatal period are used as reference category. Furthermore, the reference category corresponding to each categorical variable included in the model is shown in parenthesis beside the name of the

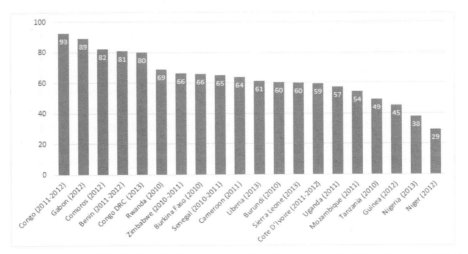

Figure 1. *Percent of live birth in the five years preceding the survey with skilled attendant at birth by country, Demographic and Health Survey (DHS, 2010–2014). Survey years are included in the parenthesis.*

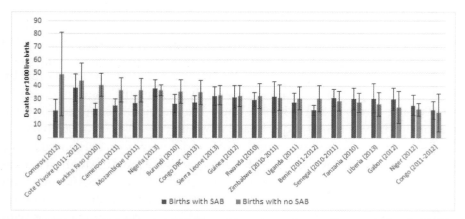

Figure 2. *Neonatal mortality rate and 95% confidence intervals according to whether the birth had a skilled attendant at birth (SAB) or not by country.*

variable in the first column. Column 2 shows the age at death, distinguishing deaths on days 0–1 and deaths on days 2–27, and column 3 shows the response category of the independent variable included in the model. Response categories with significant results are bolded. Adjusting for covariates in the model, there is no statistically significant difference in the odds of death on days 0–1 between births with SAB and births without. However, births with SAB who survived after the first day showed a statistically significant 16% lower risk of death on the period 0–27 days compared to births without SAB (OR = 0.84, 95% CI = 0709–0.996). Several demographic covariates remained statistically significant in the model. These include parity, mother's age at birth of the child, and current marital status. With regard to parity, there is no differential risk of death for first birth compared to births of parity 5 plus whether on days 0–1 or days 2–27. However, births of parity 2–4 have significantly 25% lower odds of death on the days 2–27 compared to births of parity 5 plus. Compared to births to women aged 20–29, births to older women have higher odds of death on either days 0–1 or days 2–27. Births to women aged 40 or more have respectively 72% and 62% higher odds of death on days 0–1 and days 2–27 compared to births to women aged 20–29. For births to women 30–39, the differential risk is observed only for births on days 0–1, with a 25% increased odds of death. Births to single women have 52% higher odds of death compared to births to married women. Other characteristics such as education level, residence or wealth quintile showed no significant differential risk of death on days 0–1 or days 2–27.

In **Table 3**, we present results from the multinomial mixed model regression, restricted to only births with SAB and assessing the effect of co–coverage of interventions during ANC and immediate postnatal interventions, adjusting for the same socio–demographic characteristics. Statistically significant

Table 2.Adjusted *odds ratios of death on days 0–1 or days 2–27 compared to surviving over the neonatal period among births with SAB compared to births without SAB)**

VARIABLE (REFERENCE CATEGORY)	AGE AT DEATH	CATEGORY	ODDS RATIO	95% CONFIDENCE INTERVAL		P
Skilled attendant at birth (No.)	Day 0–1	Yes	1.17	0.934	1.465	0.173
	Day 2–27	**Yes**	**0.84**	**0.709**	**0.996**	**0.045**
Parity (5 plus)	Day 0–1	1	1.35	0.919	1.984	0.127
	Day 2–27	1	1.03	0.708	1.506	0.870
	Day 0–1	2–4	0.84	0.678	1.051	0.129
	Day 2–27	**2–4**	**0.75**	**0.607**	**0.931**	**0.009**
Mother's age at birth (20–29)	Day 0–1	15–19	0.91	0.757	1.106	0.358
	Day 2–27	15–19	1.15	0.879	1.517	0.301
	Day 0–1	**30–39**	**1.25**	**1.052**	**1.488**	**0.011**
	Day 2–27	30–39	1.14	0.937	1.376	0.194
	Day 0–1	**≥40**	**1.72**	**1.349**	**2.187**	**<0.0001**
	Day 2–27	**≥40**	**1.62**	**1.247**	**2.099**	**<0.0001**
Current marital status (Married)	Day 0–1	Other	1.01	0.871	1.172	0.896
	Day 2–27	Other	1.15	0.939	1.414	0.175
	Day 0–1	Single	1.08	0.811	1.427	0.611
	Day 2–27	**Single**	**1.52**	**1.218**	**1.906**	**<0.0001**
Education level (No education)	Day 0–1	Primary	1.04	0.896	1.215	0.585
	Day 2–27	Primary	1.04	0.92	1.171	0.545
	Day 0–1	Secondary or higher	0.92	0.704	1.202	0.542
	Day 2–27	Secondary or higher	0.84	0.649	1.089	0.189
Residence (Rural)	Day 0–1	Urban	1.01	0.837	1.218	0.920
	Day 2–27	Urban	1.14	0.92	1.401	0.237
Wealth quintile (Poorest)	Day 0–1	Poorer	1.03	0.852	1.239	0.776
	Day 2–27	Poorer	1.05	0.893	1.241	0.542
	Day 0–1	Middle	1.04	0.911	1.180	0.585
	Day 2–27	Middle	1.00	0.805	1.234	0.973
	Day 0–1	Richer	1.04	0.877	1.224	0.678
	Day 2–27	Richer	0.94	0.755	1.173	0.590
	Day 0-1	Richest	1.05	0.828	1.323	0.705
	Day 2-27	Richest	0.91	0.619	1.328	0.614

SAB – skilled attendant at birth
*Analysis based on generalized linear mixed model; pooled DHS 2010-2014 from 20 countries in Africa.

Table 3. *Adjusted odds ratios of death on days 0–1 or days 2–27 compared to surviving over the neonatal period by number of ANC interventions received by mother and immediate postnatal interventions received by newborn (among births with SAB)**

Independent variable	Age at death	Category	Odds ratio	95% confidence interval		P-value
Number of seven ANC interventions received by mother	**Day 0–1**	**Continuous**	**1.02**	**1.000**	**1.044**	**0.0545**
	Day 2–27	**Continuous**	**0.95**	**0.927**	**0.979**	**0.0005**
Newborn weighed at birth (No.)	**Day 0–1**	**Yes**	**0.42**	**0.292**	**0.615**	**<.0001**
	Day 2–27	**Yes**	**0.60**	**0.450**	**0.809**	**0.0007**
Newborn initiated early on breastfeeding (No)	**Day 0–1**	**Yes**	**0.24**	**0.184**	**0.310**	**<.0001**
	Day 2–27	**Yes**	**0.59**	**0.473**	**0.744**	**<.0001**
Parity (5 plus)	**Day 0–1**	**1**	**1.54**	**1.030**	**2.307**	**0.0356**
	Day 2–27	1	1.19	0.817	1.728	0.3668
	Day 0–1	2–4	0.91	0.723	1.151	0.4372
	Day 2–27	**2–4**	**0.80**	**0.645**	**1.002**	**0.0518**
Mother's age at birth (20-29)	Day 0–1	15–19	0.86	0.702	1.043	0.1225
	Day 2–27	15–19	1.04	0.790	1.361	0.7941
	Day 0–1	**30–39**	**1.27**	**1.056**	**1.519**	**0.011**
	Day 2–27	30–39	1.16	0.941	1.432	0.1633
	Day 0–1	**≥40**	**1.80**	**1.376**	**2.364**	**<.0001**
	Day 2–27	**≥40**	**1.60**	**1.192**	**2.142**	**0.0017**
Current marital status (Married)	Day 0–1	Other	1.02	0.874	1.179	0.8458
	Day 2–27	Other	1.09	0.898	1.318	0.3867
	Day 0–1	Single	1.05	0.799	1.389	0.7119
	Day 2–27	**Single**	**1.47**	**1.162**	**1.861**	**0.0013**
Education level (No education)	**Day 0–1**	**Primary**	**1.23**	**1.064**	**1.417**	**0.0051**
	Day 2–27	**Primary**	**1.14**	**0.990**	**1.304**	**0.0695**
	Day 0–1	Secondary or higher	1.17	0.883	1.549	0.2734
	Day 2–27	Secondary or higher	0.97	0.770	1.215	0.7736
Residence (Rural)	Day 0–1	Urban	1.13	0.917	1.401	0.2456
	Day 2–27	**Urban**	**1.27**	**1.030**	**1.559**	**0.0254**
Wealth quintile (Poorest)	Day 0–1	Poorer	1.14	0.937	1.378	0.1945
	Day 2–27	Poorer	1.11	0.944	1.304	0.2079
	Day 0–1	**Middle**	**1.27**	**1.096**	**1.463**	**0.0014**
	Day 2–27	Middle	1.08	0.888	1.323	0.4300
	Day 0–1	**Richer**	**1.42**	**1.155**	**1.736**	**0.0008**
	Day 2–27	Richer	1.07	0.850	1.338	0.5777
	Day 0–1	**Richest**	**1.68**	**1.267**	**2.225**	**0.0003**
	Day 2–27	Richest	1.08	0.767	1.527	0.6531

ANC – antenatal care, SAB – skilled attendant at birth
Analysis based on generalized linear mixed model; pooled DHS 2010–2014 data from 18 countries in Africa.

variables are shown in bold. Adjusting for the socio–demographic variables included in the model and immediate postnatal interventions, there is a strong and negative significant association between the number of ANC interventions received and the odds of death on days 2–27. The odds of death on days 2–27 are reduced by 5% for each additional ANC intervention received. However, this advantage was not observed on days 0–1 and in fact there appeared to be a marginal positive association between number of ANC interventions and risk of death. Regarding immediate postnatal interventions, newborns weighed at birth or those initiated early on breastfeeding were significantly less likely to die either on days 0–1 or days 2–27. Newborns weighed at birth were 58% less like die on days 0–1 and 40% less likely to die on days 2–27. Similarly, newborns initiated early on breastfeeding were respectively 76% and 41% less likely to die on days 0–1 and days 2–27. The demographic characteristics such as parity, mother's age and marital status remained significant and in the similar direction as described for the model in **Table 2**. However, urban–rural residence, education level and wealth quintile became statistically significant in this model in somewhat unexpected direction.

DISCUSSION

Access to skilled attendant at birth during antenatal care and delivery is promoted as a key strategy for improving maternal and newborn care in low and middle–income countries. The importance of skilled personnel at the time of birth is widely acknowledged, such that the proportion of births attended by skilled health personnel has been adopted as a key coverage monitoring indicator for the Sustainable Development Goal 3.1. However, we showed in this study that the survival benefits expected for newborns delivered with skilled health personnel are not being observed in sub–Saharan Africa. We demonstrated in the analysis that there is no survival benefit on days 0–1 for newborns, whether they are delivered by a skilled birth attendant or not. Only when they survive day 1 does such benefit occur. These results are consistent with previous studies and call once again for greater attention to the fragility of care around the time around of delivery [3,4,11]. The results suggest that skilled birth attendants, and most health facilities, are not yet equipped enough to save newborns at highest risk of death immediately after birth. These results were further corroborated by assessing effects of quality of care immediately after birth on the risk of death among births with skilled attendant. Among these births, simple interventions such as being weighed at birth or being initiated on breastfeeding early showed strong and significant benefits for survival chances during the neonatal period. It may be that these interventions are also good proxy for quality of care during the immediate postnatal period. Using the number of antenatal care interventions that the mother received did not show survival benefits for births attended by skilled personnel on days 0–1, but only on days 2–27, reinforcing the finding that interventions delivered immediately after birth are most critical for the survival of the newborn during the immediate periods following birth.

In **Table 4**, we estimated, based on annual births, stillbirth and number of skilled health professionals, the number of deliveries per skilled health professional given current coverage, and for 100% coverage. The estimated number of deliveries per skilled health professional ranges from 8 in Nigeria to 120 in Guinea. While these are average estimates and do not account for highly unequal distribution of skilled health professional within countries or that some health professional may not conduct deliveries at all, and there is highly unequal distribution of deliveries for each provider, their level is not extremely high as to overwhelm the health system. Lack of significantly improved survival among those who access these professionals during the immediate postnatal period may suggest that the system is not sufficiently equipped and strong enough to deal with high–risk obstetric conditions and/or a substantial portion of these health personnel is not skilled enough to prevent such risks from leading to death. It also suggests highly inequitable distribution of SAB or facilities with lower access in higher risk populations. Even with 100% coverage of skilled delivery, a country like Nigeria will see only an average of 20 deliveries per skilled health personnel, and in most countries skilled health personnel will perform on average fewer than 100 deliveries per year.

In such conditions, it is not entirely inappropriate to question whether it still makes sense to continue to advocate for increased skilled delivery when this strategy is not producing the expected survival advantage in resource constrained countries. The answer from our study would be yes, because, at least beyond the first two days of life, there is significant survival advantage for newborns delivered with skilled birth attendants. Nevertheless, the question underscores the tremendous missed opportunities for the health system when women are encouraged to deliver in health facilities with skilled attendant, yet do not receive needed quality of care when they show up. The lack of survival advantage during the first days of life for the newborn, even when delivery occur with skilled personnel or in health facility can reinforce barriers to facility use.

Our results raise three main implications, which are also generally raised to explain the lack of significant improvement in survival of newborns delivered with skilled attendants compared those without. First is the need for improving access to equitable high–quality maternal and delivery care in African countries. Many studies have demonstrated the low level of quality of care, including low access to basic and emergency obstetric services. Nesbitt and

Table 4. *Estimated average annual deliveries per skilled health professional by country*

Country	Total Population 2015 (in 1000s)^	Births in 2015 (in 1000s)*	Number of Still-Births in 2015†	Skilled Health Professionals Density (per 10 000 Population)‡	Estimated No. of Skilled Health Professionals	Percentage of Births with Skilled Health Professional	Number of Annual Deliveries per Skilled Health Professional §	Number of Annual Deliveries per Skilled Health Professional if 100% Coverage
Benin	10 880	388	11 700	8.3	9030	80.9	36	44
Burkina Faso	18 106	717	14 900	6.1	11 044	65.9	44	66
Burundi	11 179	488	12 700	–	–	60.3	–	–
Cameroon	23 344	847	16 400	5.2	12 139	63.6	45	71
Comoros	788	26	800	–	–	82.2	–	–
Congo	4620	167	2500	9.2	4251	92.5	37	40
Cote d'Ivoire	22 702	838	22 800	6.3	14 302	59.4	36	60
Democratic Republic of the Congo	77 267	3217		–	–	80.1	–	–
Gabon	1725	51	700	–	–	89.3	–	–
Guinea	12 609	460	9900	1.4	1765	45.3	120	266
Liberia	4503	156	3300	2.9	1306	61.1	75	122
Mozambique	27 978	1087	20 700	4.5	12 590	54.3	48	88
Niger	19 899	983	36 200	1.6	3184	29.3	94	320
Nigeria	182 202	7133	313 700	20.1		38.1	8	20
Rwanda	11 610	363	5900	7.5	8707	69.0	29	42
Senegal	15 129	567	14 500	4.8	7262	65.1	52	80
Sierra Leone	6453	229	5400	1.9	1226	59.7	114	191
Uganda	39 032	1665	34 200	14.2	55 426	57.4	18	31
United Republic of Tanzania	53 470	2064	47 100	4.7	25 131	48.9	41	84
Zimbabwe	15 603	539		14.2	22 156	66.2	16	25

*Source: United Nations, Department of Economic and Social Affairs, Population Division [22].
†Source: Lawn et al [23].
‡Source: WHO [24].
§Assumed same coverage level of skilled health personnel for stillbirths.

colleagues showed a quality gap, defined as the difference between the crude coverage of SAB and the coverage of SAB with high quality of care, as large as 50 percentage points in health facilities in several districts in Ghana. Marchant raised the concern that contacts with the health system are not used sufficiently to deliver life–saving, timely interventions. While these studies have either assessed readiness of health facilities or delivery of interventions according to international or WHO–recommended standards, another important knowledge gap remains, namely an accurate assessment of care provision decision–making process based on obstetric risk to the woman or her newborn in resource–constrained settings. In an environment where there are not enough equipment, drugs or human resources, how health professionals decide on who should get what interventions and who should not, is not always factored in the measure of quality of care. It is clear that if, given such shortages, only a few patients can receive an intervention, some triage process will need to be in place based on obstetric risk. Under such circumstances, measures of quality of care based on optimal international standards applicable to every woman regardless of risk, or a sum of required interventions that every pregnant woman must receive will always yield low quality of care. The understanding of care provision and triage decision–making process that health care workers are forced to make when faced with a shortage of essential equipment and drugs will allow an appropriate and contextualized remedy on how countries should adapt international standards to their specific resource constrained contexts. For example, to tackle the shortage of qualified health professionals, countries have resorted to task–shifting, with increasing reliance on lower level health professionals, including in some cases community health workers. However, it is essential that countries which adopt such strategies ensure that it is accompanied with the appropriate education, skill upgrade training, and necessary equipment within a mentorship and supportive environment. Another critical aspect is the extent to which quality of care is equitable across facilities, regions and population groups. Equitable access to quality care is closely linked to population level effective coverage, a proximal determinant of survival impact. In a context of equitable access, results shown in **Table 4** would not imply overburdened delivery system, in terms of human resources.

Second, while there is a standard definition of skilled health personnel, its application at country level and its measurement remain a challenge at country level [5]. While WHO and UNICEF are rallying the midwifery and newborn communities to revise the current definition, its applicability at country level will always face contextual challenges, where most of qualified health personnel do not work where the need for them is highest. Rural, poor and difficult access areas will remain disadvantaged since no doctors or qualified personnel will opt to go there without substantial benefits. Countries will therefore continue to use task shifting strategy to address accessibility issues in poor areas. Under such conditions, expanding the training of all those involved in maternal and newborn care to raise their skills, and equipping facilities for basic and emergency obstetric and newborn care would be a reasonable strategy. Furthermore, the measurement of skilled birth attendant through household surveys is also challenged with misclassification and inaccuracy. Low literacy mothers delivering in facilities do not always know the cadre of health professional in charge of their delivery [25,26]. In addition, categories of cadres of health personnel used in survey instruments such as those in DHS or Multiple Indicator Cluster Surveys (MICS) are not consistent across time and countries. Furthermore, the type of cadres that are included as skilled varies largely within and between countries. This creates difficulties in assessing accurately, not only the coverage levels of SAB but its trends. A growing number of studies are now researching measurement approaches based on linking of household surveys to health facilities [27,28]. While findings from these studies will be very valuable, an immediate step to take is for large survey programs such as the DHS and the Multiple Indicator Cluster Surveys (MICS) to standardize their instruments across surveys and time to allow comparability of results over time. While measurement issues with skilled attendant at birth could have affected our findings above, it is important to note that the large majority of births reported being delivered with skilled personnel occurred in health facilities in these countries. The findings therefore stand for births occurring in health facilities and highlight the tremendous missed opportunities and insufficient quality of care that substantial number of pregnant women face in countries included in this study.

Finally, there has been a suggestion that lack of improved outcomes at facility levels could be due to higher obstetric risk pregnancies rushing to the facility, which increases the risk profile of births with skilled attendants vs those without [16–18]. While this may be happening, it also suggests that drastic measures to improve access to timely antenatal care, counselling on institutional delivery or access to skilled delivery and attention to quality of care, including respectful maternal care, are to be prioritized. Implementation of quality pre–delivery maternity homes may be a solution to delayed access in some contexts [29].

Ending preventable newborn death while relying on current health systems in sub–Saharan African countries will require not only improvement in access to skilled delivery but also drastic measures to ensure effective coverage by improving availability of equipment and essential medicine, and equitable distribution of health personnel that is ready to deliver lifesaving interventions especially at time around delivery.

Acknowledgements: Preliminary results of this study were presented at the Countdown technical meeting in April 2015 and at that African Population Conference in December 2015.

Ethics: The study is based on de–identified publicly available household survey data. Ethical approval was the responsibility of data collection institutions.

Funding: This work was partly funded through a sub–grant from the US Fund for UNICEF under their Countdown to 2015 grant from the Bill and Melinda Gates Foundation.

Authorship declaration: AA conceived the manuscript and developed analysis plan. ZM & AA carried out analysis. LC and JQ reviewed earlier drafts of the manuscript. All authors reviewed and approved final version of the manuscript.

Competing interest: All authors have completed the Unified Competing Interest form at www.icmje.org/coi_disclosure.pdf (available on request from the corresponding author). We declare that we have no conflicts of interest.

References

1 You D, Hug L, Ejdemyr S, Idele P, Hogan D, Mathers C, et al. Global, regional, and national levels and trends in under-5 mortality between 1990 and 2015, with scenario-based projections to 2030: a systematic analysis by the UN Inter-agency Group for Child Mortality Estimation. Lancet. 2015;386:2275-86. Medline:26361942 doi:10.1016/S0140-6736(15)00120-8

2 UNICEF. WHO. Every Newborn: An action plan to end preventable newborn deaths. Geneva: World Health Organization; 2014.

3 Bhutta ZA, Das JK, Bahl R, Lawn JE, Salam RA, Paul VK, et al. Can available interventions end preventable deaths in mothers, newborn babies, and stillbirths, and at what cost? Lancet. 2014;384:347-70. Medline:24853604 doi:10.1016/S0140-6736(14)60792-3

4 Lawn JE, Blencowe H, Oza S, You D, Lee ACC, Waiswa P, et al. Every Newborn: progress, priorities, and potential beyond survival. Lancet. 2014;384:189-205. Medline:24853593 doi:10.1016/S0140-6736(14)60496-7

5 World Health Organization. Making pregnancy safer: the critical role of the skilled attendant: a joint statement by WHO, ICM and FIGO. Geneva: World Health Organization; 2004.

6 World Health Organization. Competent attendance in maternal and newborn health: the definition of the competent health care provider in maternal and newborn health. A joint statement by WHO, UNFPA, UNICEF, ICM, ICN, FIGO and IPA. Available: http://www.who.int/reproductivehealth/skilled-birth-attendant/en/. Accessed: 19 September 2017.

7 United Nations. The Millennium Development Goals Report 2015. Available: http://www.un.org/millenniumgoals/2015_MDG_Report/pdf/MDG%202015%20rev%20(July%201).pdf. Accessed: 19 September 2017.

8 World Health Organization. Strategies toward ending preventable maternal mortality (EPMM). Geneva: World Health Organization; 2015.

9 Nesbitt RC, Lohela TJ, Manu A, Vesel L, Okyere E, Edmond K, et al. Quality along the Continuum: A Health Facility Assessment of Intrapartum and Postnatal Care in Ghana. PLoS One. 2015;10:e0141517. Medline:26485127 doi:10.1371/journal.pone.0141517

10 Marchant T, Tilley-Gyado RD, Tessema T, Singh K, Gautham M, Umar N, et al. Adding Content to Contacts: Measurement of High Quality Contacts for Maternal and Newborn Health in Ethiopia, North East Nigeria, and Uttar Pradesh, India. PLoS One. 2015;10:e0126840. Medline:26000829 doi:10.1371/journal.pone.0126840

11 Hodgins S, D'Agostino A. The quality–coverage gap in antenatal care: toward better measurement of effective coverage. Glob Health Sci Pract. 2014;2:173-81. Medline:25276575 doi:10.9745/GHSP-D-13-00176

12 Singh K, Brodish P, Suchindran C. A Regional Multilevel Analysis: Can Skilled Birth Attendants Uniformly Decrease Neonatal Mortality? Matern Child Health J. 2014;18:242-9. Medline:23504132 doi:10.1007/s10995-013-1260-7

13 Dickson KE, Kinney MV, Moxon SG, Ashton J, Zaka N, Simen-Kapeu A, et al. Scaling up quality care for mothers and newborns around the time of birth: an overview of methods and analyses of intervention-specific bottlenecks and solutions. BMC Pregnancy Childbirth. 2015;15 Suppl 2:S1. Medline:26390820 doi:10.1186/1471-2393-15-S2-S1

14 Sharma G, Mathai M, Dickson KE, Weeks A, Hofmeyr GJ, Lavender T, et al. Quality care during labour and birth: a multicountry analysis of health system bottlenecks and potential solutions. BMC Pregnancy Childbirth. 2015;15 Suppl 2:S2. Medline:26390886 doi:10.1186/1471-2393-15-S2-S2

15 Blanc AK, Warren C, McCarthy KJ, Kimani J, Ndwiga C. RamaRao S. Assessing the validity of indicators of the quality of maternal and newborn health care in Kenya. J Glob Health. 2016;6:010405. Medline:27231541 doi:10.7189/jogh.06.010405

16 Paul BK, Rumsey DJ. Utilization of health facilities and trained birth attendants for childbirth in rural Bangladesh: An empirical study. Soc Sci Med. 2002;54:1755-65. Medline:12113433 doi:10.1016/S0277-9536(01)00148-4

17 Ronsmans C, Chowdhury ME, Koblinsky M, Ahmed A. Care seeking at time of childbirth, and maternal and perinatal mortality in Matlab, Bangladesh. Bull World Health Organ. 2010;88:289-96. Medline:20431793 doi:10.2471/BLT.09.069385

18 Ronsmans C, Scott S, Qomariyah SN, Achadi E, Braunholz D, Marshall T, et al., et al. Midwife-led community care and maternal mortality in Indonesia. Bull World Health Organ. 2009;87:416-23. Medline:19565119 doi:10.2471/BLT.08.051581

19 Demographic and health surveys. Available: https://www.dhsprogram.com/. Accessed: 18 October 2017.

20 Preston SH, Heuveline P, Guillot M. Demography: Measuring and modeling population processes. Oxford: Blackwell Publishers; 2001.

21 Lohr SL. Sampling: design and analysis. Boston: Cengage Learning; 2010.

22 United Nations, Department of Economic and Social Affairs, Population Division. World Population Prospects: The 2015 Revision. New York: UN; 2015.

23 Lawn JE, Blencowe H, Waiswa P, Amouzou A, Mathers C, Hogan D, et al. Stillbirths: rates, risk factors, and acceleration towards 2030. Lancet. 2016;387:587-603. Medline:26794078 doi:10.1016/S0140-6736(15)00837-5

24 WHO. World Health Statistics 2016. Monitoring Health for the SDGs. Geneva: WHO; 2016.

25 Blanc AK, Warren C, McCarthy KJ, Kimani J, Ndwiga C. RamaRao S. Assessing the validity of indicators of the quality of maternal and newborn health care in Kenya. J Glob Health. 2016;6:010405. Medline:27231541 doi:10.7189/jogh.06.010405

26 McCarthy KJ, Blanc AK, Warren C, Kimani J, Mdawida B, Ndwidga C. Can surveys of women accurately track indicators of maternal and newborn care? A validity and reliability study in Kenya. J Glob Health. 2016;6:020502. Medline:27606061 doi:10.7189/jogh.06.020502

27 Do M, Micah A, Brondi L, Campbell H, Marchant T, Eisele T, et al. Linking household and facility data for better coverage measures in reproductive, maternal, newborn, and child health care: Systematic review. J Glob Health. 2016;6:020501. Medline:27606060 doi:10.7189/jogh.06.020501

28 Carvajal-Aguirre L, Mehra V, Amouzou A, Khan SM, Vaz L, Guenther T, et al. Does health facility service environment matter for the receipt of essential newborn care? Linking health facility and household survey data in Malawi. J Glob Health. 2017;76:020509. doi:10.7189/jogh.07.020509

29 van Lonkhuijzen L, Stekelenburg J, van Roosmalen J. Maternity waiting facilities for improving maternal and neonatal outcome in low-resource countries. Cochrane Database Syst Rev. 2009;10:CD006759. Medline:19588403

The importance of skin–to–skin contact for early initiation of breastfeeding in Nigeria and Bangladesh

Kavita Singh[1,2], Shane M Khan[3], Liliana Carvajal–Aguirre[3], Paul Brodish[1], Agbessi Amouzou[4], Allisyn Moran[5]

[1] MEASURE Evaluation/Carolina Population Center, University of North Carolina at Chapel Hill, Chapel Hill, North Carolina, USA
[2] Department of Maternal and Child Health, Gillings School of Global Public Health, University of North Carolina at Chapel Hill, Chapel Hill, North Carolina, USA
[3] Data and Analytics, Division of Data, Research and Policy, UNICEF, New York, New York, USA
[4] Institute for International Programs, Department of International Health, Johns Hopkins Bloomberg School of Public Health, Baltimore, Maryland, USA
[5] Global Health Fellows Program II, United States Agency for International Development (USAID), Washington, D.C., USA

Background Skin–to–skin contact (SSC) between mother and newborn offers numerous protective effects, however it is an intervention that has been under–utilized. Our objectives are to understand which newborns in Bangladesh and Nigeria receive SSC and whether SSC is associated with the early initiation of breastfeeding.

Methods Demographic and Health Survey (DHS) data were used to study the characteristics of newborns receiving SSC for non–facility births in Nigeria (DHS 2013) and for both facility and non–facility births in Bangladesh (DHS 2014). Multivariable logistic regression was used to study the association between SSC and early initiation of breastfeeding after controlling for key socio–demographic, maternal and newborn–related factors.

Results Only 10% of newborns in Nigeria and 26% of newborns in Bangladesh received SSC. In the regression models, SSC was significantly associated with the early initiation of breastfeeding in both countries (OR = 1.42, 95% CI 1.15–1.76 for Nigeria; OR = 1.27, 95% CI 1.04–1.55, for Bangladesh). Findings from the regression analysis for Bangladesh revealed that newborns born by Cesarean section had a 67% lower odds of early initiation of breastfeeding than those born by normal delivery (OR = 0.33, 95% CI 0.26–0.43). Also in Bangladesh newborns born in a health facility had a 30% lower odds of early initiation of breastfeeding than those born in non–facility environments (OR = 0.70, 95% CI 0.53–0.92). Early initiation of breastfeeding was significantly associated with parity, urban residence and wealth in Nigeria. Geographic area was significant in the regression analyses for both Bangladesh and Nigeria.

Conclusions Coverage of SSC is very low in the two countries, despite its benefits for newborns without complications. SSC has the potential to save newborn lives. There is a need to prioritize training of health providers on the implementation of essential newborn care including SSC. Community engagement is also needed to ensure that all women and their families regardless of residence, socio–economic status, place or type of delivery, understand the benefits of SSC and early initiation of breastfeeding.

Globally there were an estimated 5.9 million deaths to children under–five in the year 2015, and 45% of these deaths occurred during the neonatal period, the first month of life [1]. While there have been substantial reductions in under–five mortality, reductions in neonatal mortality have been less pronounced. From 1990 to 2015 under–five mortality fell by 52% compared to 42% for neonatal mortality [1]. The main causes of under–five mortality are now prematurity, pneumonia; and intrapartum–related conditions including birth asphyxia [2]. Notably two of the top three main causes of death occur either exclusively in the neonatal period (birth asphyxia) or mostly in the neonatal period (prematurity), while pneumonia is a cause of death for both neonates and children 1–59 months. The global health community has provided specific recommendations on essential newborn care (ENC), which refers to care provided to the newborn within the first moments to days of life [3]. Components of ENC include thermal care, early and exclusive breastfeeding, appropriate cord care and monitoring/early treatment for low birth weight or sick newborns. ENC is intended to enable countries to protect newborns through the implementation of simple, yet, life–saving interventions.

The ENC interventions focused on thermal care are intended to ensure that newborns do not develop hypothermia (state of being too cold) or hyperthermia (state of being too hot). Newborns regulate temperature less effectively and lose heat more easily compared to adults. These issues are intensified for low birth weight and premature newborns [4]. Interventions for thermal care include immediate drying, delayed bathing, head covering and skin–to–skin contact (SSC), which is the placement of a naked newborn baby prone on the mother's bare chest soon after birth [5]. The mother and baby may be covered loosely with a blanket or cloth, preferable pre–warmed [6]. The newborn baby should remain in that position until the end of the first successful breastfeeding [5,7]. In addition to providing warmth, SSC also has numerous other benefits including improved attachment between mother and newborn [8–10] and the reduction of infant stress [5,11,12]. A Cochrane Review of randomized trials including mother–baby dyads, found that SSC at birth was associated with breastfeeding at one to four months post–birth with a risk ratio of 1.25. A total of 13 trials, composing of 702 mother–baby dyads, were included in the review for the breastfeeding outcomes [5]. Despite the benefits and the simplicity of SSC as a natural intervention, over time it became common practice to separate newborns from their mothers after delivery often due to routine procedures [5,13–5]. In 2012, the American Academy of Pediatrics stated that many maternal and newborn assessments can be done during SSC or can be delayed until after the critical SSC period, so long as the mother and newborn do not have any complications [16].

There is an increased focus on newborn health interventions among the global health community and recently some large–scale household surveys have included measures of such interventions. The use of population–based data are important, as it can provide some indication of how well a country is implementing SSC in real–life settings. Data on SSC are only currently available from a few household surveys, most recently the Nigeria Demographic and Health Survey (DHS) 2013 [17] and the Bangladesh DHS 2014 [18]. These two countries together accounted for 12% of the world's neonatal deaths [1].

The first objective of this analysis is to assess the level of practice of SSC in Nigeria and Bangladesh and to examine the characteristics of newborns who are receiving SSC. Understanding SSC by key factors is essential in efforts to improve coverage of this intervention. The second objective is to determine whether SSC is associated with the early initiation of breastfeeding, defined as breastfeeding within the first hour of life. Early initiation of breastfeeding is an important outcome to study for several reasons. First milk or colostrum is rich in protective factors including antibodies and vitamin A, and early breastfeeding is a pivotal step towards longer–term and exclusive breastfeeding [19]. Trials in Nepal and Ghana have found that early initiation of breastfeeding could prevent 19% and 22%, respectively, of neonatal deaths [20,21].

METHODS

Data sources

We used data from the 2013 Nigeria DHS and the 2014 Bangladesh DHS. The DHS are a source of nationally representative data for monitoring socio–economic and health indicators at the population level. In sampled households women age 15–49 are eligible to participate, but in some countries, such as

Bangladesh, only ever–married women 15–49 are eligible to participate. The sample is based on a stratified two–stage cluster design. The first stage is the sample enumeration area (SEA), and the second stage is a list of households from each SEA. The samples are representative at the national, urban/rural residence and regional levels. For both Nigeria and Bangladesh we restricted our sample to women with a live birth. For Nigeria the question on SSC was asked of the most recent birth in the past five years for non–facility births only. For Bangladesh the question on SSC was asked of the most recent birth in the past three years for both facility and non–facility births. (The specific questions are described in the section on the key independent variable.) The sample sizes were 11 966 mother–newborn pairs in Nigeria and 4444 mother–newborn pairs in Bangladesh.

Outcome variable

The dependent variable was early initiation of breastfeeding, defined as breast-feeding within one hour of birth. The question was worded the same in both Bangladesh and Nigeria: *How long after birth did you first put (NAME) to the breast?*

The variable was coded as "0" if more than 1 hour and "1" if one hour or less.

Key independent variable

The key independent variable was a dichotomous indicator of SSC for the most recent birth in the past three (Bangladesh) or five (Nigeria) years. The questions were slightly different between the two surveys as shown below.

Nigeria (non–facility births only): *Was (Name) placed on your belly/breast before delivery of the placenta?*

Bangladesh (facility and non–facility births): *After the birth was (Name) put directly on the bare skin of your chest?*

Another difference is that in Bangladesh the interviewers were trained to show the respondent a picture of the SSC position.

Control variables

Several maternal health variables were studied including mother's age in years by the following age groups: 15–19, 20–24, 25–34, 35+; education (none, primary, secondary or higher); current marital status (married, not married) and parity (1, 2–3, 4+). The analysis included two socio–economic variables – urban residence and wealth quintile and a demographic variable–subnational region of residence (which were zones for Nigeria and divisions for Bangladesh). Several delivery–rated factors were studied including Cesarean delivery (yes/ no: Bangladesh only); facility delivery (yes/no Bangladesh only; facility vs non–facility) and type of delivery attendant [skilled birth attendant (SBA) vs unskilled birth attendant]. SBA was defined as a doctor, nurse or midwife in accordance with the global definition. We included mother's perceptions of her baby's birthweight (small, average, large, large) to understand any differentials in SSC by perceived size of the baby.

Analysis

The analysis was carried out separately for each country. Bivariate analyses (using Pearson χ^2 test) compared several control variables for mothers reporting SSC immediately after birth to those who did not. In multivariate logistic regressions, early breastfeeding was regressed on SSC, controlling for all of the maternal and infant–related variables mentioned in the section above.

RESULTS

Table 1 shows column percentages of SSC by key characteristics of the mother and newborn in Nigeria. Only about 10% of mothers (1217/12 265) reported SSC, and there was little difference between mothers whose newborns received SSC and mothers whose newborns did not receive SSC. However, there was one significant difference. Newborns who were perceived to be large were significantly more likely to experience SSC than smaller newborns. About 55% of the newborns who received SSC were perceived to be large, compared to 29% and 16% for those perceived to be average and small, respectively.

Table 2 shows column percentages of SSC by key characteristics for the Bangladesh sample. Overall, about 26% of mothers (1210/4586) reported SSC with their newborn, and once again there was little difference between mothers whose newborns received SSC vs those that did not. The only significant finding was that newborns of parity 2–3 were significantly more likely to have experienced SSC with their mothers compared to newborns of parity one and higher parity. Of the newborns receiving SSC 50% were of parity 2–3 compared to 39% for newborns of parity one and 11% for newborns of parity 4 and higher. This finding, however was only significant at $P < 0.10$.

Table 1. *Skin-to-skin contact by key characteristics in Nigeria: Last non–facility birth in past five years (survey–weighted column percentages and counts)*

	Skin–to–skin contact						P
	Yes		No		Total		
	10%	(n = 1217)	90%	(n = 11 048)	100.0%	(N = 12 265)	
	%	n	%	n	%	n	
Mother's age:							
15–19	7.9	96	7.7	850	7.7	946	
20–24	20.3	248	20.9	2305	20.8	2551	
25–34	45.2	551	44.9	4964	45.0	5515	
35–49	26.6	323	26.5	2929	26.5	3249	
Parity:							
1	13.8	168	14.6	1616	14.6	1784	
2–3	26.4	321	29.2	3223	28.9	3545	
4+	59.8	728	56.2	6204	56.5	6932	
Mother's education:							
None	70.3	856	68.2	7538	68.5	8394	
Primary	17.8	217	17.0	1877	17.1	2093	
Secondary+	11.8	144	14.8	1633	14.5	1774	
Zone:							
North Central	16.3	198	11.1	1227	11.6	1425	
North East	33.8	412	20.4	2253	21.7	2665	
North West	42.9	523	52.6	5809	51.6	6332	
South East	1.2	14	2.7	297	2.5	312	
South South	4.1	50	7.3	806	7.0	856	
South West	1.7	21	5.9	651	5.5	672	
Residence:							
Urban	18.7	228	20.4	2263	20.3	2486	
Rural	81.3	990	79.6	8785	79.7	9775	
Wealth:							
Poorest	38.6	470	34.8	3843	35.2	4313	
Second	27.2	331	29.8	3294	29.6	3624	
Middle	18.2	221	18.6	2057	18.6	2279	
Fourth	11.5	140	11.8	1300	11.7	1438	
Richest	4.6	56	5.0	553	4.9	606	
Estimated size at birth:							
Small	16.0	193	18.0	1973	17.8	2167	
Average	29.4	355	42.2	4630	40.9	4985	
Large	54.7	662	39.9	4378	41.3	5040	<0.001
Attendant at delivery:							
Doctor/midwife/Nurse	5.5	67	3.8	417	4.0	484	
Unskilled provider/ friend/family member/ other	94.5	1141	96.2	10 588	96.0	11 729	

Table 2. *Skin–to–skin contact by key characteristics in Bangladesh: last birth in past three years (survey–weighted column percentages and counts)*

	SKIN–TO–SKIN CONTACT						P
	Yes		No		Total		
	26%	(n = 1210)	84%	(n = 3376)	100.0%	(N = 4586)	
Mother's age:	%	n	%	n	%	n	
15–19	19.7	238	21.3	718	20.9	957	
20–24	33.2	401	33.7	1138	33.6	1540	
25–34	41.9	506	38.7	1305	39.5	1812	
35–49	5.2	63	6.3	214	6.0	277	
Parity:							
1	38.5	465	40.1	1352	39.6	1818	
2–3	50.3	609	45.1	1524	46.5	2132	
4+	11.2	136	14.8	500	13.9	636	<0.1
Mother's education:							
None	11.8	143	15.1	508	14.2	651	
Primary	28.6	346	27.7	936	28.0	1283	
Secondary+	59.6	721	57.2	1931	57.8	2652	
Division:							
Barisal	6.1	74	5.7	192	5.8	267	
Chittagong	17.5	212	23.4	791	21.9	1003	
Dhaka	40.2	486	33.6	1135	35.4	1621	
Khulna	8.6	104	7.7	259	7.9	363	
Rajshahi	9.0	109	10.5	353	10.1	462	
Rangpur	9.5	114	9.8	332	9.7	446	
Sylhet	9.1	110	9.3	314	9.2	424	
Residence:							
Urban	26.2	317	26.1	881	26.1	1198	
Rural	73.8	893	73.9	2495	73.9	3388	
Wealth:							
Poorest	22.1	268	21.6	730	21.8	997	
Second	17.6	213	19.5	659	19.0	872	
Middle	19.7	238	18.7	632	19.0	870	
Fourth	22.0	266	20.0	675	20.5	942	
Richest	18.6	225	20.2	680	19.7	905	
Estimated size at birth:							
Small	22.7	275	18.9	637	19.9	912	
Average	65.5	793	67.9	2291	67.3	3084	
Large	11.7	142	13.2	447	12.8	589	
Delivery location:							
Home	58.0	701	62.8	2121	61.6	2822	
Health facility	38.6	466	34.8	1175	35.8	1641	
Public	15.5*	187	12.1	409	13.0	596	
Private	23.1*	279	22.7	767	22.8	1046	
Other	3.4	41	2.4	80	2.6	121	

Table 2. *Continued*

	SKIN–TO–SKIN CONTACT						
	Yes		No		Total		P
	26%	(n = 1210)	84%	(n = 3376)	100.0%	(N = 4586)	
Attendant at delivery:							
Doctor/midwife/nurse	33.3	402	31.7	1064	32.1	1465	
Unskilled provider/ friend/family member/ other	66.7	803	68.3	2293	67.9	3096	
Caesarean delivery:							
Yes	23.3	281	24.2	817	24.0	1099	
No	76.7	928	75.8	2558	76.0	3486	

*Percentages of total deliveries.

Table 3 shows results from regression analyses of early breastfeeding on SSC, controlling for key characteristics of mothers and newborns. In both Nigeria and Bangladesh, SSC was associated with significantly increased odds of early breastfeeding, controlling for all other variables in the models. The odds of early breastfeeding was 42% for newborns receiving SSC in Nigeria and 27% for newborns receiving SSC in Bangladesh (odds ratio (OR) = 1.42, 95% confidence interval (CI) 1.15–1.76; OR = 1.27, 95% CI 1.04–1.55, respectively). Also, in Nigeria several maternal demographic variables were associated with increased odds of early breastfeeding. Newborns of parity 2 or 3 had a 23% increased odds of SSC than newborns of parity 1 (OR = 1.23, 95% CI 1.02–1.50). Compared to North Central, the referent region, the odds of early breastfeeding were significantly lower for newborns in North West, South East and Southwest. Newborns from wealthier households were significantly more likely to experience early breastfeeding than newborns from the very poorest households. The odds ranged from 30% to 59% depending on the specific wealth quintile.

The results for Bangladesh indicated that Cesarean delivery was associated with a 67% lower odds of early breastfeeding (OR = 0.33, 95% CI 0.26–0.43), and facility delivery was associated with a 30% lower odds of early breastfeeding (OR = 0.70, 95% CI 0.53–0.92). There were also two significant effects for division. Compared to the referent division, Barisal, residence in Rangpur was associated with a 50% higher odds of early breastfeeding (OR = 1.50, 95% CI 1.03–2.17) and in Sylhet with a 42% higher odds of early breastfeeding (OR = 1.42, 95% CI 1.02–1.96).

Table 3. *Survey–weighted logistic regression analysis of early breastfeeding on skin–to–skin contact for the most recent birth, controlling for maternal and infant characteristics*

CHARACTERISTIC	NIGERIA (N = 11 419)		BANGLADESH (N = 4262)	
Predictor variable	OR	95% CI	OR	95% CI
Skin–to–skin contact	1.42‡	1.15, 1.76	1.27*	1.04, 1.55
Delivery characteristics				
Facility delivery:				
No	NA		1.00	
Yes			0.70*	0.53, 0.92
Caesarean delivery:				
No	NA		1.00	
Yes			0.33‡	0.26, 0.43
Estimated size at birth:				
Small	1.00		1.00	
Average	1.10	0.94, 1.28	1.06	0.87, 1.31
Large	1.08	0.92, 1.26	0.96	0.68, 1.35
Attendant at delivery:				
Unskilled provider/friend/family member/other	1.00		1.00	
Doctor/midwife/nurse	1.03	(0.78, 1.37)	1.43	0.98, 2.09
Maternal demographic characteristics				
Age:				
15–19	1.00		1.00	
20–24	1.07	0.86, 1.32	1.14	0.92, 1.42
25–34	1.15	0.92, 1.45	0.94	0.73, 1.20
35–49	1.23	1.02, 1.50	0.74	0.44, 1.25
Parity:				
1	1.00		1.00	
2–3	1.23*	1.02, 1.50	1.08	0.90, 1.31
4+	1.18	0.95, 1.47	1.04	0.75, 1.43
Zone/Division:				
Nigeria Bangladesh				
North Central Barisal	1.00		1.00	
North East Chittago	1.21	0.95, 1.55	0.83	0.60, 1.14
North West Dhaka	0.58‡	0.46, 0.73	1.15	0.80, 1.64
South East Khulna	0.45†	0.28, 0.71	0.81	0.57, 1.14
South South Rajshahi	0.92	0.71, 1.18	1.22	0.88, 1.70
South West Rangpur	0.40‡	0.28, 0.57	1.50*	1.03, 2.17
Sylhet			1.42*	(1.02, 1.96)
Residence:				
Rural	1.00		1.00	
Urban	1.91‡	1.49, 2.43	0.85	0.67, 1.08

Table 3. *Continued*

Characteristic	Nigeria (N = 11 419)		Bangladesh (N = 4262)	
Predictor variable	OR	95% CI	OR	95% CI
Education:				
None	1.00		1.00	
Primary	1.07	0.91, 1.26	0.90	0.66, 1.22
Secondary+	1.05	0.86, 1.28	0.86	0.65, 1.13
Wealth:				
Poorest	1.00		1.00	
Second	1.30‡	1.08, 1.58	0.85	0.66, 1.10
Middle	1.37*	1.08, 1.75	0.93	0.70, 1.26
Fourth	1.59†	1.20, 2.11	1.13	0.84, 1.52
Richest	1.47*	1.00, 2.16	1.06	0.75, 1.51
Marital status:				
Not married	1.00		1.00	
Married	0.96	0.76, 1.21	1.00	0.41, 2.44

*$P < 0.05$.
†$P < 0.01$.
‡$P < 0.001$.

DISCUSSION

SSC is a natural intervention with numerous benefits, yet it is under–practiced as many mothers and newborns are separated after birth often due to routine procedures [5,13–15]. SSC has been studied as part of trials, but this is the first analysis to use population–level data to look at coverage and factors related to coverage. Associations between SSC with the early initiation of breastfeeding were also studied given the numerous benefits of early breastfeeding, including reduced infant mortality [20,21]. SSC is also considered step 4 of 10 Steps to Successfully Breastfeeding promoted by the Baby Friendly Hospital Initiative [22].

In our study, we found low coverage of SSC in both Nigeria (10%) and Bangladesh (26%) and few differences between newborns receiving SSC and those not receiving SSC. Though an uncommon intervention, in the regression models SSC was significantly associated with early initiation of breastfeeding in both Nigeria and Bangladesh. Thus, our results support findings from trials indicating that SSC is associated with improved breastfeeding outcomes [5] and specifically with early breastfeeding.

Another key finding from the first regression models was that in Bangladesh newborns born in a health facility were less likely to experience early breastfeeding than those born in non–facility environments. There are several plausible explanations for this finding. Some of the mothers and babies may have gone to the facility because of a complication, and this complication may have required separation beyond one hour. A second possible explanation involves health facility procedures, which often require the immediate separation of mother and newborns, which in turn prevents both SSC and early breastfeeding. Many maternal and newborn assessments can actually be done during SSC or can be delayed until after the critical SSC period, so long as the mother and newborn do not have any complications [16,23–25]. Findings from Bangladesh revealed that newborns of mothers who had a Cesarean section were significantly less likely to be breastfed early. Other studies have found the same results [26,27], but there is an increasing recognition that health facilities must implement protocols that allow mothers who have a Cesarean section to breastfeed early. The Baby Friendly Hospital Initiative recommends that SSC can actually begin in the operating theater (after a Cesarean section) when the mother is alert [22,25].

Skilled delivery in a health facility is promoted as an essential strategy to improve both maternal and newborn health [28,29]. The ideal situation would be for women to deliver in a health facility with a SBA who can oversee SSC, as mother and baby should be monitored in case any complication or safety concerns should arise [30].

Other significant findings from the regression analyses are also worthy to note. In both countries there were some differences by zone or division. In Nigeria the northern zones are generally poorer than the southern zones. However early breastfeeding was less common in the southern zones than in the North Central zone. A study by Berde and Yalcin also found variation in the early initiation of breastfeeding by zone [31]. Our results from Bangladesh indicated that early breastfeeding was more common in Rangpur and Sylhet, the poorest divisions, compared to Barisal. A systematic review of early breastfeeding in South Asia also found geographic differences in the early initiation of breastfeeding within countries and also highlighted the influence of traditional practices, which may vary within countries [32]. Another systematic review highlighted the importance of the knowledge and beliefs of family members, particularly for women who deliver at home [33]. A study from Nepal attributed variations in early breastfeeding to many factors including socioeconomic factors, geographic terrain and the availability of formula [34]. Our findings from Nigeria suggested that wealthier and urban women as well as those of parity 2 or 3, had increased odds of having their newborns initiate breastfeeding early. These women may have greater knowledge than their counterparts and some previous experience with breastfeeding. Perceived size at birth was not significant in our regression analyses, but other studies have found that low birthweight and premature newborns are less likely to be breastfed early than normal weight and term newborns [32,33]. Taken together, these comprehensive findings suggest that there is a need to ensure equitable diffusion of knowledge on the importance of early breastfeeding and SSC to all delivery attendants and to all women and families regardless of wealth, parity or geographic residence.

There are several limitations to this analysis. The questions on SSC were not the same for the two countries, and SSC was only asked to women who had a non–facility delivery in Nigeria. More broadly additional work may be needed to validate measures of SSC. A validation study by Blanc et al. 2016 [35] in Kenya found that questions on SSC (newborn placed against mother's chest after delivery and newborn was naked on skin, not wrapped in towel) did not perform well in terms of individual–level reporting accuracy and population–level accuracy. In this study women's reports before discharge were compared to direct observation in two hospitals. However, Stanton et al. 2013 [36] found that a question on SSC met the criteria for quality reporting in study in Mozambique, which compared women's reporting in household surveys (8 to 10 months after delivery) to direct observations. Further work may be needed on exact wording for questions on SSC and for appropriate probes. Another limitation is that the DHS data did not yield complete information on actual birthweight, which is often unknown for newborns who are born at home and not weighed. Also lacking were information on maternal and newborn complications as well as quality of care at the facilities and characteristics of providers. Recall bias could also be an issue in that mothers were asked to recall an event that occurred in a one–hour period. Some of the mothers had births several years (three to five) before the survey.

In terms of program recommendations, training of SBAs on proper thermal care for newborns including SSC is a key step in improving newborn health. The WHO's Essential Newborn Training Guide includes modules on thermal care including SSC [6]. Manasyan et al. 2011 found this training to be cost–effective for midwives at first level health facilities in Zambia [37]. Trainings will need to be done on a large scale to ensure that all healthy newborns, regardless of delivery type (vaginal vs Cesarean), size or socioeconomic status, receive SSC. At the same time community engagement is needed to enable more mothers and families to learn about the protective effects of SSC. More research is needed on exact timing of initiation of SSC, frequency and duration as well as measures to ensure SSC is as safe as possible [5]. SSC is an intervention with the potential to save newborn lives.

Acknowledgements: We are grateful to the Carolina Population Center and its NIH Center grant (P2C HD050924) for general support.

Disclaimers: The views expressed are those of the authors and do not necessarily reflect the views of the United States Agency for International Development (USAID), the United States Government or those of UNICEF.

Funding: This study was carried out with support provided by the United States Agency for International Development (USAID) through MEASURE Evaluation (cooperative agreement AID–OAA–L–14–00004). The views expressed are not necessarily those of USAID or the United States government.

Authorship declaration: KS, SK, LCV and AA led the development of ideas for the paper. KS led the writing and analysis plan, and PB led the data management. SK, LCV, AA and AM provided substantial inputs and ideas into all drafts of the paper.

Competing interests: The authors have completed the Unified Competing Interest form at www.icmje.org/coi_disclosure.pdf (available on request from the corresponding author) and declare no competing interests.

References

1 UNICEF. Levels and trends in under-five mortality. Estimates developed by the UN Interagency Group for Child Mortality Estimation. New York: UNICEF; 2015.

2 WHO. MCEE-WHO methods and data sources for child causes of death 2000-2015. Global Health Estimates Technical Paper WHO/HIS/IER/GHE/2016.1 Geneva: WHO; 2016.

3 WHO. Every newborn: An action plan to end preventable deaths. Geneva:WHO; 2014.

4 WHO. Thermal Protection of the Newborn: A practical guide. The Safe Motherhood Initiative. Geneva: WHO; 1997.

5 Moore ER, Anderson G, Bergman N, Doswell T. Early skin-to-skin contact for mothers and their healthy infants. Cochrane Database Syst Rev. 2012;5:CD003519. Medline:22592691

6 WHO. Essential newborn care training module. 2010. Available: http://www.who.int/maternal_child_adolescent/documents/newborncare_course/en/. Accessed: 6 February 2017.

7 Widström AM, Lilja G, Aaltomaa-Michalias P, Dahllöf A, Lintula M, Nissen E. Newborn behaviour to locate the breast when skin-to-skin: a possible method for enabling early self-regulation. Acta Paediatr. 2011;100:79-85. Medline:20712833 doi:10.1111/j.1651-2227.2010.01983.x

8 Nahidi F, Tavafian SS, Heidarzadeh M, Hajizadeh E, Montazeri A. The Mother-Newborn Skin-to-Skin Contact Questionnaire (MSSCQ): development and psychometric evaluation among Iranian midwives. BMC Pregnancy Childbirth. 2014;14:85. Medline:24564830 doi:10.1186/1471-2393-14-85

9 Saastad E, Ahlborg T, Froen JF. Low maternal awareness of fetal movement is associated with small for gestational age infants. J Midwifery Womens Health. 2008;53:345-52. Medline:18586188 doi:10.1016/j.jmwh.2008.03.001

10 Mikiel-Kostyra K, Mazur J, Bołtruszko I. Effect of early skin-to-skin contact after delivery on duration of breastfeeding: a prospective cohort study. Acta Paediatr. 2002;91:1301-6. Medline:12578285 doi:10.1111/j.1651-2227.2002.tb02824.x

11   Thukral A, Sankar MJ, Agarwal R, Gupta N, Deorari AK, Paul VK. Early skin-to-skin contact and breastfeeding behaviors in term neonates: A randomized controlled trial. Neonatology. 2012;102:114-9. Medline:22699241 doi:10.1159/000337839

12   Bornstein MH. Sensitive periods in development: Structural characteristics and casual intrepretations. Psychol Bull. 1989;105:179-97. Medline:2648441 doi:10.1037/0033-2909.105.2.179

13   Anderson GC. The mother and newborn: Mutual caregivers. JOGN Nurs. 1977;6:50-7. Medline:242611 doi:10.1111/j.1552-6909.1977.tb02181.x

14   Odent M. New reasons and new ways to study birth physiology. Int J Gynaecol Obstet. 2001;75 Suppl 1:S39-45. Medline:11742641 doi:10.1016/S0020-7292(01)00512-4

15   Winberg J. Examining breast-feeding performance: forgotten influencing factors. Acta Paediatr. 1995;84:465-7. Medline:7633136 doi:10.1111/j.1651-2227.1995.tb13675.x

16   American Academy of Pediatrics Section on Breastfeeding. Breastfeeding and the use of human milk. Pediatrics. 2012;129:e827-41. Medline:22371471 doi:10.1542/peds.2011-3552

17   National Population Commission (NPC) [Nigeria] and ICF International. Nigeria Demographic and Health Survey 2013. Abuja, Nigeria, and Rockville, Maryland, USA: NPC and ICF International; 2014.

18   National Institute of Population Research and Training (NIPORT), Mitra and Associates, and ICF International. Bangladesh Demographic and Health Survey 2014. Dhaka, Bangladesh, and Rockville, Maryland, USA: NIPORT, Mitra and Associates, and ICF International; 2016.

19   Begum K, Dewey K. Impact of early initiation on breastfeeding on neonatal deaths. A&T Technical Brief. Issue 1. FHI 360. Washington, DC: FHI 360, Alive and Thrive; 2010.

20   Edmond KM, Zandoh C, Quigley MA, Amenga-Etego S, Owusu-Agyei S, Kirkwood BR. Delayed breastfeeding initiation increases risk of neonatal mortality. Pediatrics. 2006;117:e380-6. Medline:16510618 doi:10.1542/peds.2005-1496

21   Mullany LC, Katz J, Li YM, Khatry SK, LeClerq SC, Darmstadt GL, et al. Breast-feeding patterns, time to initiation, and mortality risk among newborns in southern Nepal. J Nutr. 2008;138:599-603. Medline:18287373

22   World Health Organization, United Nations Children's Fund. Baby-Friendly Hospital Initiative: Revised, updated, and expanded for integrated care. Geneva: WHO; 2009.

23   American College of Obstetrics and Gynecologists Committee on Obstetrics Practice, Committee on Health Care for Underserved. Special report from ACOG. Breastfeeding: Maternal and infant aspects. ACOG Clin Rev. 2013;12 Suppl. 1:1S-16S.

24   Sobel HL, Silvestre MAA, Mantaring JBV III, Oliveros YE, Nyunt US. Immediate newborn care practices delay thermoregulation and breastfeeding initiation. Acta Paediatr. 2011;100:1127-33. Medline:21375583 doi:10.1111/j.1651-2227.2011.02215.x

25   Crenshaw JT. Healthy Birth Practice #6: Keep mother and baby together—it's best for mother, baby and breastfeeding. J Perinat Educ. 2014;23:211-7. Medline:25411542 doi:10.1891/1058-1243.23.4.211

26   Hobbs AJ, Mannion CA, McDonald SW, Brockway M, Tough SC. The impact of caesarean section on breastfeeding initiation, duration and difficulties in the first four months postpartum. BMC Pregnancy Childbirth. 2016;16:90. Medline:27118118 doi:10.1186/s12884-016-0876-1

27   Rowe-Murray HJ, Fisher JRW. Baby friendly hospital practices: cesarean section is a persistent barrier to early initiation of breastfeeding. Birth. 2002;29:124-31. Medline:12000413 doi:10.1046/j.1523-536X.2002.00172.x

28 Kerber KJ, de Graft J, Bhutta Z, Okong P, Starrs A, Lawn J. Continuum of care for mater-
    nal, newborn,and Child health: from slogan to service delivery. Lancet. 2007;370:1358-
    69. Medline:17933651 doi:10.1016/S0140-6736(07)61578-5

29 Campbell OMR, Calvert C, Testa A, Strehlow M, Benova L, Keyes E, et al. The scale,
    scope, coverage, and capability of childbirth care. Lancet. 2016;388:2193-208. Med-
    line:27642023 doi:10.1016/S0140-6736(16)31528-8

30 Feldman-Winter L, Goldsmith JP; AAP Committee on Fetus and Newborn, AAP Task
    Force on Sudden Infant Death Syndrome. Safe sleep and skin-to-skin care in the neona-
    tal period for healthy term newborns. Pediatrics. 2016;138:e20161889. Medline:27550975
    doi:10.1542/peds.2016-1889

31 Berde AS, Yalcin SS. Determinants of early initiation of breastfeeding in Nigeria: A
    population-based study using the 2013 demographic and health survey data. BMC
    Pregnancy Childbirth. 2016;16:32. Medline:26852324 doi:10.1186/s12884-016-0818-y

32 Sharma IK, Bryne A. Early initiation of breastfeeding: A systematic literature review
    of factors and barriers in South Asia. Int J Breastfeed. 2016;11:17. Medline:27330542
    doi:10.1186/s13006-016-0076-7

33 Esteves TMB, Daumas RP, Couto de Oliveira MI, de Ferreira de Andrade CA, Leite IC.
    Factors associated to breastfeeding in the first hour of life: Systematic review. Rev Saude
    Publica. 2014;48:697-708. Medline:25210829 doi:10.1590/S0034-8910.2014048005278

34 Adhikari M, Khanal V, Karkee R, Gavidia T. Factors associated with EIBF among Nep-
    alese mothers: further analysis of Nepal Demographic and Health Survey, 2011. Int
    Breastfeed J. 2014;9:21. Medline:25493094 doi:10.1186/s13006-014-0021-6

35 Blanc AK, Warren C, McCarthy KJ, Kimani J, Ndwiga C. RamaRao S. Assessing the
    validity of indicators of the quality of maternal and newborn health care in Kenya. J
    Glob Health. 2016;6:010405. Medline:27231541 doi:10.7189/jogh.06.010405

36 Stanton CK, Rawlins B, Drake M, dos Anjos M, Cantor D, Chongo L, et al. Measuring
    coverage in MNCH: Testing the validity of women's self-report of key maternal and
    newborn health interventions during the peripartum period in Mozambique. PLoS
    One. 2013;8:e60694. Medline:23667427 doi:10.1371/journal.pone.0060694

37 Manasyan A, Chomba E, McClure EM, Wright LL, Krzywanski S, Carlo WA. Cost-
    effectiveness of essential newborn care training in urban first-level facilities. Pediatrics.
    2011;127:e1176-81. Medline:21502223 doi:10.1542/peds.2010-2158

Does postnatal care have a role in improving newborn feeding? A study in 15 sub–Saharan African countries

Shane M Khan[1], Ilene S Speizer[2,3], Kavita Singh[2,3], Gustavo Angeles[2,3], Nana AY Twum–Danso[2], Pierre Barker[2]

---

[1] Data and Analytics, Division of Data, Research and Policy, United Nations Children's Fund (UNICEF), New York, New York, USA
[2] Department of Maternal and Child Health, Gillings School of Global Public Health, University of North Carolina at Chapel Hill, Chapel Hill, North Carolina, USA
[3] Carolina Population Center, University of North Carolina at Chapel Hill, Chapel Hill, North Carolina, USA

Background Breastfeeding is known as a key intervention to improve newborn health and survival while prelacteal feeds (liquids other than breastmilk within 3 days of birth) represents a departure from optimal feeding practices. Recent programmatic guidelines from the WHO and UNICEF outline the need to improve newborn feeding and points to postnatal care (PNC) as a potential mechanism to do so. This study examines if PNC and type of PNC provider are associated with key newborn feeding practices: breastfeeding within 1 day and prelacteal feeds.

Methods: We use data from the Demographic and Health Surveys for 15 sub–Saharan African countries to estimate 4 separate pooled, multilevel, logistic regression models to predict the newborn feeding outcomes.

Findings: PNC is significantly associated with increased breastfeeding within 1day (OR = 1.35, $P < 0.001$) but is not associated with PLFs (OR = 1.04, $P = 0.195$). PNC provided by nurses, midwives and untrained health workers is also associated with higher odds of breastfeeding within 1 day of birth (OR = 1.39, $P < 0.001$, (OR = 1.95, $P < 0.001$) while PNC provided by untrained health workers is associated with increased odds of PLFs (OR = 1.20, $P = 0.017$).

Conclusions: PNC delivered through customary care may be an effective strategy to improve the breastfeeding within 1 day but not to discourage PLFs. Further analysis should be done to examine how these variables operate at the country level to produce finer programmatic insight.

Breastfeeding is recognized as a key intervention to improve the health and survival of children and the use of optimal breastfeeding practices such as exclusive breastfeeding is one of the most effective means to reduce under-nutrition, an underlying cause of under–five mortality [1]. The World Health Organization (WHO) and the United National Children's Fund (UNICEF) recommend early initiation of breastfeeding [2] which refers to breastfeeding of a newborn within an hour of birth. Global monitoring efforts by UNICEF also include initiation of breastfeeding within one day of birth which pro-vides additional information on the feeding patterns of newborns and the behaviors of women. Early initiation of breastfeeding has a number of health benefits, one of which is to reduce neonatal mortality [3–5]. The early inges-tion of breastmilk can have positive effects on a newborn's immune systems such as the provision of immunoglobulins and lymphocytes [6–8], priming of the gastrointestinal tract and decreasing the permeability of the tract to pathogens, including HIV [9,10]. Another health benefit of early initiation of breastfeeding is reduced rates of diarrhea among infants, as demonstrated in Egypt and Pakistan [11,12].

Early initiation of breastfeeding is also associated with a number of factors. One such factor is skin–to–skin contact with the mother [13,14], a form of thermal care which is a recommended means to reduce neonatal mortality [15]. Early breastfeeding is also associated with a number of factors related to contact with the health system. For example, in Brazil, early initiation is associated with vaginal delivery as well as other factors such as antenatal guidance on breastfeeding and having a full term pregnancy [16]. Other studies point out that breastfeeding within an hour of birth is less likely to occur when women have caesarian sections, even in the presence of hospital practices that favor breastfeeding [17,18]. In a review article, authors find that higher socio–eco-nomic status is associated with lower odds of breastfeeding initiation but this pattern is only seen in developing countries [19].

Prelacteal feeds (PLFs) represent a departure from optimal newborn feeding practices. PLFs are any liquid other than breast milk that is given to the new-born before breastfeeding is established between the mother and newborn. The WHO and UNICEF outline that for successful breastfeeding, PLFs should be avoided and PLFs should not be encouraged unless medically indicated [20]. These feeds usually occur within the first few days of life and are associated with a number of negative health outcomes for the newborn and mother. These include insufficient maternal milk production, newborn diarrhea and reduced length of breastfeeding duration [21,22]. PLFs can also expose newborns to infections through the ingestion of contaminated food and liquids which can act on the GI tract to increase permeability to pathogens, and hence, increase newborn infections [9,11].

A number of studies have shown factors related to PLFs. For example, PLFs are negatively associated with early initiation of breastfeeding (within an hour of birth) [23]. In India, PLFS were associated with lower maternal education among hospital–delivered infants [24]. However, in rural, Western Uganda, more educated women were more prone to provide PLFs to newborns [25]. In low socio–economic settlements in Karachi, Pakistan, PLFs were associated with having a birth attendant [26]. In a national study in Nepal, women without education, who were not working, who had no antenatal care and were first time mothers were more likely to provide PLFs [27]. Both in India and Vietnam, newborns of women with a cesarean section were more likely to ingest PLFs [24,28].

In a recent joint statement, the WHO and UNICEF recommend that all newborns, regardless of place of birth (whether in a facility or not), should receive a basic package of care, including postnatal care which includes the promotion and support of exclusive breastfeeding and the early initiation of breastfeeding [29]. Interventions such as thermal care, hygienic cord care, examination for danger signs and improving parental knowledge of care seeking are also recommended. The evidence on the importance of PNC from developing countries comes mainly from South Asian countries (India, Bangladesh and Pakistan) and are from interventions and trials at sub–national levels (such as districts, villages and communities) [30–32].

Currently, there is a gap in the literature on how interventions such as PNC are associated with newborn feeding practices at the national level, when delivered through usual services of the government and non–governmental sources of care ie, outside of an intervention setting. The literature is especially sparse for sub–Saharan Africa. The only study we found was a small, cross–sectional study in Ethiopia [33] where PNC was associated with increased odds of timely initiation of breastfeeding. Apart from the issue of generalizability of PNC interventions, we currently do not know which type of provider of PNC is best suited to improve the newborn feeding outcomes. The WHO–UNICEF PNC recommendation acknowledges that skilled and unskilled health workers can provide PNC though skilled providers are better suited [29]. However, in the literature on newborn feeding, we find varying opinions on if skilled or unskilled care can improve breastfeeding. In Bangladesh, for example, specially trained peer counselors can improve initiation and duration of exclusive breastfeeding [34]. However, a literature review finds that trained health care workers (physicians, nurses etc.) were found to be a barrier to providing quality information, counseling and care to women on early breastfeeding [19].

The main objective of this paper is to examine the association between PNC within 1 day and two key newborn feeding practices: breastfeeding within 1 day and prelacteal feeds. Given that WHO–UNICEF recommends both skilled and unskilled health workers to provide PNC and that there are mixed results regarding the association of provider type on newborn feeding, we also examine if the type of provider of PNC is important for the two stated outcomes. We use data from nationally representative surveys in 15 sub–Saharan African countries in a pooled, multi–level analysis, controlling for a number of individual and country–level variables. The results of this paper can provide indications on which types of providers are best suited for the delivery of PNC as it relates to newborn feeding.

METHODS

Data and variables

Data for this study are from the USAID–supported Demographic and Health Surveys (DHS). DHS surveys collect data from nationally–representative probability samples of households. Households are selected using a two–stage sample design where census enumeration areas are first selected and then a random sample of households is selected in the second stage. Within selected households, all women ages 15–49 are interviewed and provide information on themselves and their children on various health, population and nutrition issues. Women also provide informed consent to the survey prior to the start of questions. All data are anonymized. This analysis focuses on the last birth in the last two years before the surveys for which information on PNC is provided. We include Benin 2011–2012, Burkina Faso 2010, Comoros 2012, Congo Brazzaville 2012, Cote d'Ivoire 2012, Gabon 2012, Guinee 2012, Mali 2012–2013, Namibia 2013, Niger 2012, Nigeria 2013, Sierra Leone 2013, Tanzania 2010, Uganda 2011 and Zimbabwe 2011, based on the availability of comparable data on PNC.

There are two outcome variables. The first is the percentage of newborns who were breastfed within 1 day of birth among all newborns. The second outcome variable is the percentage of newborns who received a PLF ie, a feed that occurs within 3 days of births that is not breastmilk. The measure of PLFs is based on asking the mother if, within the first 3 days after delivery, the newborn was given anything to drink, other than breast milk. This is only asked for newborns who were ever breastfed.

The key independent variable is PNC within 1 day which refers to any check within 1 day to a newborn following birth. The question also provides examples of what a check may entail (checking temperature, cord etc.). We exclude a check by 'others' (such as friends or relatives as these are not likely to be medical). Women were also asked, if for the last birth in the 2 years before the survey, what provider or traditional birth attendant performed the check on the newborn's health. Qualitative work confirms that women are able to tell coherent narratives about the moments around birth and recognize checks on the health of a child [35]. Given that PLFs can occur anytime within 3 days, we attempt to establish PNC preceding PLFs by defining PNC as a check within 1 day of birth instead of 3 days. Both of these outcomes are binary. To investigate if PNC provider is associated with the outcomes, we create a variable for PNC provided by three categories of caregivers: physicians, nurses/midwives/auxiliary midwives and finally, traditional birth attendants/community health workers/other.

In our models, we introduce a number of statistical controls based on the literature, classified as individual–level controls or country–level controls. We include: age of the mother, previous birth interval, parity, caesarian section of birth, use of antenatal care (ANC), receipt of tetanus toxoid vaccination, skilled delivery, educational level of the woman, marital status, media access (regular access to print and mass media), place of residence and a wealth index of household goods and assets (provided in the DHS data files), constructed using Principal Component Analysis of household–level ownership of goods and assets.

We include 4 binary, country–level variables to account for the variation in the supply of PNC. The five country–level variables are: Gross Domestic Product (GDP) per capita ("high" when US$ 1000 or greater per capita or "low" when below US$ 1000 per capita), per capita government expenditure on health ("high" when US$ 100 or greater per capita and "low" when below US$ 100 per capita), number of physicians per 1000 population ("high" when the value is 0.1 or greater and "low" when the value is below 0.1) and finally, the number of nurses per 1000 population ("high" when the value is 1 and greater and "low" when the value is less than 1). Finally, since there are prominent recommendations on newborn feeding practices in areas of high HIV prevalence, we included a dummy variable for HIV prevalence ("high" when 5% or greater and "low" when less than 5%) as an explanatory variable in the models.

Statistical analysis

We use descriptive statistics and multivariate models to examine the association between the main predictors and the outcomes. First, we describe the sample using frequencies of the variables and then produce cross–tabulations of key variables by the outcome variables using chi–square tests. Finally, we model the outcome variables on the key variables (in separate models), with a number of statistical controls. Univariate analysis is done at the country level to provide an indication of the contribution of each country to overall sample but as the aim of the analysis is cross–country, the remainder of the analysis is done at the aggregate level.

As breastfeeding within 1 day and PLFs are binary outcomes, a logistic regression model can be used, assuming that the error term follows a logistic distribution. However, as we study individual–level data from different countries, this suggest that these data are clustered and as a consequence, a multilevel model may be required (MLM). To verify if MLM is needed, we compared all MLMs to single level logistic regressions using a Likliehood–ratio (LR) test. These results should that the data are clustered at the country level and that MLMs perform better than the single–level logistic regressions. In our models, country–level variance was between 4 to 11 percent. Multilevel models and bivariate table are run without sample weights while univariate are weighted using DHS sample weights provided in datafiles.

RESULTS

Breastfeeding within a day of birth is high (81 percent) and varies considerably across the countries, ranging from 66 percent in Cote d'Ivoire to 94 percent in Mali (**Table 1**). Levels of prelacteal feeds are lower (39 percent overall), ranging from 11 percent in Namibia to 65 percent in Cote d'Ivoire. PNC is low overall; only 15 percent of the sample received PNC within a day, of which the vast majority was provided by a nurse (12 percent) and only 2 and 1 percent provided by physicians and by traditional birth attendants/community health workers/others (TBA/CHWs/others) respectively. In the sample, about half of the women had 3 or fewer children. Caesarian sections are uncommon (4 percent). More than half of the women had contact with the health system through ANC care (52 percent), receipt of tetanus toxoid (56 percent) and had a skilled delivery (62 percent). The majority of the sample is married, has no education, no regular access to media and about 40 percent is classified into the poorest or second lowest wealth quintiles.

In 7 of the 15 countries, newborns who receive PNC were more likely to be breastfed within 1 day compared with newborns who did not receive PNC but in several countries (eg, Comoros, Congo (Brazzaville), Uganda), the opposite occurs (**Figure 1**). **Figure 2** shows that while overall newborns receiving PNC are significantly less likely to receive a prelacteal feed, patterns by country vary considerably; 5 countries show a statistically significant relationship but 4 show the opposite pattern.

Table 1. *Weighted distribution of sample for 15 countries*

	Benin 2011–2012	Burkina Faso 2010	Comoros 2012	Congo Brazzaville 2012	Cote d'Ivoire 2012	Gabon 2012	Guinee 2012	Mali 2012–2013
Outcomes								
Breastfeeding within 1 d of birth:								
Yes	80.9	80.5	76.3	69.8	66.2	70.0	73.1	94.0
No	19.1	19.5	23.7	30.2	33.8	30.0	26.9	6.0
Prelacteal feeding:*								
Yes	18.1	35.9	37.5	36.1	65.6	41.3	59.1	21.1
No	81.9	64.1	62.5	63.9	34.4	58.7	40.9	78.9
Key variables								
PNC within 1 d:								
Yes:	20.6	18.0	10.3	15.4	24.8	12.7	16.7	13.5
By Physician	2.0	0.2	1.6	2.7	2.7	1.2	4.4	1.7
By Nurse/Midwife/Aux. midwife	17.4	17.5	8.2	12.6	17.5	11.2	9.5	7.2
By TBA/CHW/Other	1.1	0.2	0.6	0.1	4.6	0.2	2.8	4.5
No	79.4	82.0	89.7	84.6	75.2	87.3	83.3	86.5
Maternal factors								
Age of mother:								
15–19	6.2	8.6	8.5	14.0	12.2	14.9	14.3	11.3
20–24	22.1	26.6	22.7	25.8	26.3	25.8	23.1	22.9
25–29	31.8	25.3	24.4	25.8	27.3	24.3	25.4	28.6
30–34	22.1	19.9	23.5	18.1	18.7	18.3	17.1	19.2
35–39	12.0	12.9	15.1	12.6	10.1	11.1	12.8	12.1
40–49	5.7	6.8	5.8	3.8	5.4	5.6	7.3	5.8
Previous birth interval:								
First birth (and twins)	20.8	17.6	22.4	23.7	22.5	27.9	21.2	17.1
<18 months	2.6	1.9	9.2	3.4	3.1	4.8	1.4	3.9
18–23 months	6.5	6.0	12.4	7.3	6.1	8.7	5.7	8.1
24–29 months	13.8	13.2	13.7	12.6	13.1	11.7	9.5	14.4
30–35 months	14.0	17.7	10.7	10.2	13.2	8.1	15.7	14.2
36–47 months (ref)	20.3	23.4	13.6	15.0	16.4	12.0	21.1	20.2

Table 1. *Continued*

	Benin 2011–2012	Burkina Faso 2010	Comoros 2012	Congo Brazza-ville 2012	Cote d'Ivoire 2012	Gabon 2012	Guinee 2012	Mali 2012–2013
48–53 months	6.2	6.0	4.9	6.1	5.3	4.7	7.2	5.7
54+ months	15.7	14.2	13.1	21.7	20.3	22.1	18.3	16.4
Parity:								
1	20.5	17.5	22.1	23.4	22.1	27.6	21.1	17.0
2–3	38.7	33.8	35.3	42.4	37.3	38.2	33.0	33.4
4–5	24.5	23.3	23.6	22.9	22.8	20.1	23.5	27.1
6+	16.3	25.3	19.0	11.2	17.7	14.1	22.4	22.5
Cesarean section:								
Yes	6.1	2.1	11.4	6.6	3.0	10.6	3.0	3.0
No	93.9	97.9	88.6	93.4	97.0	89.4	97.0	97.0
Personal illness control factors								
Antenatal care (4+ with any provider):								
Yes	58.7	32.5	47.6	76.0	42.8	75.6	56.2	41.0
No	41.3	67.5	52.4	24.0	57.2	24.4	43.8	59.0
Tetanus toxoid (2+ during last pregnancy):								
Yes	59.4	70.3	36.2	59.9	52.1	66.5	70.1	36.8
No	40.6	29.7	63.8	40.1	47.9	33.5	29.9	63.2
Skilled delivery:								
Yes	85.6	74.2	85.6	94.1	61.4	91.2	46.2	61.2
No	14.4	25.8	14.4	5.9	38.6	8.8	53.8	38.8
Socio–economic factors								
Education of mother:								
None	69.7	83.4	43.3	7.0	62.4	5.8	75.5	81.6
Primary	16.7	10.8	24.9	31.1	26.5	25.9	13.6	9.1
Secondary+	13.6	5.7	31.8	61.9	11.2	68.3	10.9	9.3
Marital status:								
Married/cohabiting	93.6	97.1	94.5	78.3	83.4	70.3	92.3	96.7
Not currently married/cohabiting	6.4	2.9	5.5	21.7	16.6	29.7	7.7	3.3
Media access:								

Table 1. *Continued*

	Benin 2011–2012	Burkina Faso 2010	Comoros 2012	Congo Brazza-ville 2012	Cote d'Ivoire 2012	Gabon 2012	Guinee 2012	Mali 2012–2013
Yes	22.5	9.2	26.6	25.9	17.0	46.7	17.0	23.7
No	77.5	90.8	73.4	74.1	83.0	53.3	83.0	76.3
Household wealth status:								
Poorest quintile	20.3	20.2	23.0	22.2	24.3	21.3	22.9	20.4
Second quintile	20.5	21.9	20.8	23.0	20.4	21.6	21.4	20.2
Middle quintile	19.4	22.0	21.1	20.2	20.7	22.5	20.7	19.4
Fourth quintile	19.7	21.0	18.5	19.0	18.6	19.3	19.1	22.1
Richest quintile	20.1	14.9	16.6	15.5	15.9	15.2	15.9	17.8
Residence:								
Urban	41.3	17.0	28.4	61.4	38.7	84.3	26.5	20.3
Rural	58.7	83.0	71.6	38.6	61.3	15.7	73.5	79.7
Country-level characteristics								
GDP per capita (US$):								
High (1000 per capita and greater)	–	–	–	–	–	–	–	–
Low (less than 1000 per capita)	–	–	–	–	–	–	–	–
Per capita government expenditure on health at average exchange rate (US$):								
High (100 per capita and greater)	–	–	–	–	–	–	–	–
Low (less than 100 per capita)	–	–	–	–	–	–	–	–
No. physicians per 1000 population:								
High (0.1 or greater)	–	–	–	–	–	–	–	–
Low (less than 0.1)	–	–	–	–	–	–	–	–
No. nurses per 1000 population:								
High (1 or greater)	–	–	–	–	–	–	–	–
Low (less than 1)	–	–	–	–	–	–	–	–
HIV prevalence:								
High (5%+)	–	–	–	–	–	–	–	–
Low (<5%)	–	–	–	–	–	–	–	–
Total	5130	5988	1298	3426	3039	2102	2818	3965

Table 1. *Continued*

	Namibia 2013	Niger 2012	Nigeria 2013	Sierra Leone 2013	Tanzania 2010	Uganda 2011	Zimbabwe 2011	All Countries
Outcomes								
Breastfeeding within 1 d of birth:								
Yes	89.1	78.6	73.7	89.1	90.5	88.7	91.7	80.1
No	10.9	21.4	26.3	10.9	9.5	11.3	8.3	19.8
Prelacteal feeding:*								
Yes	10.2	49.1	58.4	20.7	30.8	41.1	13.1	39.1
No	89.8	50.9	41.6	79.3	69.2	58.9	86.9	60.9
Key variables								
PNC within 1 d:								
Yes:								
By Physician	15.3	10.7	11.4	26.4	1.2	8.8	9.5	14.6
By Nurse/Midwife/Aux. midwife	5.6	0.2	4.5	1.5	0.1	1.8	1.6	2.3
By TBA/CHW/Other	9.5	8.8	5.9	21.0	0.9	6.7	7.7	10.9
	0.2	1.7	1.0	3.9	0.2	0.3	0.2	1.5
No	84.7	89.3	88.6	73.6	98.8	91.2	90.5	85.4
Maternal factors								
Age of mother:								
15–19	10.7	9.6	8.5	13.5	10.2	10.3	12.4	10.4
20–24	25.5	23.1	22.7	23.0	27.1	28.2	31.2	24.5
25–29	25.5	27.4	28.0	26.1	25.4	27.5	27.6	27.1
30–34	20.1	20.8	20.1	18.0	17.5	16.2	16.3	19.3
35–39	12.3	13.0	13.4	12.9	14.2	12.5	9.0	12.6
40–49	5.9	6.1	7.3	6.5	5.5	5.4	3.5	6.1
Previous birth interval:								
First birth (and twins)	32.2	13.6	20.3	22.0	19.9	17.2	29.3	20.7
<18 months	2.4	4.1	4.1	2.5	3.6	6.1	2.4	3.5
18–23 months	4.9	11.3	9.9	6.9	8.0	12.9	3.6	8.1
24–29 months	8.2	20.6	15.7	12.0	16.9	20.5	6.8	14.3
30–35 months	7.7	18.1	15.1	13.9	15.6	13.7	8.7	14.2
36–47 months (ref)	9.8	18.3	18.1	16.7	16.0	15.0	14.9	17.8

Table 1. *Continued*

	Namibia 2013	Niger 2012	Nigeria 2013	Sierra Leone 2013	Tanzania 2010	Uganda 2011	Zimbabwe 2011	All Countries
48–53 months	4.9	4.3	4.4	5.7	5.0	3.4	5.8	5.2
54+ months	29.8	9.7	12.4	20.4	14.9	11.1	28.5	16.3
Parity:								
1	31.7	13.4	20.1	21.7	19.6	17.1	29.0	20.4
2–3	42.7	27.4	32.3	35.0	35.7	31.5	47.4	35.1
4–5	17.4	24.6	22.6	24.8	23.2	22.4	16.6	23.1
6+	8.2	34.5	25.0	18.6	21.5	29.0	6.9	21.4
Cesarean section:								
Yes	15.7	1.4	2.2	4.0	5.2	5.5	4.5	4.3
No	84.3	98.6	97.8	96.0	94.8	94.5	95.5	95.7
Personal illness control factors								
Antenatal care (4+ with any provider):								
Yes	62.0	33.1	51.1	76.0	38.4	46.2	59.2	51.4
No	38.0	66.9	48.9	24.0	61.6	53.8	40.8	48.6
Tetanus toxoid (2+ during last pregnancy):								
Yes	33.9	50.2	48.7	86.7	44.1	52.2	42.8	55.4
No	66.1	49.8	51.3	13.3	55.9	47.8	57.2	44.6
Skilled delivery:								
Yes	89.0	33.4	42.4	62.6	49.7	60.9	64.9	61.6
No	11.0	66.6	57.6	37.4	50.3	39.1	35.1	38.4
Socio–economic factors								
Education of mother:								
None	5.6	85.3	47.6	64.7	25.6	12.9	1.1	51.8
Primary	22.5	9.6	18.1	15.3	67.0	63.9	31.3	22.7
Secondary+	71.9	5.1	34.3	20.1	7.4	23.2	67.5	25.5
Marital status:								
Married/cohabiting	44.2	98.3	95.6	84.7	84.0	85.5	87.3	89.3
Not currently married/cohabiting	55.8	1.7	4.4	15.3	16.0	14.5	12.7	10.7
Media access:								
Yes	34.9	7.4	22.2	7.5	18.0	16.0	19.8	19.1

Table 1. *Continued*

	Namibia 2013	Niger 2012	Nigeria 2013	Sierra Leone 2013	Tanzania 2010	Uganda 2011	Zimbabwe 2011	All Countries
No	65.1	92.6	77.8	92.5	82.0	84.0	80.2	80.9
Household wealth status:								
Poorest quintile	21.3	19.3	23.2	23.0	21.0	22.4	22.2	21.8
Second quintile	22.6	20.5	22.8	21.0	23.9	22.0	21.1	21.7
Middle quintile	21.7	20.8	18.9	21.9	21.7	19.5	19.5	20.4
Fourth quintile	20.0	21.1	18.0	19.1	18.8	18.1	21.2	19.5
Richest quintile	14.4	18.3	17.1	14.9	14.6	18.0	16.0	16.6
Residence:								
Urban	47.5	13.5	35.3	25.7	20.9	14.6	29.3	31.5
Rural	52.5	86.5	64.7	74.3	79.1	85.4	70.7	68.5
Country-level characteristics								
GDP per capita (US$):								
High (1000 per capita and greater)	–	–	–	–	–	–	–	37.7
Low (less than 1000 per capita)	–	–	–	–	–	–	–	62.3
Per capita government expenditure on health at average exchange rate (US$):								
High (100 per capita and greater)	–	–	–	–	–	–	–	50.7
Low (less than 100 per capita)	–	–	–	–	–	–	–	49.3
No. physicians per 1000 population:								
High (0.1 or greater)	–	–	–	–	–	–	–	43.9
Low (less than 0.1)	–	–	–	–	–	–	–	56.1
No. nurses per 1000 population:								
High (1 or greater)	–	–	–	–	–	–	–	36.2
Low (less than 1)	–	–	–	–	–	–	–	63.8
HIV prevalence:								
High (5%+)	–	–	–	–	–	–	–	17.6
Low (<5%)	–	–	–	–	–	–	–	82.4
Total	1947	5143	12473	4820	3266	3092	2448	60956

PNC – postnatal care, TBA – Traditional Birth Attendant, CHW – Community Health Worker
*Denominator is ever–breast fed newborns.

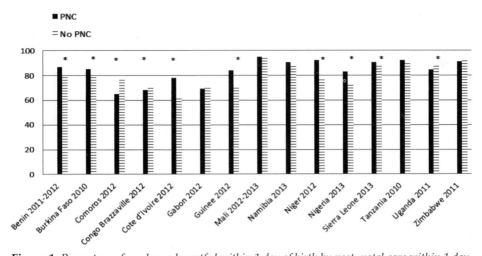

Figure 1. *Percentage of newborns breastfed within 1 day of birth by post–natal care within 1 day. Asterisk indicates P < 0.05.*

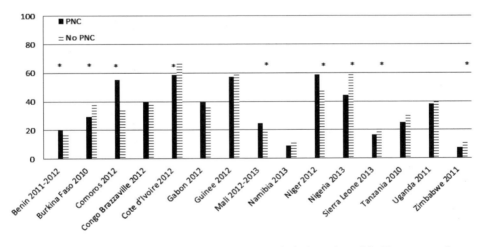

Figure 2. *Among ever breast–fed newborns, percentage who had a prelacteal feed by post–natal care within 1 day of birth. Asterisk indicates P < 0.05.*

In the bivariate analysis, newborns receiving PNC within 1 day are significantly more likely to initiate breastfeeding within a day and less likely to receive a prelacteal feed (**Table 2**). Women receiving antenatal care, tetanus toxoid and skilled delivery are significantly more likely to breastfeed within a day and less likely to provide a prelacteal feed to the newborn. A caesar-

Table 2. *Percentage of all newborns breastfed within 1 day and percentage of newborns receiving prelacteal feeds among ever breastfed newborns, by key characteristics (unweighted), 15 countries*

	ALL NEWBORNS		EVER BREASTFED NEWBORNS	
	Breastfeeding within:		Prelacteal feed	
	1 day	P		P
Key dependent variables				
PNC within 1 day:				
Yes	84.2	<0.001	35.3	<0.001
No	79.8		39.3	
Maternal factors				
Age of mother:				
15–19	76.3	<0.001	42.5	<0.001
20–24	80.1		38.9	
25–29	81.9		37.0	
30–34	81.4		37.7	
35–39	80.8		38.6	
40–45	80.4		40.7	
45–49	79.9		45.3	
Previous birth interval:				
First birth (and twins)	81.8	<0.001	38.7	<0.001
<18 months	76.8		39.6	
18–23 months	78.2		41.6	
24–29 months	80.5		41.6	
30–35 months	82.1		40.7	
36–47 months	81.8		39.7	
48–53 months	81.5		35.7	
54+ months	81.5		33.7	
Parity:				
1	77.0	<0.001	39.6	<0.001
2–3	81.9		35.6	
4–5	82.2		38.2	
6+	79.9		43.2	
Cesarean section:				
Yes	62.4	<0.001	38.3	0.710
No	81.3		38.7	
Breastfed within 1 hour:				
Yes	–		28.0	<0.001
No	–		47.3	
Personal illness control factors				
Antenatal care (4+ with any provider):				
Yes	82.0	<0.001	33.9	<0.001
No	78.9		43.8	
Tetanus toxoid (2+ during last pregnancy):				
Yes	81.5	<0.001	35.5	<0.001
No	79.2		42.7	

Table 2. *Continued*

	ALL NEWBORNS		EVER BREASTFED NEWBORNS	
	Breastfeeding within:		**Prelacteal feed**	
Skilled delivery:				
Yes	82.8	<0.001	30.9	<0.001
No	76.7		51.4	
Socio–economic factors				
Education of mother:				
None	79.3	<0.001	42.7	<0.001
Primary	82.4		37.1	
Secondary+	81.2		32.2	
Marital status:				
Married/cohabiting	80.7	0.001	39.4	<0.001
Not currently married/cohabiting	79.0		33.2	
Media access:				
Yes	81.6	0.001	33.6	<0.001
No	80.3		39.8	
Household wealth status:				
Poorest quintile	77.2	<0.001	43.2	<0.001
Second quintile	79.2		40.8	
Middle quintile	82.1		38.1	
Fourth quintile	82.3		35.7	
Richest quintile	83.1		33.3	
Residence:				
Urban	81.7	<0.001	34.2	<0.001
Rural	80.0		40.6	
Country characteristics				
GDP per capita (US$):				
High (1000+ per capita)	74.0	<0.001	49.7	<0.001
Low (<1000 per capita)	84.7		31.6	
Per capita government expenditure on health at average exchange rate (US$):				
High (100+ per capita)	77.5	<0.001	44.3	<0.001
Low (<100 per capita)	83.7		32.7	
No. physicians per 1000 population.				<0.001
High (0.1+)	75.7	<0.001	50.6	
Low (<0.1)	84.3		29.2	
No. nurses per 1000 population:				
High (1+)	79.1	<0.001	44.1	<0.001
Low (<1)	81.4		35.6	
HIV prevalence:				
High (5%+)	90.2	<0.001	24.9	<0.001
Low (<5%)	78.5		41.6	
Total	61018		59309	

PNC – postnatal care

ian birth is significantly associated with breastfeeding within 1 day but not with PLFs. Women with no education are less likely to breastfeed early and more likely to provide a prelacteal feed. While household wealth is positively associated with breastfeeding within 1 day, the association is negative with prelacetal feeds. Women in urban areas are more likely than rural women to initiate breastfeeding within 1 day and less likely to give a prelacetal feed. Bivariate analysis of the country–level variables also shows lower levels of GDP, expenditures, and physician and nurse density are associated with greater initiation of breastfeeding within 1 day and lower levels of prelacteal feeds. In countries with higher HIV prevalence, breastfeeding within 1 day is higher and prelacteal feeds are lower.

Table 3 shows that after controlling for individual and country–level variables, PNC within 1 day is significantly associated with higher odds of breastfeeding within 1 day (OR = 1.35, 95% CI 1.27–1.44). The odds of breastfeeding within 1 day are significantly lower for women who had a caesarian section compared with those that did not have a caesarian section (OR = 0.26, 95% CI 0.23–0.28). Many of the variables related to contact with the health care system that are significant at the bivariate level are also significant in the multilevel model. These include ANC (OR = 1.07, 95% CI 1.02–1.12), tetanus coverage (OR = 1.10, 95% CI 1.05–1.15) and skilled delivery (OR = 1.48, 95% CI 1.40–1.56). Several socio–economic variables are significantly associated with breastfeeding within 1 day. Compared to women with no education, women with primary education are significantly more likely to initiate breastfeeding within 1 day (OR = 1.10, 95% CI 1.04–1.17) though the association with secondary or higher education is not significant (OR = 1.06, 95% CI 0.99–1.14). Women in rural areas are significantly less likely to initiate breastfeeding within a day than those in urban areas (OR = 0.92, 95% CI 0.87–0.98). Of the country–level controls in the model, higher HIV prevalence is associated with increased odds of breastfeeding within 1 day (OR = 2.13, 95% CI 1.19–3.82).

Model 2 shows that the provider of PNC is significantly associated with breastfeeding within 1 day. PNC from physicians is not associated with breastfeeding within 1 day but PNC provided by nurses/midwives/auxiliary midwives and TBA/CHW/others is associated with higher odds of breastfeeding within 1 day (nurses/midwives/aux. midwives OR = 1.39, 95% CI 1.29–1.50, TBA/CHW/others OR = 1.95, CI 1.60–2.36).

Table 3 shows that after controlling for individual and country–level variables, PNC within 1 day is not significantly associated with prelacteal feeds (OR = 1.04, 95% CI 0.98–1.09). Age is significantly associated with the outcome

Table 3. Multilevel logistic regression for breastfeeding within 1 d among all newborns and prelacteal feeds among ever breastfed newborns, 15 countries

	ALL NEWBORNS, BREASTFEEDING WITHIN 1 D							AMONG EVER BREASTFED NEWBORNS, PRELACTEAL FEEDS						
	Model 1	P	95% CI		Model 2	P	95% CI		Model 3	P	95% CI		Model 4	P	95% CI	
Fixed Effects																
Key variables																
PNC within 1 d:																
Yes	1.35	<0.001	1.27	1.44	–	–	–	–	1.04	0.195	0.98	1.09	–	–	–	–
No	1.00	–	–	–	–	–	–	–	1.00	–	–	–	–	–	–	–
Provider of PNC within 1 d:																
By Physician	–	–	–	–	0.93	0.269	0.81	1.06	–	–	–	–	0.94	0.343	0.83	1.07
By Nurse/Midwife	–	–	–	–	1.39	<0.001	1.29	1.50	–	–	–	–	1.03	0.315	0.97	1.09
By TBA/CHW/Other	–	–	–	–	1.95	<0.001	1.60	2.36	–	–	–	–	1.20	0.017	1.03	1.39
No	–	–	–	–	1.00	–	–	–	–	–	–	–	1.00	–	–	–
Maternal factors																
Age of mother:																
15–19	1.00	–	–	–	1.00	–	–	–	1.00	–	–	–	1.00	–	–	–
20–24	1.08	0.049	1.00	1.17	1.09	0.043	1.00	1.17	0.93	0.038	0.86	1.00	0.93	0.040	0.86	1.00
25–29	1.15	0.002	1.05	1.26	1.16	0.001	1.06	1.26	0.84	<0.001	0.78	0.91	0.85	<0.001	0.78	0.92
30–34	1.13	0.020	1.02	1.25	1.14	0.014	1.03	1.26	0.85	<0.001	0.77	0.93	0.85	<0.001	0.77	0.93
35–39	1.12	0.050	1.00	1.26	1.13	0.038	1.01	1.27	0.85	0.002	0.77	0.94	0.85	0.002	0.77	0.94
40–49	1.16	0.027	1.02	1.33	1.17	0.020	1.03	1.34	0.91	0.117	0.81	1.02	0.91	0.127	0.81	1.03
Previous birth interval:																
First birth (and twins)	0.35	<0.001	0.24	0.49	0.35	<0.001	0.24	0.50	1.19	0.374	0.81	1.77	1.20	0.374	0.81	1.77
<18 months	0.78	<0.001	0.69	0.88	0.78	<0.001	0.69	0.88	1.07	0.181	0.97	1.19	1.07	0.185	0.97	1.19
18–23 months	0.92	0.070	0.84	1.01	0.92	0.069	0.84	1.01	1.04	0.332	0.96	1.12	1.04	0.332	0.96	1.12
24–29 months	1.01	0.733	0.94	1.09	1.01	0.721	0.94	1.09	1.03	0.399	0.96	1.10	1.03	0.400	0.96	1.10
30–35 months	1.01	0.805	0.94	1.09	1.01	0.813	0.94	1.09	0.98	0.624	0.92	1.05	0.98	0.623	0.92	1.05
36–47 months (ref)	1.00	–	–	–	1.00	–	–	–	1.00	–	–	–	1.00	–	–	–

Table 3. *Continued*

	All newborns, breastfeeding within 1 d								Among ever breastfed newborns, prelacteal feeds							
48–53 months	0.93	0.190	0.84	1.04	0.93	0.194	0.84	1.04	0.97	0.457	0.88	1.06	0.97	0.455	0.88	1.06
54+ months	0.89	0.003	0.83	0.96	0.89	0.003	0.83	0.96	0.96	0.231	0.90	1.03	0.96	0.230	0.90	1.03
Parity:																
1	1.00	–	–	–	1.00	–	–	–	1.00	–	–	–	1.00	–	–	–
2–3	0.48	<0.001	0.34	0.68	0.48	<0.001	0.34	0.69	0.97	0.868	0.65	1.43	0.97	0.869	0.65	1.43
4–5	0.49	<0.001	0.34	0.70	0.49	<0.001	0.34	0.71	1.03	0.889	0.69	1.53	1.03	0.891	0.69	1.53
6+	0.45	<0.001	0.32	0.65	0.45	<0.001	0.32	0.65	1.05	0.794	0.71	1.57	1.05	0.797	0.71	1.57
Cesarean section																
Yes	0.26	<0.001	0.23	0.28	0.26	<0.001	0.24	0.29	1.60	<0.001	1.46	1.76	1.61	<0.001	1.47	1.77
No	1.00	–	–	–	1.00	–	–	–	1.00	–	–	–	1.00	–	–	–
Breastfed within 1 h:																
Yes	–	–	–	–	–	–	–	–	0.57	<0.001	0.55	0.59	0.57	<0.001	0.55	0.59
No	–	–	–	–	–	–	–	–	1.00	–	–	–	1.00	–	–	–
Personal illness control factors																
Antenatal care (4+ with any provider):																
Yes	1.07	0.009	1.02	1.12	1.07	0.008	1.02	1.12	0.90	<0.001	0.87	0.94	0.90	<0.001	0.87	0.94
No	1.00	–	–	–	1.00	–	–	–	1.00	–	–	–	1.00	–	–	–
Tetanus toxoid (2+ during last pregnancy):																
Yes	1.10	<0.001	1.05	1.15	1.10	<0.001	1.05	1.15	0.87	<0.001	0.83	0.90	0.87	<0.001	0.83	0.90
No	1.00	–	–	–	1.00	–	–	–	1.00	–	–	–	1.00	–	–	–
Skilled delivery:																
Yes	1.48	<0.001	1.40	1.56	1.50	<0.001	1.42	1.59	0.58	<0.001	0.56	0.61	0.59	<0.001	0.56	0.62
No	1.00	–	–	–	1.00	–	–	–	1.00	–	–	–	1.00	–	–	–
Socio-economic factors																

Table 3. *Continued*

	All newborns, breastfeeding within 1 d								Among ever breastfed newborns, prelacteal feeds							
	OR	P	95% CI		OR	P	95% CI		OR	P	95% CI		OR	P	95% CI	
Education of mother:																
None	1.00	–	–	–	1.00	–	–	–	1.00	–	–	–	1.00	–	–	–
Primary	1.10	0.002	1.04	1.17	1.10	0.002	1.04	1.17	0.86	<0.001	0.82	0.91	0.86	<0.001	0.82	0.91
Secondary+	1.06	0.081	0.99	1.14	1.07	0.061	1.00	1.15	0.78	<0.001	0.73	0.83	0.78	<0.001	0.73	0.83
Marital status:																
Married/cohabiting	1.13	0.001	1.05	1.21	1.13	0.001	1.05	1.21	1.02	0.624	0.95	1.09	1.02	0.622	0.95	1.09
Not currently married/cohabiting	1.00	–	–	–	1.00	–	–	–	1.00	–	–	–	1.00	–	–	–
Media access:																
Yes	0.96	0.221	0.90	1.02	0.96	0.260	0.91	1.03	0.99	0.777	0.94	1.05	0.99	0.796	0.94	1.05
No	1.00	–	–	–	1.00	–	–	–	1.00	–	–	–	1.00	–	–	–
Household wealth status:																
Poorest quintile	1.00	–	–	–	1.00	–	–	–	1.00	–	–	–	1.00	–	–	–
Second quintile	1.05	0.084	0.99	1.12	1.05	0.115	0.99	1.11	0.98	0.418	0.93	1.03	0.98	0.386	0.93	1.03
Middle quintile	1.19	<0.001	1.12	1.28	1.19	<0.001	1.11	1.27	0.95	0.116	0.90	1.01	0.95	0.102	0.90	1.01
Fourth quintile	1.09	0.023	1.01	1.17	1.08	0.030	1.01	1.17	1.01	0.836	0.94	1.07	1.01	0.866	0.94	1.07
Richest quintile	1.10	0.040	1.00	1.21	1.11	0.031	1.01	1.22	1.04	0.309	0.96	1.13	1.04	0.296	0.96	1.13
Residence:																
Urban	1.00	–	–	–	1.00	–	–	–	1.00	–	–	–	1.00	–	–	–
Rural	0.92	0.006	0.87	0.98	0.92	0.004	0.86	0.97	1.04	0.125	0.99	1.10	1.04	0.143	0.99	1.09
Country characteristics																
GDP per capita (US$):																
High (1000+ per capita)	0.60	0.137	0.30	1.18	0.60	0.138	0.30	1.18	1.14	0.765	0.48	2.68	1.14	0.762	0.48	2.69
Low (<1000 per capita)	1.00	–	–	–	1.00	–	–	–	1.00	–	–	–	1.00	–	–	–

Table 3. *Continued*

	ALL NEWBORNS, BREASTFEEDING WITHIN 1 D								AMONG EVER BREASTED NEWBORNS, PRELACTEAL FEEDS							
Per capita government expenditure on health at average exchange rate (US$):																
High (100+ per capita)	1.08	0.800	0.58	2.03	1.08	0.819	0.57	2.02	1.11	0.803	0.50	2.45	1.10	0.809	0.50	2.44
Low (<100 per capita)	1.00	–	–	–	1.00	–	–	–	1.00	–	–	–	1.00	–	–	–
No. physicians per 1000 population:																
High (0.1+)	0.62	0.052	0.38	1.00	0.62	0.054	0.38	1.01	2.26	0.009	1.22	4.17	2.26	0.009	1.22	4.18
Low (<0.1)	1.00	–	–	–	1.00	–	–	–	1.00	–	–	–	1.00	–	–	–
No. nurses per 1000 population:																
High (1+)	1.36	0.348	0.72	2.57	1.37	0.338	0.72	2.59	0.63	0.266	0.28	1.42	0.63	0.269	0.28	1.42
Low (<1)	1.00	–	–	–	1.00	–	–	–	1.00	–	–	–	1.00	–	–	–
HIV prevalence:																
High (5%+)	2.13	0.011	1.19	3.82	2.14	0.011	1.19	3.83	0.60	0.168	0.29	1.24	0.60	0.171	0.29	1.25
Low (<5%)	1.00	–	–	–	1.00	–	–	–	1.00	–	–	–	1.00	–	–	–
Random effects																
Country–level variance (SE):	0.147(0.055)				0.147(.055)				0.237(0.09)				0.238(0.09)			
Log–likelihood	–28 043.57				–28 021.71				–34 632.369				–34 629.4			
AIC	56 159.13				56 119.41				69 338.7				69 336.8			
Log–likelihood ratio test (Chi–square)	715.1*				712.06*				1803.4*				1808.2*			
Total	61 018				61 018				59 309				59 309			

PNC – postnatal care, TBA – Traditional Birth Attendant, CHW – Community Health Worker
*P<0.01.

in the model with older women tending to have lower odds of providing pre-lacteal feeds to newborn while birth spacing and parity were not associated with prelacteal feeds. Newborns who had a Caesarian section delivery are significantly more likely to have PLFs (OR = 1.60, 95% CI 1.46–1.76). Contact with the health care system through ANC, tetanus toxoid vaccination and skilled delivery are significantly associated with lower odds of prelacteal feeds (see **Table 3**). For example, skilled delivery is associated with a 42% reduction in odds of prelacteal feeding (OR = 0.58, 95% CI 0.56–0.61). Education shows a clear gradient with prelacteal feeds; as the educational level of the woman in-creases, the odds of prelacteal feeding decreases (see **Table 3**). Of the country–level characteristics, only the density of physicians is significantly associated with prelacteal feeds in the models: higher density of physicians is associated with higher odds of prelacteal feeds (OR = 2.26, CI 1.22–4.17). In model 4 of **Table 3**, the type of provider of PNC is not associated with prelacteal feeds. Other results remain similar to model 2 of the second panel of **Table 3**.

DISCUSSION

PNC is one of the current strategies recommended for scale–up and imple-mentation in many developing countries to improve health outcomes for new-borns and mothers. While several trials and intervention studies show that PNC can improve newborn feeding patterns [30–32], this is the first study to demonstrate this association using national–level data for multiple countries in sub–Saharan Africa.

The major findings are that PNC is associated with breastfeeding within 1 day though not with prelacteal feeds. These findings are important as they suggest that PNC when delivered through customary care (as opposed to intervention and trial conditions) can be a useful strategy to improve breast-feeding (within 1 day) but not to reduce PLFs. These findings highlight the need to strengthen clinical practice so that providers of PNC can move be-yond promoting timely initiation of breastfeeding to providing more empha-sis on the avoidance of PLFs, which by definition would improve exclusive breastfeeding rates in these countries.

Our findings also indicate that both trained medical personal (nurses, mid-wives and auxiliary midwives) and untrained providers of PNC are associ-ated with increased odds of breastfeeding within 1 day though the type of provider of PNC is not associated with PLFs. Given that all of the countries that we studied are developing countries, use of untrained persons for this type of intervention may be a useful implementation approach as the promotion of optimal newborn feeding does not require high levels of specialized training.

A third important finding from this study is that, with the exception of caesarian section, contact with the formal health care system is associated with improved newborn feeding practices. This is seen in other studies eg, Nepal [27] and India [24]. This underscores the utility of the continuum of care and reinforces the need to implement around this framework. Delivery mode by caesarian section, however, is associated with poorer newborn feeding outcomes, a finding that is reflected in a number of other studies [16,24,28,36,37], even in the presence of baby–friendly policies [17].

Our study has a number of limitations. DHS data do not include any information on what procedures were done during a check and therefore cannot control for content of care. We also use cross–sectional data where PNC was not randomly assigned to individuals. As such, we are not able to provide causal linkages between PNC and the outcomes though we are able to examine associations. One of the more studied variables on breastfeeding initiation is breastfeeding within 1 hour of birth. With our data, we could study the association of PNC within an hour and breastfeeding within the same time period. However, we considered that a short time period of 1 hour does not provide sufficient time for PNC to be provided (given that in these settings, even PNC within 1 day is low). The literature also identifies a number of additional factors that predict early initiation of breastfeeding and PLFs which were not available for analysis. For example, intention to breastfeed [38] is an important predictor of initiation and duration of breastfeeding but was not available in DHS data. Dealing with sample weights is a challenge for analysis of this kind. Different countries contribute varying proportions of the overall sample and do not reflect the relative population size of the country. Appropriate sample weight can be constructed though the sample weights must be de–normalized. However, the appropriate sampling fraction for each country and their population sizes used to create these weights are not publicly available.

Despite these limitations, our findings are consistent with trials and intervention studies, and overall, PNC policy and practice can be further tailored to reduce PLFs rates. Further research at a country–level is needed to understand if the results of this aggregate, multi–country study are reflected within each of these countries.

Disclaimer: *The findings and conclusions in this report are those of the authors and do not necessarily represent the official position of their respective organizations.*

Funding: None.

Authorship contributions: *SMK conceived and operationalized the analysis and first draft of the paper. All authors discussed the paper, contributed to the final content, and writing of the paper and approved the final version.*

Competing interests: *The authors have completed the Unified Competing Interest form at www.icmje.org/coi_disclosure.pdf (available on request from the corresponding author) and declare no competing interests.*

References

1 Bhutta ZA, Ahmed T, Black RE, Cousens S, Dewey K, Giugliani E, et al. What works? Interventions for maternal and child undernutrition and survival. Lancet. 2008a;371. doi:10.1016/S0140-6736(07)61693-6. Medline:18206226

2 World Health Organization, United Nations Children's Fund. Global strategy for infant and young child feeding. Geneva: World Health Organization, 2003.

3 Edmond KM, Zandoh C, Quigley MA, Amenga-Etego S, Owusu-Agyei S, Kirkwood BR. Delayed breastfeeding initiation increases risk of neonatal mortality. Pediatrics. 2006;117:e380-6. doi:10.1542/peds.2005-1496. Medline:16510618

4 Huffman SL, Zehner ER, Victora C. Can improvements in breast-feeding practices reduce neonatal mortality in developing countries? Midwifery. 2001;17:80-92. doi:10.1054/midw.2001.0253. Medline:11399129

5 Mullany LC, Katz J, Li YM, Khatry SK, LeClerq SC, Darmstadt GL, et al. Breast-feeding patterns, time to initiation, and mortality risk among newborns in southern Nepal. J Nutr. 2008;138:599-603. Medline:18287373

6 Goldman AS. The immune system of human milk: antimicrobial, antiinflammatory and immunomodulating properties. Pediatr Infect Dis J. 1993;12:664-71. Medline:8414780 doi:10.1097/00006454-199308000-00008

7 Goldman AS, Garza C, Nichols BL, Goldblum RM. Immunologic factors in human milk during the first year of lactation. J Pediatr. 1982;100:563-7. Medline:6977634 doi:10.1016/S0022-3476(82)80753-1

8 Brandtzaeg P. Mucosal immunity: integration between mother and the breast-fed infant. Vaccine. 2003;21:3382-8. Medline:12850345 doi:10.1016/S0264-410X(03)00338-4

9 Goldman AS. Modulation of the gastrointestinal tract of infants by human milk. Interfaces and interactions. An evolutionary perspective. J Nutr. 2000;130:426S-31S. Medline:10721920

10 Rollins NC, Filteau SM, Coutsoudis A, Tomkins AM. Feeding mode, intestinal permeability, and neopterin excretion: a longitudinal study in infants of HIV-infected South African women. J Acquir Immune Defic Syndr. 2001;28:132-9. Medline:11588506 doi:10.1097/00126334-200110010-00004

11 Badruddin SH, Islam A, Hendricks KM, Bhutta ZA, Shaikh S, Snyder JD, et al. Dietary risk factors associated with acute and persistent diarrhea in children in Karachi, Pakistan. Am J Clin Nutr. 1991;54:745-9. Medline:1897481

12 Clemens J, Elyazeed RA, Rao M, Savarino S, Morsy BZ, Kim Y, et al. Early initiation of breastfeeding and the risk of infant diarrhea in rural Egypt. Pediatrics. 1999;104:e3. Medline:10390289 doi:10.1542/peds.104.1.e3

13 Sinusas K, Gagliardi A. Initial management of breastfeeding. Am Fam Physician. 2001;64:981-8. Medline:11578034

14 World Health Organization. Pregnancy, childbirth, postpartum and newborn care: A guide for essential practice. Geneva: World Health Organization, 2003.

15 Darmstadt GL, Bhutta ZA, Cousens S, Adam T, Walker N, de Bernis L, et al. Evidence-based, cost-effective interventions: how many newborn babies can we save? Lancet. 2005;365:977-88. Medline:15767001 doi:10.1016/S0140-6736(05)71088-6

16 Vieira TO, Vieira GO, Giugliani ERJ, Mendes CM, Martins CC, Silva LR. Determinants of breastfeeding initiation within the first hour of life in a Brazilian population: cross-sectional study. BMC Public Health. 2010;10:760. Medline:21143893 doi:10.1186/1471-2458-10-760

17 Rowe-Murray HJ, Fisher JRW. Baby friendly hospital practices: cesarean section is a persistent barrier to early initiation of breastfeeding. Birth. 2002;29:124-31. Medline:12000413 doi:10.1046/j.1523-536X.2002.00172.x

18 Boccolini CS, de Carvalho ML, de Oliveira MIC, Leal Mdo C, Carvalho MS. Factors that affect time between birth and first breastfeeding. [Article in Portuguese] Cad Saude Publica. 2008;24:2681-94. Medline:19009148

19 Dennis C-L. Breastfeeding initiation and duration: a 1990-2000 literature review. J Obstet Gynecol Neonatal Nurs. 2002;31:12-32. Medline:11843016 doi:10.1111/j.1552-6909.2002.tb00019.x

20 World Health Organization. Evidence for the ten steps to successful breastfeeding. Geneva: World Health Organization, 1998.

21 Hossain MM, Radwan MM, Arafa SA, Habib M, DuPont HL. Prelacteal infant feeding practices in rural Egypt. J Trop Pediatr. 1992;38:317-22. Medline:1844092 doi:10.1093/tropej/38.6.317

22 Lakati AS, Makokha OA, Binns CW, Kombe Y. The effect of pre-lacteal feeding on full breastfeeding in Nairobi, Kenya. East Afr J Public Health. 2010;7:258-62. Medline:21516965

23 El-Gilany AH, Sarraf B, Al-Wehady A. Factors associated with timely initiation of breastfeeding in Al-Hassa province, Saudi Arabia. East Mediterr Health J. 2012;18:250-4. Medline:22574479

24 Patel A, Banerjee A, Kaletwad A. Factors associated with prelacteal feeding and timely initiation of breastfeeding in hospital-delivered infants in India. J Hum Lact. 2013;29:572-8. Medline:23427115 doi:10.1177/0890334412474718

25 Wamani H, Astrřm AN, Peterson S, Tylleskär T, Tumwine JK. Infant and young child feeding in western Uganda: knowledge, practices and socio-economic correlates. J Trop Pediatr. 2005;51:356-61. Medline:15947011 doi:10.1093/tropej/fmi048

26 Fikree FF, Ali TS, Durocher JM, Rahbar MH. Newborn care practices in low socioeconomic settlements of Karachi, Pakistan. Soc Sci Med. 2005;60:911-21. Medline:15589663 doi:10.1016/j.socscimed.2004.06.034

27 Khanal V, Adhikari M, Sauer K, Zhao Y. Factors associated with the introduction of prelacteal feeds in Nepal: findings from the Nepal Demographic and Health Survey 2011. Int Breastfeed J. 2013;8:9. Medline:23924230 doi:10.1186/1746-4358-8-9

28 Nguyen PH, Keithly SC, Nguyen NT, et al. Prelacteal feeding practices in Vietnam: challenges and associated factors. BMC Public Health. 2013;13:932. doi:10.1186/1471-2458-13-932. Medline:24099034

29 World Health Organization, United Nations Children's Fund. Home visits for the newborn child. Geneva: World Health Organization, 2009.

30 Bhutta ZA, Memon ZA, Soofi S, Salat MS, Cousens S, Martines J. Implementing community-based perinatal care: results from a pilot study in rural Pakistan. Bull World Health Organ. 2008;86:452-9. Medline:18568274 doi:10.2471/BLT.07.045849

31 Kumar V, Mohanty S, Kumar A, Misra RP, Santosham M, Awasthi S, et al. Effect of community-based behaviour change management on neonatal mortality in Shivgarh, Uttar Pradesh, India: a cluster-randomised controlled trial. Lancet. 2008;372:1151-62. Medline:18926277 doi:10.1016/S0140-6736(08)61483-X

32 Baqui AH, Ahmed S, El Arifeen S, Darmstadt GL, Rosecrans AM, Mannan I, et al. Effect of timing of first postnatal care home visit on neonatal mortality in Bangladesh: a observational cohort study. BMJ. 2009;339:b2826. Medline:19684100 doi:10.1136/bmj.b2826

33 Setegn T, Gerbaba M, Belachew T. Determinants of timely initiation of breastfeeding among mothers in Goba Woreda, South East Ethiopia: a cross sectional study. BMC Public Health. 2011;11:217. Medline:21473791 doi:10.1186/1471-2458-11-217

34 Haider R, Ashworth A, Kabir I, Huttly SR. Effect of community-based peer counsellors on exclusive breastfeeding practices in Dhaka, Bangladesh: a randomised controlled trial [see commments]. Lancet. 2000;356:1643-7. Medline:11089824 doi:10.1016/S0140-6736(00)03159-7

35 Yoder P. Stanley, Mikey Risato, Riad Mahmud, Alfredo Fort, Fazlur Rahman, Avril Armstrong, and Sayed Rubayet. Women's recall of delivery and neonatal care in Bangladesh and Malawi: A study of terms, concepts, and survey questions. DHS Qualitative Research Studies No. 17. Calverton, Maryland, USA: ICF Macro. 2010. Available: http://dhsprogram.com/pubs/pdf/QRS17/QRS17.pdf. Accessed: 1 August 2017.

36 Chien L-Y, Tai C-J. Effect of delivery method and timing of breastfeeding initiation on breastfeeding outcomes in Taiwan. Birth. 2007;34:123-30. Medline:17542816 doi:10.1111/j.1523-536X.2007.00158.x

37 El-Gilany A-H, Abdel-Hady DM. Newborn first feed and prelacteal feeds in Mansoura, Egypt. BioMed Res Int. 2014;2014:258470. Medline:24895560 doi:10.1155/2014/258470

38 Donath SM, Amir LH; ALSPAC Study Team. The relationship between prenatal infant feeding intention and initiation and duration of breastfeeding: a cohort study. Acta Paediatr. 2003;92:352-6. Medline:12725552 doi:10.1111/j.1651-2227.2003.tb00558.x

Postnatal care for newborns in Bangladesh: The importance of health–related factors and location

Kavita Singh[1,2], Paul Brodish[1], Mahbub Elahi Chowdhury[3], Taposh Kumar Biswas[3], Eunsoo Timothy Kim[2], Christine Godwin[2], Allisyn Moran[4]

[1] MEASURE Evaluation/Carolina Population Center, University of North Carolina at Chapel Hill, Chapel Hill, North Carolina, USA
[2] Department of Maternal and Child Health, Gillings School of Global Public Health, University of North Carolina at Chapel Hill, Chapel Hill, North Carolina, USA
[3] International Centre for Diarrhoeal Disease Research, Bangladesh (icddr,b), Dhaka, Bangladesh
[4] Global Health Fellows Program II, United States Agency for International Development (USAID), Washington, D.C., USA, and Abuja, Nigeria

Background Bangladesh achieved Millennium Development Goal 4, a two thirds reduction in under–five mortality from 1990 to 2015. However neonatal mortality remains high, and neonatal deaths now account for 62% of under–five deaths in Bangladesh. The objective of this paper is to understand which newborns in Bangladesh are receiving postnatal care (PNC), a set of interventions with the potential to reduce neonatal mortality.

Methods Using data from the Bangladesh Maternal Mortality Survey (BMMS) 2010 we conducted logistic regression analysis to understand what socio–economic and health–related factors were associated with early postnatal care (PNC) by day 2 and PNC by day 7. Key variables studied were maternal complications (during pregnancy, delivery or after delivery) and contact with the health care system (receipt of any antenatal care, place of delivery and type of delivery attendant). Using data from the BMMS 2010 and an Emergency Obstetric and Neonatal Care (EmONC) 2012 needs assessment, we also presented descriptive maps of PNC coverage overlaid with neonatal mortality rates.

Results There were several significant findings from the regression analysis. Newborns of mothers having a skilled delivery were significantly more likely to receive PNC (Day 7: OR = 2.16, 95% confidence interval (CI) 1.81, 2.58; Day 2: OR = 2.11, 95% CI 1.76). Newborns of mothers who reported a complication were also significantly more likely to receive PNC with odds ratios varying between 1.3 and 1.6 for complications at the different points along the continuum of care. Urban residence and greater wealth were also significantly associated with PNC. The maps provided visual images of wide variation in PNC coverage and indicated that districts with the highest PNC coverage, did not necessarily have the lowest neonatal mortality rates.

Conclusion Newborns of mothers who had a skilled delivery or who experienced a complication were more likely to receive PNC than newborns of mothers with a home delivery or who did not report a complication. Given that the majority of women in Bangladesh have a home delivery, strategies are needed to reach their newborns with PNC. Greater focus is also needed to reach poor women in rural areas. Engaging community health workers to conduct home PNC visits may be an interim strategy as Bangladesh strives to increase skilled delivery coverage.

The prevention of neonatal mortality has become a global priority because of the high mortality experienced by newborns and the difficulty in achieving improvements in their survival. Neonatal mortality now accounts for 45% of under–five mortality which translates to 2.8 million deaths within the first 28 days of life. On a global level neonatal mortality rates have declined from 33 to 19 deaths per 1000 live births (from 1990 to 2015), but this 47% reduction is much less than the 58% reduction seen in deaths among post–neonatal children under–five [1]. In addition, an estimated 2.6 million stillbirths occur each year, though only a fraction of these deaths are recorded in vital registration systems [2–4]. An estimated 46% of stillbirths are intrapartum or "fresh" indicating that the fetus died after the onset of labor and perhaps could have been saved with appropriate interventions at delivery [3].

Every Newborn is an action plan focused on enabling countries to prevent neonatal deaths and stillbirths [4]. The plan emphasizes the critical periods of labor, birth and the first week of life as time points when interventions can achieve maximum impact on saving newborn lives. The plan is an extension of the United Nation's *Every Woman Every Child* movement and includes a vision, goals, strategies, and priorities for reducing newborn and stillbirth deaths. To achieve these goals, *Every Newborn* lays out key strategic objectives: 1. Improving care at birth, 2. Improving the quality and equity of maternal and newborn care, 3. Reaching every woman and newborn and achieving impact at scale, 4. Harnessing the power of parents, families and communities, and 5. Counting every newborn through measurement, program–tracking and accountability. Referral and follow–up care for low birth weight and sick newborns is also crucial given that prematurity and low birth weight are major predicators of neonatal mortality.

A continuum of services is needed to enhance newborn survival. Essential newborn care (ENC) involves care soon after birth and includes hygienic care, thermal control, support for breastfeeding and resuscitation with bag and mask, if needed [4]. Such interventions can address the main causes of neo-natal mortality such as intrapartum related birth asphyxia and complications due to prematurity and low birth weight, which account for more than half of neonatal deaths [5]. Complementing essential newborn care is postnatal care (PNC) for the newborn, a package of interventions delivered after birth that includes the promotion of immediate and exclusive breastfeeding (for children less than 6 months of age), hand–washing, examination of mother and child for danger signs and appropriate referral for medical care [6]. Interventions provided as part of PNC can prevent some newborn complications such as sepsis, meningitis, pneumonia and diarrhea. PNC could be a means of pro-viding follow–up care to newborns who were born premature and/or of low birth weight and provides an opportunity to check all newborns for illnesses that may have arisen since delivery [4].

Under–five mortality in Bangladesh has been steadily declining from 144 deaths per 1000 live births to 38 deaths per 1000 live births in the period between 1990 and 2015 [1]. Though Bangladesh laudably achieved the Mil-lennium Development Goal (MDG) 4 target of a two–thirds reduction in un-der–five mortality, the burden of neonatal mortality continues to remain a concern. Neonatal mortality also declined from 63/1000 to 23/1000 during the same time period, but the magnitude of the decline was not as great as for under–five mortality. The proportion of neonatal deaths out of all under–five deaths actually increased from 44% to 62% from 1990 to 2015 [1].

Promotion of PNC has been emphasized in the National Neonatal Health Strategy and Guidelines (NNHS) of Bangladesh, and PNC is provided free of charge at government health facilities. PNC is provided both at health facilities and during home visits by community health workers in efforts to make the service accessible from the community to tertiary level. During home visits community health workers focus on the i) promotion of newborn care (early/ exclusive breastfeeding, warmth, hygiene); ii) promotion of nutrition & family planning counseling to mothers; iii) providing information about danger signs of both mother and newborn; iv) Identification of danger signs in newborn and referral; v) support for breastfeeding; and vi) care of low birth weight infant (feeding, skin–to–skin contact) [7,8].

Studies in Bangladesh have found that socioeconomic factors such as education [9,10] and wealth have an influence on PNC coverage for newborns [11–16]. A study by Anwar et al. 2008 found that having at least one ANC visit [14] was associated with higher utilization of PNC, suggesting that prior contact with the health care system may be important. A qualitative study by Syed et al.

2008 found that mothers did not perceive PNC for themselves or their babies to be of much value unless they had a complication or their newborn was sick. The same study found that knowledge of maternal and newborn complications was often limited and initial care–seeking was often with a non–formal provider [17]. No quantitative studies in Bangladesh have looked at the role of complications on receipt of PNC for newborns.

The main aim of this study is to delve deeper into the question of which newborns in Bangladesh are receiving PNC by exploring not just socio–economic factors but also health–related factors, including maternal complications and contact with the health system. Our aim is to understand whether these factors, which have not been extensively studied in the literature, are associated with PNC. A secondary aim is to use maps to descriptively present geographic variability in PNC coverage and neonatal mortality. Maps can be a useful means to pinpoint geographic areas which need more programmatic focus.

METHODS

Data and sample

Data came from the 2010 Bangladesh Maternal Mortality Survey (BMMS), a large–scale survey of 175 000 households [18]. The BMMS employed a multi–stage selection procedure designed to provide representative samples for maternal mortality at the national level and representative estimates at the national, urban/rural, divisional, and district levels for most other indicators. The BMMS Women's Long Questionnaire, which collected socio–economic and health–related information from approximately 62 000 ever–married women aged 13–49, was used in this study. We also obtained information on household wealth from the BMMS Household Questionnaire. Because the primary outcome of interest was PNC for the most recent birth, we restricted the sample to those women who had a live birth in the past six years for a total sample size of 25 014 mothers.

Data for the maps came from the BMMS 2010 as well as from a 2012 Needs Assessment of Emergency Obstetric and Newborn Care (EmONC) [19]. The BMMS 2010 provided the PNC data and population–level neonatal mortality estimates for all districts while the EmONC assessment provided data on facility–level neonatal mortality for 24 of the 64 districts of Bangladesh.

This study was reviewed by the Institutional Review Board (IRB) at the University of North Carolina at Chapel Hill and was exempted from needing ethics review approval because of the secondary nature of the analysis.

Descriptive and regression analyses

Outcomes

We calculated simple weighted descriptive statistics and chi–square analyses on all predictor and demographic variables, comparing women who reported receiving PNC on or before day 7 and on or before day 2 (early PNC) to those who did not. The sample for early PNC is a subset of the larger PNC on or before day 7 sample. Early PNC was defined as within a day for facility births and within two days for non–facility births. The WHO indicates that PNC should be given to newborns within 24 hours for both facility births and as soon as possible for non–facility births [6,20]. We therefore included day 2 as relevant for early PNC for non–facility births.

Key independent variables

Our key predictor variables were focused on access to maternal health services and the presence of complications. In terms of maternal health services we included receipt of ANC, type of delivery attendant (Skilled Birth Attendant (SBA) or non–SBA), place of delivery (facility vs non–facility). A SBA was defined according to the World Health Organization's definition as "an ac-credited health professional – such as a midwife, doctor or nurse – who has been educated and trained to proficiency in the skills needed to manage normal (uncomplicated) pregnancies, childbirth and the immediate postnatal period, and in the identification, management and referral of complications in women and newborns" [21]. We, thus, defined a SBA as an accredited doctor, nurse or midwife. All others including traditional birth attendants (TBAs) were defined as non–SBAs. We looked at both the type of delivery attendant and place of delivery because Bangladesh promotes a strategy of home deliveries by SBAs when facility delivery is not feasible [22,23]. Complications reported by the mother at labor, delivery and after delivery were also key measures in our analysis. Though the BMMS included questions on timing of complication, questions on specific types of complications were not included. We were not able to include four or more ANC visits and low birth weight in our analysis because of a large amount of missing data, and data on neonatal complica-tions were not available.

Regression analysis

We performed weighted logistic regression models predicting receipt of the PNC outcomes, controlling for maternal age, parity, highest level of education, urban residence, marital status, and wealth quintile. The wealth index was constructed from data on ownership of household items including bathroom facilities, roofing, and flooring. Each asset was assigned a weight (factor score) generated through principle components analysis. Each household's scores were then summed; individuals were ranked according to the total score of the household in which they resided [18]). All analyses were performed using Stata v. 14.

Maps and chi–square comparisons

Descriptive maps of PNC by day 7 and early PNC were interposed with data on population–level neonatal mortality and facility–level neonatal mortality to present subnational level variation in PNC coverage and neonatal mortality. We also performed χ^2 analyses of the key independent variables and PNC with neonatal mortality. Studying associations between PNC and neonatal mortality, however, has its limitations. The data do not allow for a determination of whether or not deaths on the first day of life occurred to newborns before they were even eligible for PNC [9]. For example, there could be some left censoring in that some newborns might have died within minutes of birth before they could have received a PNC check, but the data does not disaggregate deaths on the first day into hours or minutes.

RESULTS

Table 1 reports sample characteristics for PNC by day 7, while **Table 2** does the same for early PNC. Given that early PNC is a subset of the PNC by day 7 outcome, the number of women who received early PNC is smaller than PNC by day 7 (7461 vs 8258). Thirty–three percent of respondents reported receipt of PNC by day 7, while 30% reported early PNC. For every characteristic except marital status, there were differences between women receiving PNC by day 7 and not receiving PNC by day 7. For example, women who reported contact with the health system in terms of ANC, facility delivery or delivery with a SBA were more likely to report PNC by day 7. Women who reported a complication during pregnancy, delivery or after delivery as well as urban, wealthier and more educated were also more likely to indicate their newborns received PNC by day 7. Results were similar when comparing women receiving early PNC to those who did not (**Table 2**).

Table 3 shows results from the logistic regressions of PNC by day 7 and by day 2. Confirming some of the findings shown in **Tables 1** and **2**, control-

Table 1. *Sample characteristics by postnatal care on or before day 7 (n = 25 014)*

Characteristic	No PNC by day 7 n	No PNC by day 7 (%)	PNC by day 7 n	PNC by day 7 (%)	P
Total	16 756	67.0	8258	33.0	
Predictor variables					
Delivery:					
– Unskilled	15 307	93.3	3489	46.0	
– Skilled	1449	6.7	4769	54.0	<0.001
Home delivery:					
– No	1078	5.2	4622	52.7	
– Yes	15 678	94.8	3636	47.3	<0.001
Any antenatal care (ANC):					
– No	6615	40.5	1135	14.8	
– Yes	10 141	59.5	7123	85.2	<0.001
Reported complications during pregnancy:					
– No	11 190	66.5	4158	49.7	
– Yes	5566	33.5	4100	50.3	<0.001
Reported complications during delivery:					
– No	13 099	78.0	5209	62.5	
– Yes	3657	22.0	3049	37.5	<0.001
Reported complications after delivery:					
– No	13 818	82.8	6270	75.9	
– Yes	2938	17.2	1988	24.1	<0.001
Demographic characteristics					
Maternal age (years):					
– 13 to 19	1950	11.7	914	11.5	
– 20 to 24	5363	32.6	2938	36.2	
– 25 to 29	4782	28.3	2329	27.9	
– 30 to 34	2677	15.9	1268	14.8	
– 35 to 39	1324	7.6	574	6.7	
– 40 to 44	485	2.9	179	2.1	
– 45 to 49	175	1.0	56	0.7	<0.001
Highest level of education (class):					
– None	4964	30.2	1269	16.0	
– 1 to 5	5658	33.3	2031	25.5	
– 6 to 8	3402	20.7	1789	22.6	
– 9+	2732	15.8	3169	35.9	<0.001
Urban residence:					
– No	10 773	81.9	3955	64.4	
– Yes	5983	18.1	4303	35.6	<0.001
Religion:					
– Islam	15 349	92.4	7334	89.8	
– Hindu/other	1407	7.6	924	10.2	<0.001
Marital status:					
– Currently not married	324	1.8	127	1.5	
– Currently married	16 432	98.2	8131	98.5	0.199
Wealth index quintile:					
– Poorest	4234	26.4	790	10.8	
– Poorer	3702	22.8	964	12.5	
– Middle	3522	21.5	1384	18.0	
– Richer	3047	17.7	1878	22.7	
– Richest	2251	11.6	3242	35.9	<0.001

Table 2. *Sample characteristics by postnatal care on or before day 2 (early PNC, n = 25 014)*

Characteristic	No PNC by day 2		PNC by day 2		P
	n	%	n	%	
Total	17 553	70.2	7461	29.8	
Predictor variables					
Delivery:					
– Unskilled	15 898	92.6	2898	42.6	
– Skilled	1655	7.4	4563	57.4	<0.001
Home delivery:					
– No	1247	5.7	4453	56.4	
– Yes	16 306	94.3	3008	43.6	<0.001
Any antenatal care (ANC):					
– No	6786	39.7	964	14.0	
– Yes	10 767	60.3	6497	86.0	
Reported complications during pregnancy:					
– No	11 584	65.7	3764	49.8	
– Yes	5969	34.3	3697	50.2	<0.001
Reported complications during delivery:					
– No	13 637	77.5	4671	61.9	
– Yes	3916	22.5	2790	38.1	<0.001
Reported complications after delivery:					
– No	14 402	82.4	5686	76.2	
– Yes	3151	17.6	1775	23.8	<0.001
Demographic characteristics					
Maternal age (years):					
– 13 to 19	2036	11.7	828	11.5	
– 20 to 24	5646	32.7	2655	36.4	
– 25 to 29	4999	28.3	2112	28.0	
– 30 to 34	2816	16.0	1129	14.5	
– 35 to 39	1371	7.5	527	6.9	
– 40 to 44	502	2.8	162	2.1	
– 45 to 49	183	1.0	48	0.7	<0.001
Highest level of education (class):					
– None	5122	29.8	1111	15.5	
– 1 to 5	5924	33.3	1765	24.7	
– 6 to 8	3567	20.8	1624	22.6	
– 9+	2940	16.1	2961	37.2	<0.001
Urban residence:					
– No	11 226	81.6	3502	63.3	
– Yes	6327	18.4	3959	36.7	<0.001
Religion:					
– Islam	16 072	92.3	6611	89.6	
– Hindu/other	1481	7.7	850	10.4	<0.001
Marital status:					
– Currently not married	340	1.8	111	1.5	
– Currently married	17 213	98.2	7350	98.5	0.2028
Wealth index quintile:					
– Poorest	4357	26.0	667	10.1	
– Poorer	3835	22.6	831	11.9	
– Middle	3697	21.6	1209	17.5	
– Richer	3213	17.9	1712	22.9	
– Richest	2451	12.0	3042	37.5	<0.001

Table 3. *Logistic regressions of postnatal care by day 7 and by day 2 on predictor variables (n = 25 014)*

Characteristic	PNC by day 7			PNC by day 2		
	Odds ratio	95% CI	P	Odds ratio	95% CI	P
Predictor variables						
Skilled delivery	2.16	1.81–2.58	<0.001	2.11	1.76–2.54	<0.001
Home delivery	0.15	0.12–0.18	<0.001	0.14	0.12–0.17	<0.001
Any antenatal care (ANC)	1.74	1.58–1.92	<0.001	1.71	1.54–1.89	<0.001
Complications during pregnancy	1.60	1.45–1.73	<0.001	1.49	1.36–1.64	<0.001
Complications at delivery	1.48	1.34–1.63	<0.001	1.53	1.38–1.69	<0.001
Complications after delivery	1.36	1.22–1.51	<0.001	1.32	1.18–1.48	<0.001
Demographic characteristics						
Maternal age (years):						
– 13 to 19	1.00					
– 20 to 24	1.12	0.98–1.27	0.110	1.10	0.96–1.27	0.172
– 25 to 29	1.07	0.91–1.25	0.431	1.06	0.90–1.26	0.478
– 30 to 34	1.02	0.84–1.23	0.856	0.98	0.81–1.19	0.841
– to 39	1.11	0.89–1.39	0.362	1.18	0.93–1.50	0.184
– 40 to 44	1.13	0.84–1.52	0.403	1.19	0.87–1.61	0.272
– to 49	1.52	1.01–2.29	0.047	1.52	0.98–2.37	0.060
Parity:						
– 1	1.00					
– 2–3	0.91	0.82–1.01	0.069	0.92	0.82–1.02	0.111
– 4+	0.94	0.80–1.11	0.450	0.91	0.76–1.08	0.278
Highest level of education (class):						
– None	1.00					
– 1 to 5	1.10	0.98–1.23	0.091	1.06	0.94–1.20	0.372
– 6 to 8	1.08	0.94–1.23	0.277	1.05	0.91–1.22	0.492
– 9+	1.14	0.99–1.31	0.073	1.11	0.95–1.29	0.174
Urban residence:						
– No	1.00					
– Yes	1.38	1.22–1.55	<0.001	1.40	1.23–1.59	<0.001
Religion:						
– Islam	1.00					
– Hindu/other	1.09	0.93–1.28	0.284	1.07	0.91–1.27	0.412
Marital status:						
– Currently not married	1.00					
– Currently married	1.04	0.77–1.41	0.791	1.04	0.76–1.44	0.793
Wealth index quintile:						
– Poorest	1.00					
– Poorer	1.15	1.00–1.32	0.058	1.14	0.98–1.32	0.090
– Middle	1.47	1.29–1.68	<0.001	1.46	1.27–1.69	<0.001
– Richer	1.65	1.42–1.91	<0.001	1.68	1.43–1.97	<0.001
– Richest	2.32	1.97–2.74	<0.001	2.35	1.97–2.80	<0.001
Constant	0.45	0.31–0.66	<0.001	0.40	0.27–0.60	<0.001

ling for maternal demographic characteristics, having had a skilled delivery significantly increased the odds of reporting PNC by day 7 and by day 2 by over 2.1 times (odds ratio (OR) = 2.16, 95% confidence interval (CI) 1.81, 2.58; OR = 2.11, 95% CI 1.76, 2.54, respectively). Having had a home delivery significantly decreased the likelihood of PNC by about 85% (OR = 0.15, 95% CI 0.12, 0.18; OR = 0.14, 95% CI 0.12, 0.17, respectively). Reporting complications during pregnancy, delivery and after delivery significantly increased the odds of reporting PNC by between 1.3 and 1.6 times. Urban residence significantly increased the odds of reporting PNC by day 7 or by day 2 by about 1.4 times (OR = 1.38, 95% CI 1.22, 1.55; OR = 1.40, 95% CI 1.23, 1.59, respectively). Being in the top three wealth quintiles also increased the odds of reporting PNC by day 7 and by day 2 by between 1.5 and 2.3 times.

Figures 1 and **2** present descriptive maps of PNC coverage interposed with population–level neonatal mortality (**Figure 1**) and facility–level neonatal mortality (**Figure 2**). Overall, there is wide variation in the PNC (from 4% to 64%) and population–level neonatal mortality rates (from 1.6 per 1000 to 96.2 per 1000) within Bangladesh. Districts with the lowest neonatal mortality do not always have the highest PNC coverage and vice versa. Chi–square statistics for key independent variables and PNC with neonatal mortality indicate significantly higher mortality for newborns receiving PNC by day 2 and for newborns of mothers having a complication and a skilled delivery. These results are presented in **Figure 3**.

DISCUSSION

PNC is a package of interventions intended for all newborns and has both a preventative focus and curative focus. In our study of PNC in Bangladesh we find that newborns whose mothers had a facility delivery or who had a complication were likely to have a PNC check than newborns of mothers who delivered at home or did not have a complication. Given that 79% of women in our sample had a home birth, efforts are needed to ensure all newborns are reached.

PNC for newborns may not always be perceived to be necessary by mothers and their families in Bangladesh [17]), unless there is a complication or the newborn appears sick. Education of families on the importance of PNC as a preventative service can lead to improvements in newborn health. Early treatment for illnesses such as pneumonia is crucial, and PNC offers an opportunity for health workers to look for signs of illnesses which may be missed by family members.

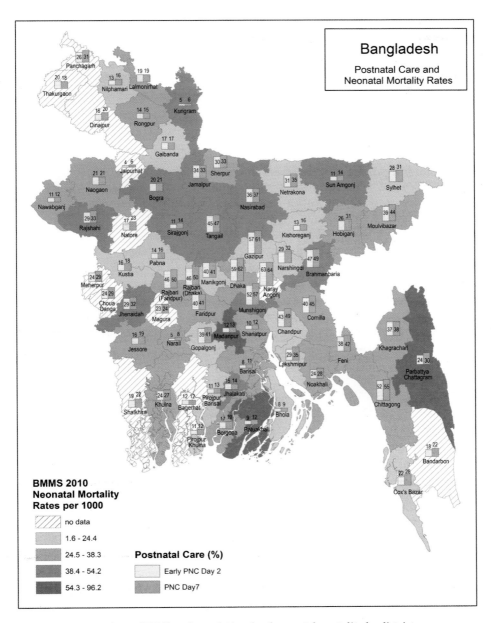

Figure 1. *Postnatal care (PNC) and population–level neonatal mortality by district.*

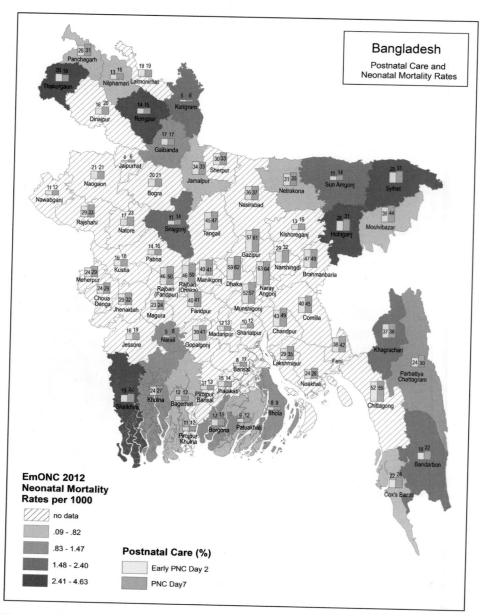

Figure 2. *Postnatal care (PNC) and facility–level neonatal mortality by district.*

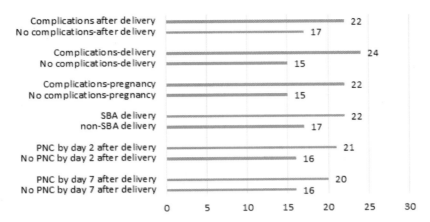

Figure 3. *Bivariate associations between selection variables and neonatal mortality (per 1000). Note: All comparisons are significant at P < 0.05 or P < 0.0001 except for PNC by Day 7 (P = 0.0635). PNC – postnatal care, SBA – skilled birth attendant.*

Traditional practices may prevent many mothers from leaving their homes for up to 40 days after delivery [24,25]. During this period of isolation, mothers are considered to be in a state of impurity and vulnerability to evil spirits [25]. Mothers often sleep on thin mats on the floor with their newborns to mini-mize the spread of pollution to others and protect themselves from spiritual attacks [16,25]. Husbands and mothers–in–law may also serve as gatekeepers to ensure minimal contact with outsiders during this period [25–28]. In light of these cultural issues, training community health workers to provide PNC for mothers and newborns at home, has surfaced as an interim solution to in-creasing the coverage of PNC [24,29,30]. Community health workers have the ability to gain the trust and support of mothers, fathers and mothers–in–law. They can engage these individuals on discussions concerning newborn care and any harmful traditional practices. For example, if newborns are sleeping on thin mats, community health workers can educate families on the risks of hypothermia. Studies conducted in rural Bangladesh have documented that community health workers are capable of correctly identifying sick newborns with a 6–sign or 7–sign clinical algorithm during their routine surveillance of newborns at home [28,31]. Home visits from community health workers by day 2 have been shown to reduce neonatal mortality [32]. Home visits have also been shown to be an effective means to assist mothers in overcoming breastfeeding problems [33].

In addition to identifying methods to reach more individual newborns, it is also important to study PNC coverage at a subnational level to enable countries to address geographic inequities. In Bangladesh there is wide variation in PNC coverage. Understanding why some districts have lower coverage than others can help inform intervention strategies. Traditional practices such as seclusion of the mother and newborn may be more prevalent in some districts than others, and thus engagement with communities on the importance of PNC (whether in a facility or in the home) may be particularly helpful.

Our maps also revealed that districts with the highest PNC coverage did not necessarily have the lowest neonatal mortality and vice versa. We further explain this finding through bivariate comparisons of our key independent variables and PNC with neonatal mortality. The findings indicated significantly higher neonatal mortality when there is a PNC by day 2 check, maternal complication and delivery with a skilled birth attendant. Families in Bangladesh seem to view PNC as a service needed only when there is a problem with the mother or newborn. According to the BMMS 2010, 56% of mothers whose newborns did not receive PNC, indicated the reason was that the service was "not needed" [18]. Unfortunately, we lacked data on newborn complications, prematurity and low birth weight.

There are several limitations to this study including our inability to include certain measures including neonatal complications, four or more ANC visits and birthweight. Though we looked at bivariate associations of PNC with neonatal mortality, there could be some left censoring of the data in that some newborns could have died before they were eligible for PNC [9]. Another limitation is the measurement of PNC itself as some women may not realize their newborn is receiving a check. Direct questions on PNC without probes, as was used in the BMMS, may lead to an underestimation of coverage [34]. The BMMS did not include questions on content or quality of the PNC check, and future research is needed to develop measures on both content and quality of PNC.

Based on the findings of this study, several programmatic recommendations can be made. Both formal health workers and community health workers should provide PNC, a service essential for both for its preventative and curative elements. Particular efforts are needed to reach rural and poor women. Bangladesh has already taken relevant steps to reduce neonatal mortality by developing a National Newborn Health Strategy, which includes PNC provided by community health workers as a national health sector program approach [35]. Important considerations for such an approach are ensuring community health workers have the proper training, supplies and supervision to conduct their work. Community health workers also need to be notified of both facility and home births so that more newborns can be reached [36].

In addition to supporting community health workers, efforts are needed to increase the quality of PNC services in health facilities and to educate families on recognizing the value of PNC for seemingly healthy newborns as well as for sick newborns.

Acknowledgments: The authors would like to thank Becky Wilkes for assistance with the maps.

Disclaimers: The views expressed are those of the authors and do not necessarily reflect the views of USAID or the United States Government.

Funding: This study was carried out with support provided by the United States Agency for International Development (USAID) through MEASURE Evaluation (cooperative agreement AID–OAA–L–14–00004). We are grateful to the Carolina Population Center and its NIH Center grant (P2C HD050924) for general support.

Author Contributions: KS led conceptualization and writing of the paper. PB led data management and analysis. MEC and TKB provided information on context and gave substantial inputs on all versions of the paper. ETK and CG assisted with the literature review, and AM provided guidance on the structure of the paper and provided suggestions on all versions of the paper.

Conflict of interest declaration: The authors completed the Unified Competing Interest form at www.icmje.org/coi_disclosure.pdf (available upon request from the corresponding author), and report no conflicts of interest.

References

1 UNICEF. Levels & trends in child mortality. Report 2015. Estimates developed by the UN Inter-agency Group for Child Mortality Estimation. New York: UNICEF; 2015.

2 Mullan Z, Horton R. Bringing stillbirths out of the shadows. Lancet. 2011;377:1291-2. Medline:21496920 doi:10.1016/S0140-6736(11)60098-6

3 Lawn JE, Blencowe H, Pattinson R, Cousens S, Kumar R, Ibiebele I, et al. Stillbirths: Where? When? Why? How to make the data count? Lancet. 2011;377:1448-63. Medline:21496911 doi:10.1016/S0140-6736(10)62187-3

4 World Health Organization. Every newborn: an action plan to end preventable deaths. Geneva: WHO; 2014.

5 Liu L, Johnson HL, Cousens S, Perin J, Scott S, Lawn J, et al. Global, regional, and national causes of child mortality: an updated systematic analysis for 2010 with time trends since 2000. Lancet. 2012;379:2151-61. Medline:22579125 doi:10.1016/S0140-6736(12)60560-1

6 World Health Organization and UNICEF Joint Statement: Home Visits for the Newborn Child: A Strategy to Improve Survival. Geneva: World Health Organization, USAID and Save the Children; 2009.

7 Health Newborn Network. Summary of Bangladesh Country experience – implementing PNC home visits: March 26, 2012. Available: http://www.healthynewbornnetwork.org/hnn-content/uploads/Country-Report-PNC-Home-Visits-Bangladesh.pdf. Accessed: 15 July 2017.

8   USAID. MCHIP and Save the Children. Postnatal Care Home Visits: A Review of the Current Status of Implementation in Five Countries. 2012. Available: http://www.mchip.net/sites/default/files/Postnatal%20Care%20Home%20Visits.pdf. Accessed: 15 July 2017.

9   Singh K, Brodish P, Haney E. Postnatal care by provider type and neonatal death in sub-Saharan Africa: a multilevel analysis. BMC Public Health. 2014;14:941. Medline:25208951 doi:10.1186/1471-2458-14-941

10 Islam MA, Chowdhury RI, Akhter HH. Complications during pregnancy, delivery, and postnatal stages and place of delivery in rural Bangladesh. Health Care Women Int. 2006;27:807-21. Medline:17060180 doi:10.1080/07399330600880368

11 Amin R, Shah NM, Becker S. Socioeconomic factors differentiating maternal and child health-seeking behavior in rural Bangladesh: a cross-sectional analysis. Int J Equity Health. 2010;9:9-12. Medline:20361875 doi:10.1186/1475-9276-9-9

12 Chakraborty N, Islam MA, Chowdhury RI, Bari W. Utilisation of postnatal care in Bangladesh: evidence from a longitudinal study. Health Soc Care Community. 2002;10:492-502. Medline:12485137 doi:10.1046/j.1365-2524.2002.00389.x

13 Rahman MM, Haque SE, Sarwar Zahan M. Factors affecting the utilisation of postpartum care among young mothers in Bangladesh. Health Soc Care Community. 2011;19:138-47. Medline:20880103

14 Anwar I, Sami M, Akhtar N, Chowdhury M, Salma U, Rahman M, et al. Inequity in maternal health-care services: evidence from home-based skilled-birth-attendant programmes in Bangladesh. Bull World Health Organ. 2008;86:252-9. Medline:18438513 doi:10.2471/BLT.07.042754

15 Mahabub-Ul-Anwar M, Rob U, Talukder MN. Inequalities in maternal health care utilization in rural Bangladesh. Int Q Community Health Educ. 2006-2007;27:281-97. Medline:18573752 doi:10.2190/IQ.27.4.b

16 Darmstadt GL, Syed U, Patel Z, Kabir N. Review of domiciliary newborn-care practices in Bangladesh. J Health Popul Nutr. 2006;24:380-93. Medline:17591335

17 Syed U, Khadka N, Khan A, Wall S. Care-seeking practices in South Asia: using formative research to design program interventions to save newborn lives. J Perinatol. 2008;28:S9-13. Medline:19057572 doi:10.1038/jp.2008.165

18 NIPORT, icddr,b. National Institute of Population Research and Training (NIPORT), MEASURE Evaluation, and icddr,b Bangladesh Maternal Mortality and Health Care Survey 2010. Dhaka, Bangladesh: NIPORT, MEASURE Evaluation, and icddr,b; 2012.

19 Chowdhury ME, Roy L, Biswas TK, Rahman M, Akhter S, Sabir AA. A needs assessment study for emergency obstetric and newborn care (EmONC) services in 24 districts of Bangladesh. Dhaka: International Centre for Diarrhoeal Disease Research, Bangladesh (icddr,b); 2014.

20 World Health Organization (WHO). Maternal, newborn, child and adolescent health –Topics at a glance – Newborn health: Postnatal care. Geneva: World Health Organization; 2013.

21 World Health Organization. Making pregnancy safer: the critical role of the skilled attendant. A joint statement by WHO, ICM and FIGO. Geneva: WHO; 2004.

22 Blum LS, Sharmin T, Ronsmans C. Attending home vs. clinic-based deliveries: Perspectives of skilled birth attendants in Matlab, Bangladesh. Reprod Health Matters. 2006;14:51-60. Medline:16713879 doi:10.1016/S0968-8080(06)27234-3

23 Huque ZA, Leppard M, Mavalankar D, Akhter HH, Chowdhury TA. Safe motherhood programmes in Bangladesh. In: Berer M, Ravindra TKS, eds. Safe motherhood initiatives: Critical issues. London: Reprod Health Matters, 1999; p.53-61.

24 Syed U, Asiruddin S, Helal MS, Mannan II, Murray J. Immediate and early postnatal care for mothers and newborns in rural Bangladesh. J Health Popul Nutr. 24:508-18. Medline:17591348

25 Winch PJ, Alam MA, Akther A, Afroz D, Ali NA, Ellis AA, et al. Local understandings of vulnerability and protection during the neonatal period in Sylhet district, Bangladesh: a qualitative study. Lancet. 2005;366:478-85. Medline:16084256 doi:10.1016/S0140-6736(05)66836-5

26 Moran AC, Winch PJ, Sultana N, Kalim N, Afzal KM, Koblinsky M, et al. Patterns of maternal care seeking behaviours in rural Bangladesh. Trop Med Int Health. 2007;12:823-32. Medline:17596248 doi:10.1111/j.1365-3156.2007.01852.x

27 Walton LM, Brown D. Cultural Barriers to Maternal Health Care in Rural Bangladesh. Online J Health Ethics. 2012. Available: https://papers.ssrn.com/sol3/papers.cfm?abstract_id=2042694.

28 Darmstadt GL, El Arifeen S, Choi Y, Bari S, Rahman SM, Mannan I, et al. Household surveillance of severe neonatal illness by community health workers in Mirzapur, Bangladesh: coverage and compliance with referral. Health Policy Plan. 2010;25:112-24. Medline:19917652 doi:10.1093/heapol/czp048

29 Choudhury N, Moran AC, Alam MA, Ahsan KZ, Rashid SF, Streatfield PK. Beliefs and practices during pregnancy and childbirth in urban slums of Dhaka, Bangladesh. BMC Public Health. 2012;12:791. Medline:22978705 doi:10.1186/1471-2458-12-791

30 Dynes M, Rahman A, Beck D, Moran A, Rahman A, Pervin J, et al. Home-based life saving skills in Matlab, Bangladesh: a process evaluation of a community-based maternal child health programme. Midwifery. 2011;27:15-22. Medline:19783081 doi:10.1016/j.midw.2009.07.009

31 Darmstadt GL, Baqui AH, Choi Y, Bari S, Rahman SM, Mannan I, et al. Validation of a clinical algorithm to identify neonates with severe illness during routine household visits in rural Bangladesh. Arch Dis Child. 2011;96:1140-6. Medline:21965811 doi:10.1136/archdischild-2011-300591

32 Baqui AH, Ahmed S, Arifeen SE, Darmstadt G, Rosecran A, Mannan I, et al. Effect of timing of first postnatal care home visit on neonatal mortality in Bangladesh: a observational cohort study. BMJ. 2009;339:b2826. Medline:19684100 doi:10.1136/bmj.b2826

33 Mannan I, Rahman SM, Sania A, Seraji HR, Arifeen S, Winch P, et al. Can early postpartum home visits by trained community health workers improve breastfeeding of newborns? J Perinatol. 2008;28:632-40. Medline:18596714 doi:10.1038/jp.2008.64

34 Hill Z, Okyere E, Wickenden M, Tawiah-Agyemang C. What can we learn about postnatal care in Ghana if we ask the right questions? A qualitative study. Glob Health Action. 2015;8:28515. Medline:18596714 doi:10.3402/gha.v8.28515

35 Rubayet S, Shahidullah M, Hossain A, Corbett E, Moran A, Mannan I, et al. Newborn Survival in Bangladesh: a Decade of Change and Future Implications. Health Policy Plan. 2012;27:iii40-56. Medline:28156809 doi:10.1093/heapol/czs044

36 Sitrin D, Guenther T, Murray J, Piligram N, Rubayet S, Ligowe R, et al. Reaching mothers and babies with early postnatal home visits: The implementation realities of achieving high coverage in large-scale programs. PLoS One. 2013;8:e68930. Medline:23874816 doi:10.1371/journal.pone.0068930

Thermal care of newborns: drying and bathing practices in Malawi and Bangladesh

Shane M Khan[1], Eunsoo Timothy Kim[2,3], Kavita Singh[2,3], Agbessi Amouzou[4], Liliana Carvajal-Aguirre[1]

[1] Data and Analytics, Division of Data, Research and Policy, United Nations Children's Fund (UNICEF), New York, New York, USA

[2] Department of Maternal and Child Health, Gillings School of Global Public Health, University of North Carolina at Chapel Hill, Chapel Hill, North Carolina, USA

[3] MEASURE Evaluation, Carolina Population Center, University of North Carolina at Chapel Hill, Chapel Hill, North Carolina, USA

[4] Institute for International Programs, Department of International Health, Johns Hopkins Bloomberg School of Public Health, Baltimore, Maryland, USA

Background Thermal care of newborns is one of the recommended strategies to reduce hypothermia, which contributes to neonatal morbidity and mortality. However, data on these two topics have not been collected at the national level in many surveys. In this study, we examine two elements of thermal care: drying and delayed bathing of newborns after birth with the objectives of examining how two countries collected such data and then looking at various associations of these outcomes with key characteristics. Further, we examine the data for potential data quality issues as this is one of the first times that such data are available at the national level.

Methods We use data from two nationally-representative household surveys: the Malawi Multiple Indicator Cluster Survey 2014 and the Bangladesh Demographic and Health Survey 2014. We conduct descriptive analysis of the prevalence of these two newborn practices by various socio-demographic, economic and health indicators.

Results Our results indicate high levels of immediate drying/drying within 1 hour in Malawi (87%). In Bangladesh, 84% were dried within the first 10 minutes of birth. Bathing practices varied in the two settings; in Malawi, only 26% were bathed after 24 hours but in Bangladesh, 87% were bathed after the same period. While in Bangladesh there were few newborns who were never bathed (less than 5%), in Malawi, over 10% were never bathed. Newborns delivered by a skilled provider tended to have better thermal care than those delivered by unskilled providers.

Conclusion These findings reveal gaps in coverage of thermal care and indicate the need to further develop the role of unskilled providers who can give unspecialized care as a means to improve thermal care for newborns. Further work to harmonize data collection methods on these topics is needed to ensure comparable data across countries.

Globally, under-five mortality has declined between 1990 and 2015, from 91 deaths per 1000 live births to 43 deaths per 1000 live births [1]. While neonatal mortality also declined during this period, the share of neonatal deaths among under-five deaths increased to approximately 45% in 2015 [1]. In the neonatal period (the first 28 days of life), nearly 1 million newborns die on the first day (37% of all neonatal deaths) and approximately 2 million newborns die in the first week (74% of all neonatal deaths) [1,2]. Of these deaths, the majority are preventable using simple and effective life-saving interventions [3].

The "Every Newborn Action Plan" which is supported by the World Health Organization (WHO) and the United Nations Children's Fund (UNICEF) and various other institutions emphasizes the critical period of labour, birth and the first week of life as a period that can be targeted to prevent newborn deaths [4]. An important set of interventions designed to minimize preventable deaths during this critical period is essential newborn care (ENC), which broadly includes hygienic cord care, thermal protection and early initiation of breastfeeding [4]. Thermal protection and care of newborns is recommended as it reduces hypothermia, a condition in which the body temperature falls below normal levels [5] and which is known to contribute to global neonatal mortality either directly or indirectly as a comorbidity of other major causes of death [6]. A recent systematic review of low- and middle-income countries found that the prevalence of hypothermia ranged between 32% and 85% for newborns delivered at hospitals and between 11% and 92% for newborns delivered at homes [6]. The review suggests that the wide-ranging prevalence of hypothermia may be associated with different risk factors including low environmental temperatures, early bathing, low socioeconomic status of the mother/family and newborn complications such as low birth weight, prematurity, intrauterine growth restriction and birth asphyxia [6].

Key interventions to prevent newborn hypothermia and its associated mortality risk are described as a chain of interlinked operations. The WHO practical guide for thermal protection of newborns recommends several key interventions to ensure that the newborn is kept warm. This includes that the place of delivery is warm, newborns are immediately dried and either wrapped or placed on the mother for skin-to-skin contact. The recommendation also states that bathing should be delayed for at least 24 hours following birth, or six hours, if culturally appropriate, and that breastfeeding is initiated within one hour after delivery [5].

A 2013 WHO recommendation on postnatal thermal care for newborns refers to the timing of first bath and echoes the same recommendation the timing of bathing [7]. The integrated management of pregnancy and childbirth provides similar advice on drying and placing the baby on the mother's chest with skin-to-skin contact right after birth [8]. In addition, the recently released "Standards for improving quality of maternal and newborn care in health facilities" [9] includes immediate and thorough drying of the newborn as a quality measure. Drying and rubbing are also an essential step in newborn resuscitation used with newborns who do not breathe spontaneously after birth [9].

Several studies in the past have examined the use of protective thermal care practices for newborns. Many have found that there is low use of adequate thermal care practices across South Asia and sub-Saharan Africa. For example, Pagel et al. reports that newborn wrapping or skin-to-skin contact within 10 minutes was relatively low for both home and facility deliveries in Eastern India and Bangladesh [10]. Coverage of bathing after 6 hours, varied widely by study location and delivery types [10]. Another study in Bangladesh reports that only 5.1% of newborns received complete thermal protection, defined as drying and wrapping within 10 minutes and bathing after 72 hours of birth [11]. A study in western Uganda had higher proportions of wrapping the newborn (85.1%) and delaying bathing until after 24 hours (66.3%) [12]. Key findings from qualitative and mixed-method studies have also shown that newborn bathing practices varied across studies but were mostly favouring early bathing due to strong cultural and traditional beliefs [13–16].

Among the recommended thermal care practices, there are few countries with national data on the topics. However, two recent national surveys in Malawi and Bangladesh have included new questions on newborn drying and bathing. There are two primary objectives of this study. The first is to describe the approaches used to collect data on these topics and then to describe associations between these two thermal care practices and key variables. As this is one of the first time that these data are being examined at the national level in the Malawi Multiple Indicator Cluster Survey (MICS) 2014 and the Bangladesh Demographic and Health Survey (DHS) 2014, we also examine potential data quality issues which can inform the development of future data collection on drying and bathing using household surveys.

METHODS

Data source

We searched the UNICEF-supported Multiple Indicator Cluster Surveys (MICS) and the USAID-supported Demographic and Health Surveys (DHS) for data on newborn drying and bathing. Data were available from the Malawi

MICS 2014 and the Bangladesh DHS 2014. The surveys used a similar two-stage sampling methodology, where census enumeration areas were first selected and then households were selected in the second stage. In the households, all women age 15-49 were interviewed in Malawi while in Bangladesh, only ever-married women were interviewed. In the Malawi MICS 2014, questions on drying and bathing were asked about the last birth in the last 2 years, while in Bangladesh, questions were asked about the last birth in the last 3 years. The sample sizes were 7490 in Malawi and 4626 in Bangladesh.

Questions on drying

The Malawi MICS 2014 asked "Was (name) dried or wiped after delivery?" The question provided response categories of 'yes', 'no', 'don't know' and 'missing' and among those who said yes, "How soon after birth was (name) dried or wiped?" recording the time in hours, with additional categories for immediate drying/less than 1 hour and another category for don't know/don't remember.

The Bangladesh DHS 2014 asked one question on drying, "How long after birth was (NAME) dried?" providing categorical response categories of <5 minutes, 5-9 minutes, 10+ minutes, not dried, and don't know.

Questions on bathing

The question on bathing in the Malawi MICS 2014 was, "How soon after birth was (name) bathed for the first time?" recording the time in hours, with additional categories for immediate bathing (less than an hour), never bathed and don't know/don't remember. It should be noted that in this survey, newborns who were not dried were skipped out of the question on bathing.

The Bangladesh DHS 2014 asked, "How long after delivery was (NAME) bathed for the first time?" recording the time in hours (if less than 1 day), days (if less than 1 week), weeks, not bathed, and don't know.

Variables and analysis

As the aim of this analysis is to understand patterns of drying and bathing across the two countries, the analysis is descriptive. Questions on drying are not comparable across the two surveys and do not allow the calculation of a comparable 'immediate drying' variable. Therefore, in both data sets, we dichotomized the variable as 'dried' or 'not dried' without regard for the timing of drying. Missing and don't know cases were minimal and treated as "not bathed" in **Table 1** and **Table 2**.

For the bathing variables, we created a variable to measure bathing after 24 hours. These data were only collected in hours in the Malawi MICS 2014, and were categorized according to the definition of above 24 hours, less than 24 hours, and cases of never bathed, don't know or missing were coded as missing for the tables. For the Bangladesh DHS 2014, we coded bathing at day 1 as bathing after 24 hours (as values over 24 hours were collected in days), coding not bathed, don't know and missing as missing values for the tables. We stratified the analysis by facility vs non-facility births given that the recommendations on thermal care can theoretically differ across these strata. In both surveys, facility births included hospitals, clinics and health centres while non-facility births were all other locations.

In the analysis, we used a number of background variables to examine drying and bathing. Mother's age in years was categorized as less than 20, 20 to 34 and 35 to 49. Birth order referred to the order of the birth of the newborn, categorized as 1 which refers to the first birth, 2-3 (the second and third births), 4-5 (fourth and fifth births) and 6+ which referred to sixth and higher order births. Mother's education was categorized as no education, primary, and a third category of secondary and higher (including university). Size of birth is based on the mother's perception of how large or small the newborn was (at birth). Attendant at delivery was categorized as either skilled or unskilled. Skilled in Malawi referred to births delivered by a doctor or nurse/midwife while skilled in Bangladesh referred to births delivered by a qualified doctor, nurse/midwife/paramedic while unskilled referred to the residual categories in each country. C-section referred to Caesarean section for delivery of the newborn. Residence referred to the type of location where the woman lived and was categorized as urban or rural. The wealth variable was calculated using Principal Component Analysis (PCA). The PCA assigned overall scores to households based on household ownership of goods and assets. The PCA ranked households and then categorized them into five categories: poorest, second, middle, fourth and richest households. Antenatal care referred to the number of times a woman visited any provider during the pregnancy of the newborn for antenatal care. This variable was categorized into no visits (labelled "none"), 2, 3 and 4 or more visits (labelled "4+").

Sampling weights supplied with the data sets were used in all analyses.

RESULTS

Figure 1 and **Figure 2** present the distribution of newborn drying in the two countries. An overwhelming majority of women (87%) said that their newborns

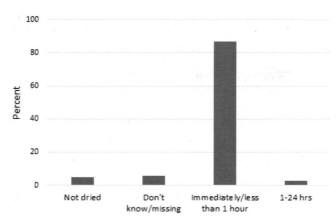

Figure 1. *Newborn drying in Malawi.*

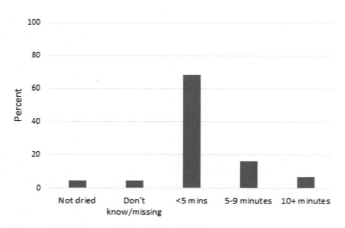

Figure 2. *Newborn drying in Bangladesh.*

were dried immediately or within 1 hour in Malawi. In Bangladesh, 68% of women said that their newborns were dried within 5 minutes of birth, 16% within 5-9 minutes following birth and 7%, 10 minutes or later. The percentage of newborns not dried was 5 and 6 percent in Malawi and Bangladesh respectively.

Table 1 and **Table 2** show distributions of drying of the newborn in each country and how they vary by facility and key variables. About 90% of newborns were dried in both countries. With such high coverage, differentials across socio-demographic subgroups were generally weak. However, several vari-

Table 1. *Percentage of newborns which were dried in Malawi, by place of delivery and various characteristics*

| | PLACE OF DELIVERY | | | | | |
	Facility	N	Non-facility	N	Total	N
Mother's age (years):						
<20	91.3	947	93.4	55	91.4	1002
20-34	93.5	4962	81.8	413	92.6	5375
35-49	91.3	968	86.5	145	90.7	1113
Birth order:						
1	94.2	152	94.9	16	94.3	168
2-3	91.2	553	82.7	57	90.4	610
4-5	92.9	1489	87.5	116	92.5	1605
6+	93.1	4683	82.7	424	92.2	5107
Mother's education:						
No education	92.3	743	77.2	129	90.1	872
Primary education	93.0	4866	85.5	453	92.3	5318
Secondary or higher	92.9	1268	89.3	32	92.8	1300
Size at birth:	‡					
Very small	92.7	431	61.8	61	75.2	492
Smaller than average	93.9	584	84.9	66	93.0	650
Average	94.6	3495	85.0	325	93.8	3820
Larger than average	93.2	1684	84.5	111	92.7	1795
Very large	93.6	683	87.5	50	93.2	733
Attendant at delivery:	‡				‡	
Skilled	94.5	6383	100.0	610	94.5	6386
Unskilled provider	71.6	494	90.1	3	78.4	1104
C-section:	‡				‡	
No	93.6	6482	84.0	515	92.8	7095
Yes	81.3	396	0.0	0	81.3	396
Residence:	†		‡		‡	
Urban	88.8	860	45.6	29	87.4	889
Rural	93.5	6018	85.9	584	92.8	6602
Wealth:			‡			
Poorest	93.2	1615	88.3	237	92.5	1853
Second	94.5	1522	87.5	153	93.8	1676
Middle	92.7	1425	82.0	132	91.8	1556
Fourth	92.3	1176	72.5	67	91.2	1242
Richest	91.2	1139	61.7	24	90.6	1163
Antenatal visits:	‡				‡	
None	43.9	169	75.6	68	53.3	237
1	95.8	133	83.7	41	92.9	174
2	94.5	755	84.7	121	93.1	877
3	93.1	2650	84.1	202	92.4	2852
4+	94.8	3170	86.2	181	94.4	3351
Total	92.9	6877	84.0	613	92.2	7490

*$P < 0.05$.
†$P < 0.01$.
‡$P < 0.001$.

Table 2. *Percentage of newborns which were dried in Bangladesh, by place of delivery and various characteristics*

| | PLACE OF DELIVERY | | | | | |
	Facility	N	Non-facility	N	Total	N
Mother's age (years):						
<20	89.7	351	93.1	619	91.8	970
20-34	89.9	1334	92.1	2043	91.2	3379
35-49	82.4	100	84.1	178	83.5	277
Birth order:			†		*	
1	89.0	888	93.8	956	91.4	1845
2-3	90.4	786	91.3	1355	91.0	2141
4-5	87.7	96	93.2	388	92.1	484
6+	77.5	14	79.0	141	78.8	155
Mother's education:			†		*	
No education	85.7	283	89.1	1120	88.4	1403
Primary education	89.8	955	93.1	1479	91.8	2436
Secondary or higher	90.8	545	96.1	241	92.4	786
Size at birth:						
Very small	86.3	124	91.4	191	89.4	316
Smaller than average	85.6	198	88.0	409	87.2	607
Average	90.8	1193	92.4	1911	91.8	3105
Larger than average	88.4	240	91.6	256	90.1	495
Very large	82.2	29	97.4	73	93.1	102
Attendant at delivery:						
Skilled	89.3	1740	92.9	228	89.7	1970
Unskilled provider	95.3	44	91.7	2612	91.8	2656
C-section:					†	
No	92.8	663	91.8	2840	92.0	3504
Yes	87.5	1120	0.0	0	87.4	1121
Residence:						
Urban	91.3	705	93.1	504	92.0	1209
Rural	88.3	1078	91.5	2337	90.5	3416
Wealth:			†		*	
Poorest	79.8	154	89.3	849	87.8	1003
Second	87.8	214	88.1	660	88.0	876
Middle	88.0	307	94.2	574	92.0	881
Fourth	90.8	455	95.8	500	93.4	955
Richest	92.0	654	96.6	258	93.3	912
Antenatal visits:			*		*	
None	87.6	110	88.3	886	88.2	996
1	91.1	219	90.2	608	90.4	827
2	92.5	313	93.8	435	93.2	748
3	90.2	297	96.6	315	93.5	613
4+	87.9	845	94.7	595	90.7	1442
Total	89.4	1784	91.8	2840	90.9	4626

*P < 0.05.
†P < 0.01.

ables showed notable differences. While newborns who were born in a facility in Malawi were significantly more likely to be dried compared to those born outside a facility (93% vs 84%), in Bangladesh, there is no discernible difference. Likewise, in Malawi, births with a skilled provider were more likely to be dried (95%) compared to those with an unskilled provider (78%) though this pattern was not found in Bangladesh. Women who had had no antenatal visits were least likely to have a newborn that was dried (53%) compared to others with such care (1 or more visits, >90%) in Malawi. This differential was significant in Bangladesh as well but differences in levels were not substantial. In both countries, women who had a C-section reported less drying than women with vaginal births (eg, in Bangladesh, 87% vs 92%). In addition, in Malawi, place of residence was also a marker for differences in drying with a larger proportion of mothers in rural areas reporting that the baby was dried immediately after birth. In Bangladesh, mother's education and household wealth also show significant differences in the results regarding newborn drying with mothers with no education and in the poorest households reporting lower levels of newborn drying. Despite significance, differences are not substantial.

We examined the distribution of timing of bathing of newborns for the first 100 hours of life, shown in **Figure 3** and **Figure 4** (excluding cases where newborns were not bathed, about 10% in Malawi and 5% in Bangladesh, or were missing). In both countries, there is a small but important percentage of newborns who are bathed immediately after birth (about 10% in Malawi and 8% in Bangladesh). The graphs also show clear evidence of heaping of the data. In Malawi, this is evident on hours 24, 48 and 72 which correspond to 1, 2 and 3 days. Similarly, in Bangladesh, some heaping occurs at 24 and 72 hours.

Table 3 and **Table 4** show bathing after 24 hours in Malawi and Bangladesh. In these tables, cases of never bathed, don't know and missing were removed from analysis. In Malawi, only 26% of newborns were bathed after 24 hours,

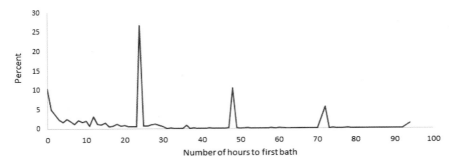

Figure 3. *Bathing of newborns in Malawi in hours.*

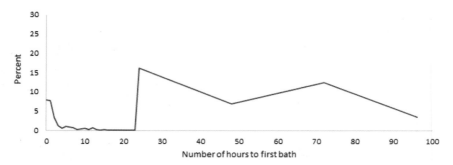

Figure 4. *Bathing of newborns in Bangladesh in hours.*

while in Bangladesh, 74% were bathed after 24 hours. In both countries, there were few missing cases (not included in the **Tables 3** and **4**). Comparing by place of birth, newborns in facilities were more likely to have a delayed bathed compared to those born outside of facilities in both countries (see **Table 3** and **4**). Newborns in Malawi and Bangladesh who were born using a skilled provider or those who were born with a C-section were more likely to have a delayed bath than those who were born to an unskilled provider or those born by a vaginal birth. For example, in Bangladesh, among all newborns, 92% born using a skilled attendant was bathed after 24 hours while only 60% born without a skilled attendant was bathed after 24 hours.

DISCUSSION

Monitoring ENC is needed to identify programmatic coverage gaps and to provide an empirical basis for policy, accountability and investment to improve newborn survival and care. The renewed emphasis on newborn survival on the global agenda has led to the inclusion of new questions and modules on ENC in survey programs for the collection of data on key indicators in a systematic manner. For instance, in the latest round of MICS surveys, launched in late 2016, questions on ENC including thermal practices, cord care and skin-to-skin contact are included for countries to use. Changes have also occurred for the DHS surveys, which has an optional newborn care module with similar topics.

Levels of drying are remarkable similar in the two countries with nearly all newborns being dried. However, bathing practices differ in the two countries, with newborns in Malawi being bathed much earlier than those of Bangladesh. These levels seen in Malawi are much lower than those seen in Uganda in other literature [12]. The analysis also shows that skilled providers are important for the delivery of timely drying in both countries and drying in Malawi. However,

Table 3. *Bathing of newborns after 24 h in Malawi by place of delivery*

	PLACE OF DELIVERY					
	Facility	N	Non-facility	N	Total	N
Mother's age (years):						
<20	28.4	738	18.3	45	27.8	783
20-34	27.5	3925	13.5	299	26.5	4224
35-49	25.0	722	10.7	119	23.0	840
Birth order:						
1	21.8	118	0.0	13	19.7	131
2-3	22.2	438	7.4	39	21.0	477
4-5	29.4	1190	12.8	89	28.3	1279
6+	27.4	3638	14.6	322	26.4	3960
Mother's education:						
No education	26.7	550	20.3	83	25.9	634
Primary education	27.8	3818	11.4	353	26.4	4171
Secondary or higher	25.7	1016	15.8	26	25.4	1042
Size at birth:					*	
Very small	34.8	253	6.2	43	30.7	296
Smaller than average	35.4	441	18.1	53	33.6	494
Average	25.2	2756	12.3	241	24.1	2997
Larger than average	28.6	1393	16.8	85	27.9	1477
Very large	24.8	542	12.2	42	23.9	583
Attendant at delivery:					‡	
Skilled	27.6	5075	0.0	3	27.6	5078
Unskilled provider	22.7	309	13.3	459	17.1	769
C-section:	‡				‡	
No	26.7	5131	0.0	0	25.6	5594
Yes	40.4	254	13.2	462	40.4	254
Residence:						
Urban	24.1	662	0.0	11	23.7	674
Rural	27.8	4722	13.6	451	26.5	5174
Wealth:			†			
Poorest	24.7	1252	13.5	190	23.3	1442
Second	30.5	1197	7.0	119	28.4	1316
Middle	28.8	1116	21.8	95	28.2	1211
Fourth	25.9	938	5.5	44	25.0	982
Richest	26.2	883	29.3	14	26.3	897
Antenatal visits:			*			
None	26.9	43	5.8	47	15.8	90
1	21.6	99	24.8	31	22.4	130
2	29.4	597	12.0	89	27.1	686
3	28.2	2094	17.2	150	27.4	2244
4+	26.3	2552	9.9	146	25.4	2697
Total	27.3	5385	13.2	462	26.2	5847

*P < 0.05.
†P < 0.01.
‡P < 0.001.

Table 4. *Bathing of newborns after 24 h in Bangladesh by place of delivery*

	Facility	N	Non-facility	N	Total	N
			PLACE OF DELIVERY			
Mother's age (years):			‡		†	
<20	94.5	337	61.0	605	73.0	942
20-34	94.9	1285	62.1	2009	74.9	3295
35-49	96.4	97	41.7	176	61.1	273
Birth order:			‡			
1	95.2	854	62.6	934	78.2	1789
2-3	94.3	760	62.6	1334	74.1	2094
4-5	95.7	92	58.7	381	66.0	473
6+	100.0	13	33.3	141	39.0	154
Mother's education:			‡		‡	
No education	95.1	272	51.2	1101	59.9	1373
Primary education	94.1	918	66.0	1452	76.9	2370
Secondary or higher	96.1	530	70.8	237	88.3	767
Size at birth:					†	
Very small	91.3	117	59.5	188	71.8	305
Smaller than average	93.8	190	57.1	402	68.8	592
Average	95.5	1164	61.2	1882	74.3	3046
Larger than average	95.1	224	67.2	247	80.5	471
Very large	88.6	25	43.9	71	55.6	96
Attendant at delivery:					‡	
Skilled	94.9	1676	67.6	226	91.7	1903
Unskilled provider	92.9	44	59.9	2564	60.5	2607
C-section:	‡				‡	
No	90.0	644	-	-	66.1	3434
Yes	97.8	1075	-	-	97.8	1076
Residence:					‡	
Urban	95.1	686	59.7	498	80.2	1184
Rural	94.7	1034	60.8	2292	71.3	3326
Wealth:	*		†		‡	
Poorest	95.5	149	54.0	832	60.3	982
Second	93.2	205	60.0	643	68.0	849
Middle	90.6	292	62.5	566	72.1	859
Fourth	96.6	439	66.6	494	80.7	932
Richest	96.1	634	67.6	254	87.9	889
Antenatal visits:			‡		‡	
None	92.1	107	49.2	870	53.9	977
1	95.1	213	62.8	602	71.2	815
2	94.8	300	64.8	428	77.2	728
3	96.6	285	72.0	313	83.7	598
4+	94.6	815	66.1	576	82.8	1392
Total	94.9	1719	60.6	2789	73.7	4510

*$P < 0.05$.
†$P < 0.01$.
‡$P < 0.001$.

given that a sizeable proportion of births occur outside of facility settings, it would be useful to ensure that unskilled providers are able to provider these two elements of thermal care. This recommendation is supported by the 2009 WHO/UNICEF joint statement on home visits for newborns, wherein both skilled and unskilled providers are endorsed for certain elements of care, including thermal care, following the time of birth [17].

Our results show that the measurement approaches used in these two surveys are not standardized. This is to be expected as these are initial efforts to measure these variables in the survey programmes. Drying data for the two surveys are largely incomparable. While the Malawi survey data allow a category of 'immediate drying', this category also includes cases of drying within 1 hour. The Bangladesh survey provides response categories using ranges of minutes and no 'immediate' drying category. As such, both cases do not allow an easy calculation of the 'immediate drying' indicator, which in part reflects the lack of clarity of what constitutes 'immediate'. These concerns are largely addressed in the latest round of MICS and the DHS optional module on newborn care. In MICS6, the relevant question asks if the newborn was wiped or dried soon after birth, while the DHS asks if the newborn was wiped dry within a few minutes. It is of course necessary to note that both question approaches allow a certain level of subjectivity to measure the immediacy of drying, an approach that is necessary until there is an agreed definition of what 'immediate drying' refers to.

With reference to newborn bathing, the major methodological issue is that the cut-off for the indicator is for values greater than 24 hours. Both surveys show heaping of data at the 24-hour mark, which is used as a cut-off for indicator calculation. Similar heaping of data exists across different health and nutrition indicators such as low birth weight (at 2500 g). Due to this issue, in the latest round of MICS, after the question on bathing is asked, an addition probe is activated if the respondent says that the newborn was bathed on the 1 day/24-hour mark to ascertain if the bath took place before, after or on that exact moment. A similar approach can be useful for surveys using the DHS approach. We also detect that in Malawi an important proportion of cases was not bathed, but in Bangladesh, there were much fewer cases. It would be important to monitor this proportion in future surveys and to understand the circumstances that produce this outcome.

There are important limitations in this paper that should be considered when interpreting the results. Data on ENC practices used in the analysis are based on mother's recall of care provided to the newborn soon after birth. Apart from recall, women not know if certain events have occurred or the exact timing, especially in the case of C-sections, where the mother and newborn may be quickly separated. This may explain why women who had a C-section reported lower levels of drying. As with other measures based on mother's recall, this could have led to differential recall bias and may not entirely reflect the level of quality of care in facilities [18]. This is particularly the case for interventions that occur during the postpartum period as it is an intense moment for mothers. The Malawi MICS 2014, newborns who were not dried were skipped out of the question on bathing which can potentially under-estimate the indicator level, given that some newborns who are not dried could have a bath later than the 24-hour period. Due to the questions asked, a comparable measure of immediate drying could not be calculated. As such, the analysis in this paper focusses on newborns who were ever dried or not.

Our findings shed light into gaps on two essential yet simple newborn care interventions, which at low cost, can help maintain the newborn in a stable condition. The results also indicate potential areas of intervention for training up of staff for implementing drying and bathing in these countries. Further research is required to study the results of the new MICS and DHS approaches to measuring drying and bathing in different countries to ensure that the intention of these questions are properly reflected.

Disclaimer: *The findings and conclusions in this report are those of the authors and do not necessarily represent the official position of their respective organizations.*

Funding: *None.*

Authorship contributions: *SMK led the development of the paper. SMK and ETK led the writing of the paper. ETK performed the data analysis. KS, AA and LCA provided substantial inputs and ideas into all drafts of the paper.*

Competing interests: *The authors has completed the Unified Competing Interest form at www.icmje.org/coi_disclosure.pdf (available on request from the corresponding author) and declare no competing interests.*

References

1 UNICEF. Committing to Child Survival: A Promise Renewed Progress Report 2015. Available: https://www.unicef.org/publications/index_83078.html. Accessed: 1 October 2017.

2 Wardlaw T, You D, Hug L, Amouzou A, Newby H. UNICEF Report: enormous progress in child survival but greater focus on newborns urgently needed. Reprod Health. 2014;11:82. Medline:25480451 doi:10.1186/1742-4755-11-82

3 UNICEF. World Health Organization, World Bank, & UN-DESA Population Division. Levels &; Trends in Child Mortality 2015.

4 World Health Organization & NICEF. EVERY NEWBORN: An Action Plan To End Preventable Deaths. 2014. Geneva. Available: http://apps.who.int/iris/bitstream/10665/127938/ 1/9789241507448_eng.pdf. Accessed: 1 October 2017.

5   World Health Organization. Maternal and Newborn Health/Safe Motherhood Unit. Thermal Protection of the Newborn: a practical guide. Geneva: World Health Organization; 1997.

6   Lunze K, Bloom DE, Jamison DT, Hamer DH. The global burden of neonatal hypothermia: systematic review of a major challenge for newborn survival. BMC Med. 2013;11:24. Medline:23369256 doi:10.1186/1741-7015-11-24

7   World Health Organization. Recommendations on Postnatal care of the mother and newborn. Available: http://apps.who.int/iris/bitstream/10665/97603/1/9789241506649_eng.pdf. Accessed: 1 April 2017.

8   World Health Organization. UNFPA, UNICEF. 2015. Integrated Management of Pregnancy and Childbirth. Pregnancy, childbirth, postpartum and newborn care: a guide for essential practice – 3rd edition. Available: http://apps.who.int/iris/bitstream/10665/249580/ 1/9789241549356-eng.pdf. Accessed: 1 October 2017.

9   World Health Organization. Standards for improving quality of maternal and newborn care in health facilities. 2016. Available: http://apps.who.int/iris/bitstream/10665/ 249155/ 1/9789241511216-eng.pdf?ua=1. Accessed: 1 October 2017.

10 Pagel C, Prost A, Hossen M, Azad K, Kuddus A, Roy SS. Is essential newborn care provided by institutions and after home births? Analysis of prospective data from community trials in rural South Asia. BMC Pregnancy Childbirth. 2014;14:99. Medline:24606612 doi:10.1186/1471-2393-14-99

11 Rahman M, Haque SE, Zahan S, Islam O. Noninstitutional births and newborn care practices among adolescent mothers in Bangladesh. J Obstet Gynecol Neonatal Nurs. 2011;40:262-73. Medline:21585526 doi:10.1111/j.1552-6909.2011.01240.x

12 Kabwijamu L, Waiswa P, Kawooya V, Nalwadda CK, Okuga M, Nabiwemba EL. Newborn care practices among adolescent mothers in Hoima District, Western Uganda. PLoS One. 2016;11: e0166405. Medline:27855186 doi:10.1371/journal.pone.0166405

13 Adejuyigbe EA, Bee MH, Amare Y, Omotara BA, Iganus RB, Manzi F, et al. "Why not bathe the baby today?": A qualitative study of thermal care beliefs and practices in four African sites. BMC Pediatr. 2015;15:156. Medline:26466994 doi:10.1186/s12887-015-0470-0

14 Moran AC, Choudhury N, Uz Zaman Khan N, Ahsan Karar Z, Wahed T, Faiz Rashid S, et al. Newborn care practices among slum dwellers in Dhaka, Bangladesh: a quantitative and qualitative exploratory study. BMC Pregnancy Childbirth. 2009;9:54. Medline:19919700 doi:10.1186/1471-2393-9-54

15 Sacks E, Moss WJ, Winch PJ, Thuma P, Van Dijk JH, Mullany LC. Skin, thermal and umbilical cord care practices for neonates in southern, rural Zambia: a qualitative study. BMC Pregnancy Childbirth. 2015;15:149. Medline:26177637 doi:10.1186/s12884-015-0584-2

16 Shamba D, Schellenberg J, Hildon ZJ, Mashasi I, Penfold S, Tanner M, et al. Thermal care for newborn babies in rural southern Tanzania: a mixed-method study of barriers, facilitators and potential for behaviour change. BMC Pregnancy Childbirth. 2014;14:267. Medline:25110173 doi:10.1186/1471-2393-14-267

17 World Health Organization. UNICEF. Joint Statement on home visits for the newborn child: a strategy to improve survival. Geneva: World Health Organization; 2009.

18 Stanton CK, Rawlins B, Drake M, Dos Anjos M, Cantor D, Chongo L, et al. Measuring coverage in MNCH: testing the validity of women's self-report of key maternal and newborn health interventions during the peripartum period in Mozambique. PLoS One. 2013;8:e60694. Medline:23667427 doi:10.1371/journal.pone.0060694

Gap between contact and content in maternal and newborn care: An analysis of data from 20 countries in sub–Saharan Africa

Liliana Carvajal–Aguirre[1], Agbessi Amouzou[2], Vrinda Mehra[1], Meng Ziqi[1], Nabila Zaka[3], Holly Newby[4]

[1] Data and Analytics, Division of Data, Research and Policy, UNICEF, New York, New York, USA
[2] Institute for International Programs, Department of International Health, Johns Hopkins Bloomberg School of Public Health, Baltimore, Maryland, USA
[3] UNICEF, Program Division, New York, New York, USA
[4] Independent consultant

Background Over the last decade, coverage of maternal and newborn health indicators used for global monitoring and reporting have increased substantially but reductions in maternal and neonatal mortality have remained slow. This has led to an increased recognition and concern that these standard globally agreed upon measures of antenatal care (ANC), skilled birth attendance (SBA) and postnatal care (PNC) only capture the level of contacts with the health system and provide little indication of actual content of services received by mothers and their newborns. Over this period, large household surveys have captured measures of maternal and newborn care mainly through questions assessing contacts during the antenatal, delivery and postnatal periods along with some measures of content of care. This study aims to describe the gap between contact and content –as a proxy for quality– of maternal and newborn health services by assessing level of co–coverage of ANC and PNC interventions.

Methods We used Demographic and Health Surveys (DHS) data from 20 countries between 2010 and 2015. We analysed the proportion of women with at least 1 and 4+ antenatal care visit, who received 8 interventions. We also assessed the percentage of newborns delivered with a skilled birth attendant who received 7 interventions. We ran random effect logistic regression to assess factors associated with receiving all interventions during the antenatal and postnatal period.

Results While on average 51% of women in the analysis received four ANC visits with at least one visit from a skilled health provider, only 5% of them received all 8 ANC interventions. Similarly, during the postnatal period though two–thirds (65%) of births were attended by a skilled birth attendant, only 3% of newborns received all 7 PNC interventions. The odds of receiving all ANC and PNC interventions were higher for women with higher education and higher wealth status.

Conclusion The gap between coverage and content as a proxy of quality of antenatal and postnatal care is excessively large in all countries. In order to accelerate maternal and newborn survival and achieve Sustainable Development Goals, increased efforts are needed to improve both the coverage and quality of maternal and newborn health interventions.

Over the past 25 years, concerted global efforts have led to dramatic reductions in maternal and under–five mortality. Globally, the maternal mortality ratio has declined by nearly 44%, [1] while the under–five mortality rate has fallen by 53% [2]. Yet, most low and middle income countries failed to attain the maternal, newborn and child health goals set out in the Millennium Development Goals (MDGs) [3] and an unacceptably large numbers of women, newborn and children are still dying. About 800 women and 7700 newborns die each day from complications during pregnancy and childbirth and in the postnatal period [4]. Increasing newborn survival is a continuing challenge that must be addressed as neonatal deaths are becoming an increasing share of under–five deaths. [3]. Thus, a major unfinished agenda is the annual toll of 2.9 million neonatal deaths which account for 45% of all under–five deaths [5,6]. It is now well established that care around the time of birth has the potential to avert more than 40% of neonatal deaths and must be prioritized as the world seek to eliminate preventable neonatal deaths [7]. Key proven interventions include care by a skilled birth attendant, emergency obstetric care, immediate care for every newborn baby including breastfeeding support and clean birth practices such as cord and thermal care and newborn resuscitation [2]. Evidence also suggests that increased coverage and quality of preconception, antenatal, intrapartum, and postnatal interventions by 2025 could avert 71% of neonatal deaths, 33% of stillbirths and 54% of maternal deaths per year [7].

Monitoring the coverage of effective and affordable maternal, newborn and child health interventions is central to assess progress [8,9]. For the purpose of global monitoring and reporting, a set of coverage indicators along the continuum of care have been adopted by global monitoring frameworks like the Global Strategy for Women's, Children's and Adolescents' Health 2016–2030 and the Every Newborn Action Plan, to mention a few [10–12]. More women are now receiving antenatal care and delivering with a skilled attendant. Globally, antenatal care coverage for 4 or more antenatal visits by any provider has increased from 35% in 1990 to 58% in 2015 [13], while the proportion of births delivered with a skilled birth attendant rose from 61 to 78% between 1990 and 2015 [14]. However, these changes in coverage of maternal and newborn health have not reflected expected progress in impact indicators related to maternal and newborn survival. It is being increasingly recognized that the global measures of coverage of maternal and newborn health capture only contacts with the health system with little information about the quality of care received. Maximizing coverage of measures focused on contacts alone is insufficient to reduce maternal, newborn and child mortality. To move towards elimination of preventable causes of maternal and newborn deaths, increased coverage of recommended contacts should be accompanied by increased focus on content of services [4,15–21]. Recent evidence shows that closure of quality gap of facility based maternal and newborn health services could prevent an estimated 113 000 maternal deaths, 531 000 stillbirths and 1.325 million neonatal deaths annually by 2020 [7].

Currently, the global indicators specific to pregnancy, delivery and postnatal periods that are common to the Global Strategy and ENAP include antenatal care (at least four visits), skilled attendant at birth and postnatal care for mothers and newborns within 48 hours following birth. These global maternal and newborn health indicators are truly the tip of the iceberg as these focus only on contacts between women or newborns with the health system and provide no indication of the content of services and quality of care delivered, which limits their usefulness for programmatic purposes [22]. A critical gap is noted in the measurement and reporting of quality of services received by women and children with the recommendation of adding core indicators assessing quality of maternal and newborn health care to the global coverage indicators [4,12,18,23,24]. Recently, the World Health Organization has proposed standards of care and measures assessing quality of maternal and newborn health care [4].

Large–scale, nationally representative household surveys such as UNICEF–supported Multiple Indicator Cluster Surveys (MICS) [25] and USAID–supported Demographic and Health Surveys (DHS) [26] are the largest source of data on maternal and child health outcomes at the population level. But, these surveys are limited in terms of providing information on content of care during the antenatal, labour, delivery and postnatal period. Data are often collected on basic services received during antenatal care such weighing, testing of urine and blood, measuring blood pressure, tetanus protection, etc. During intra and postpartum periods, information on initiation of breastfeeding, weighing, immunization and postnatal care of mother and newborn is collected. While this information does not cover the breath of all services required, and especially in cases of emergency care and treatment, together, it can allow an assessment of whether women and newborns are receiving the minimum expected services. Thus, data collected through MICS and DHS has the potential to provide an indication of level of quality of care, at least at a basic level. Unlike health facility or quality of care surveys that focus on care provided at service delivery sites, these household surveys have the advantage to provide nationally representative estimates that can also be disaggregated by relevant background characteristics including sub–national regions, mother's education, mother's age, sex of the child, wealth quintiles, etc., and allow to conduct relevant equity analyses which are a priority in the Sustainable Development Goals (SDGs) era.

In this paper, we analyse the co–coverage of content interventions used as proxy for quality of care received by women during antenatal care and by the newborn during postnatal period using data from nationally representative surveys. We then compare this co–coverage estimate with the global coverage indicators assessing contacts with health system to highlight the gap between contact and content.

METHODS

Data Source

Data for this study are from DHS surveys conducted between 2010 and 2015. We used data on interventions during the antenatal, delivery and postnatal periods from DHS surveys in 20 countries (see Table S1 in **Online Supplementary Document**). These 20 countries were included due to the availability of data on 8 antenatal care (ANC) and 7 postnatal care (PNC) interventions included in this analysis. Of the 20 countries, 18 countries had data on the full set of ANC interventions and 17 countries reported on all 7 PNC interventions included in the analysis.

Method of analysis

To assess the quality of maternal and newborn health services during pregnancy, birth and postnatal period, we analysed the co–coverage of selected interventions received by mothers and newborns. The co–coverage indicator, proposed in 2005, is a simple count of how many interventions are received by mothers and newborns out of a set of selected interventions [27].

For the purpose of this analysis, we included 8 ANC content interventions as a proxy for quality of antenatal care (**Table 1**). We first assessed the contact coverage estimates defined as (1) percent of women with a live birth in last 2

Table 1. *Set of interventions included for co–coverage analysis*

8 INTERVENTIONS DURING ANTENATAL PERIOD	7 INTERVENTIONS DURING POSTNATAL PERIOD
1. Urine test	1. Newborn weighed at birth
2. Blood pressure taken	2. Early initiation of breastfeeding
3. Blood sample	3. No pre–lacteal feed during first three days of life
4. Iron supplementation	4. BCG vaccination
5. Tetanus protection	5. Polio vaccination at birth
6. Counselled on pregnancy complications	6. Postnatal care for newborn within 2 d of birth
7. Tested for HIV and received results	7. Postnatal care for the mother within 2 d of birth
8. Intermittent preventive treatment of malaria in pregnancy (IPTP)	

years who had at least one ANC visit with a skilled provider and (2) percent of women with a live birth in previous 2 years who had four or more ANC visits with at least one visit with a skilled health personnel. We then described coverage of content among all women with a live birth in previous 2 years and also restricted to women who reported having an ANC contact as the proportion of women with at least one ANC visit and those with four or more visits who received all 8 interventions.

In order to compare the gap between contact and content at the time of birth we included 7 PNC interventions. Interventions as weighing the newborn at birth, early initiation of breastfeeding, vaccinating the newborn with Polio dose 0 and BCG were included as proxy for quality as these are directly within the control of the skilled birth attendant. No prelacteal feeds for first 3 days was included as educating and assisting women on initiating exclusive breastfeeding and maintaining successful breastfeeding has been identified as a core function of skilled health personnel [28]. Postnatal health checks within 48 hours of birth for the mother and newborn was included due to lack of data availability on content of postnatal care in the analysed household surveys. For PNC, we analysed women delivering with a skilled birth attendant (SBA) whose surviving newborn received the 7 interventions. In the present analysis, a skilled birth attendant was identified based on the database maintained by UNICEF and Countdown which validates the skill and qualifications of the health personnel. For postnatal interventions, data on immunization was collected only on surviving children. We therefore, restricted the analysis to surviving children under 2 years at the time of the survey. This may positively affect the results if it is assumed that children who have died may be more likely to have had low quality care.

To assess the factors associated with the receipt of all interventions during ANC and PNC periods, we carried out random effect logistic regression on pooled data on women who had a contact. The regression model controlled for several maternal, socio–demographic characteristics as maternal age, education status, parity, area of residence and wealth status.

RESULTS

Antenatal period

The analysis presented in **Figure 1** characterizes the quality of care received, among women who reported receiving at least one ANC visit with a skilled provider and those with four or more ANC visits. The gap between contact and content, defined as the difference between the percentage with four or more antenatal care visits and the percentage who received all 8 interventions, in the antenatal period is huge; compared to an average of 51% [range: 32%–76%] of women who received four or more ANC visits with at least one visit with a skilled health provider, only 5% (range: 0.3%–19%) of the women received all 8 ANC interventions (panel A in **Figure 1**). Among all interventions

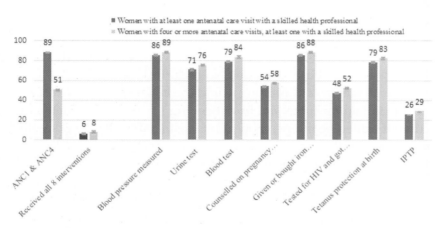

Figure 1. A. *Percentage of women with a live birth in last 2 years receiving the complete set of 8 antenatal care (ANC) interventions; average across 18 countries, Demographic and Health Surveys (DHS) 2010–2015. The analysis included 18 countries as Burundi, and Rwanda did not have information about the full set of interventions.* **B.** *Percentage of women with at least one ANC visit and women with four or more visits by ANC intervention received; average across 18 countries, DHS 2010–2015. The analysis included 18 countries as Burundi, and Rwanda did not have information about the full set of interventions.*

provided to women who had a contact during the antenatal period, receipt of three doses of intermittent preventive treatment of malaria in pregnancy was lowest (panel B in **Figure 1**). The gap between contact and content was found to be widest in case of Congo and Gabon where difference of 70 percentage points was noted between percentage of women who received 4+ ANC and the percentage of women who received all 8 ANC content interventions (see Table S2a in **Online Supplementary Document**).

The logistic regression analysis showed that women who had four or more ANC visits had 2 times higher odds of receiving all 8 interventions than those with only 1 ANC visit (odds ratio (OR) = 2.06, 95% confidence interval (CI) = 1.72–2.46). It was also found that primiparous women had 23% increased odds to receive all 8 ANC interventions compared to women with 5 or more children. The odds of receiving all ANC interventions increased significantly with greater levels of education and wealth status (**Figure 2**).

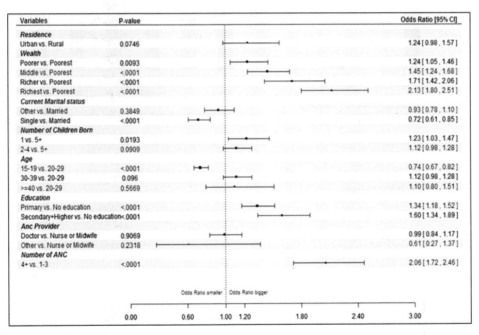

Figure 2. *Odds ratios, 95% confidence intervals and p–values of receipt of all 8 antenatal care (ANC) interventions among women with antenatal contact from random effect logistic regression, (pooled Demographic and Health Surveys (DHS) data from 18 countries, DHS 2010–2014). The analysis included 18 countries as Burundi, and Rwanda did not have information about the full set of interventions.*

Postnatal period

The gap between contact and content of care highlights that though about two–thirds (65%, range: 34% to 93%) of women and newborns had contact with the health system only a handful are able to report receiving all 7 interventions considered (3%, range: <1% to 9%). (**Figure 3**). In the postnatal period, this gap was found to be the widest for Congo and Gabon. (see Table S2b in **Online Supplementary Document**).

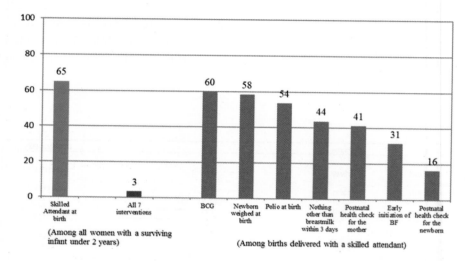

Figure 3. *Percentage of newborns/mothers by type of intervention received during postnatal period, average across 17 countries, Demographic and Health Surveys (DHS) 2010–2015. The analysis included 17 countries as Cameroon, Mozambique and Zimbabwe did not have information about the full set of interventions.*

As with ANC interventions, the likelihood of receiving all 7 PNC interventions was higher for newborns born to women with higher education (OR = 1.23, 95% CI = 1.12–1.35) and wealth status (OR = 1.31, 95% CI = 1.02–1.67). Contact during antenatal period was also found to be associated with the receipt of PNC interventions. Analysis revealed that the odds of newborns receiving all PNC interventions were 17% (OR = 1.17, 95%CI = 0.94–1.46) more for newborns whose mothers received four or more ANC visits than those who received 1–3 visits (**Figure 4**).

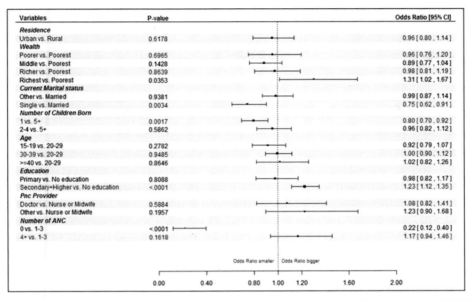

Variables	P-value		Odds Ratio [95% CI]
Residence			
Urban vs. Rural	0.6178		0.96 [0.80 , 1.14]
Wealth			
Poorer vs. Poorest	0.6965		0.96 [0.76 , 1.20]
Middle vs. Poorest	0.1428		0.89 [0.77 , 1.04]
Richer vs. Poorest	0.8639		0.98 [0.81 , 1.19]
Richest vs. Poorest	0.0353		1.31 [1.02 , 1.67]
Current Marital status			
Other vs. Married	0.9381		0.99 [0.87 , 1.14]
Single vs. Married	0.0034		0.75 [0.62 , 0.91]
Number of Children Born			
1 vs. 5+	0.0017		0.80 [0.70 , 0.92]
2-4 vs. 5+	0.5862		0.96 [0.82 , 1.12]
Age			
15-19 vs. 20-29	0.2782		0.92 [0.79 , 1.07]
30-39 vs. 20-29	0.9485		1.00 [0.90 , 1.12]
>=40 vs. 20-29	0.8646		1.02 [0.82 , 1.26]
Education			
Primary vs. No education	0.8088		0.98 [0.82 , 1.17]
Secondary+Higher vs. No education	<.0001		1.23 [1.12 , 1.35]
Pnc Provider			
Doctor vs. Nurse or Midwife	0.5884		1.08 [0.82 , 1.41]
Other vs. Nurse or Midwife	0.1957		1.23 [0.90 , 1.68]
Number of ANC			
0 vs. 1-3	<.0001		0.22 [0.12 , 0.40]
4+ vs. 1-3	0.1618		1.17 [0.94 , 1.46]

Odds Ratio smaller : Odds Ratio bigger

0.00   0.40   0.80   1.00   1.20   1.60   2.00

Figure 4. *Odds ratios, 95% confidence intervals and p–values of receipt of all postnatal care (PNC) interventions from random effect logistic regression (pooled Demographic and Health Surveys (DHS) data from 17 countries, DHS 2010–2014). The analysis included 17 countries as Cameroon, Mozambique and Zimbabwe did not have information about the full set of interventions.*

DISCUSSION

Our analysis demonstrates that there are large gaps between contact and content of care during antenatal, birth and postnatal period across all countries, as assessed using mothers' recall from household survey. Among all ANC interventions included in the analysis, measurement of blood pressure was found to be the most commonly received intervention. Our finding resonates with an earlier study which assessed the content of antenatal care when data on antenatal interventions such as h8 and weight checking, blood pressure testing, and blood and urine testing was first available in Demographic and Health surveys [29]. The findings of the present study are also consistent with other studies that examined coverage of high quality contacts during the antenatal and postnatal period [24,29–31]. A recent study noted a substantial decline in the coverage of at least one antenatal contact and skilled birth attendance on adding content in Nigeria, Ethiopia and India [30]. Such gaps between globally recommended coverage indicators measuring contacts and actual content indicate ineffective care resulting in lack of accelerated progress towards maternal and newborn survival.

A limitation of this analysis is that we were able to analyse only interventions that were available in household surveys across the countries included in the analysis. We recognize that the scope of essential newborn care is broader and encompasses a range of interventions. Additional essential newborn care interventions such as thermal care and cord care have recently started to be included in household surveys. However, at the time of analysis data on additional newborn care interventions was available for only a few countries. Thus, our analysis included a subset of interventions in the antenatal and postnatal period for which data were available for a larger number of countries. Another limitation is that all measures included in the analysis are based on mother's recall of care during the antenatal and postnatal period and therefore may be subject to differential recall bias. Further, only few studies have assessed the validity of coverage indicators for MNCH interventions measured through household surveys. A recent series on "Measuring Coverage in MNCH" found that the sensitivity and specificity of coverage indicators is highly variable across interventions and women report less accurately about interventions that occurred immediately following childbirth [9].

An area of further research would be linking data from facilities surveys with population based data in order to better understand the quality of available services. Recent studies linking these two sources have found an association between service readiness in health facilities and the likelihood of receiving an appropriate set of essential newborn care interventions, as well as highlighted important gaps in service delivery as obstacles to universal access to health services [32,33]. The current global maternal, newborn and child health coverage indicators for pregnancy, labour and postnatal period focus merely on contacts with the health system with no information on quality and process of care. These measures of MNCH coverage only show whether services are reaching intended beneficiaries but do not assess the effectiveness or actual content of the care received. Our analysis establishes that focusing on merely contacts with health system rather than on content of care is a critical gap in assessing the true effectiveness of maternal and child health interventions. For example, we observed that although 2 in 3 births were attended by a skilled birth attendant, only 3% of the births received all 7 interventions recommended during the immediate postnatal period.

There is increasing evidence to support that increased coverage of recommended contacts alone is insufficient to reduce maternal and neonatal mortality and morbidity [4,7,15–21,24]. Quality of care is being internationally recognized as a critical aspect of the unfinished maternal and newborn health agenda [4,15]. Our findings also highlight the need to include elements of quality of care for regular monitoring through health management information systems (HMIS), household and facility surveys in other to identify the real gaps in effective coverage. Periodic program assessments can include a measure for content analysis of ANC and PNC visits in a given sample of mothers and newborns and explore reasons of omitting certain interventions which can vary from lack of competency to stock–outs of urine and haemoglobin test kits. Further research is also required to identify more sensitive indicators on quality of care and including these in future household surveys.

Acknowledgements: The authors acknowledge the support from the Countdown group in terms of financing this work and facilitating presentation of preliminary results at a technical Countdown meeting in April 2015. Comments received during the meeting have helped improve the analysis. Kim Dickson was also part of the initial discussion on design and analysis plan, authors are also grateful for her contribution.

Disclaimer: The findings and conclusions in this report are those of the authors and do not necessarily represent the official position of the respective organization.

Funding: This work was funded through a Sub–grant from the US Fund for UNICEF under their Countdown to 2030 grant from the Bill and Melinda Gates Foundation.

Authorship contributions: HN, AA and LCV conceived and designed the analysis plan. ZM and AA carried out the analysis. LCV and VM composed the initial draft. LCV, AA, VM and NZ reviewed early drafts. All authors approved the final draft.

Competing interests: The authors have completed the Unified Competing Interest form at www.icmje.org/coi_disclosure.pdf (available on request from the corresponding author) and declare no conflict of interest.

References

1 World Health Organization, UNICEF, UNFPA, World Bank and UNPD. Trends in maternal mortality: 1990 to 2015: estimates by WHO, UNICEF, UNFPA, World Bank Group and the United Nations Population Division. Geneva; World Health Organization: 2015.

2 UNICEF. Committing to Child Survival: A promise renewed – Progress report 2015. New York: UNICEF: 2015.

3 Victora CG, Requejo JH, Barros AJ, Berman P, Bhutta Z, Boerma T, et al. Countdown to 2015: a decade of tracking progress for maternal, newborn, and child survival. Lancet. 2016;387:2049-59. Medline:26477328 doi:10.1016/S0140-6736(15)00519-X

4 World Health Organization. Standards for improving quality of maternal and newborn care in health facilities. Geneva; World Health Organization: 2016.

5 United Nations Inter-agency Group for Child Mortality Estimation (IGME). Levels and Trends in Child Mortality: Report 2015. New York: UNICEF; 2015.

6 Lawn JE, Blencowe H, Oza S, De Y, Lee AC, Waiswa P, et al. Progress, priorities, and potential beyond survival. Lancet. 2014;384:189-205. Medline:24853593 doi:10.1016/S0140-6736(14)60496-7

7   Bhutta ZA, Das JK, Bahl R, Lawn JE, Salam RA, Paul VK, et al. Can available interventions end preventable deaths in mothers, newborn babies, and stillbirths, and at what cost? Lancet. 2014;384:347-70. Medline:24853604 doi:10.1016/S0140-6736(14)60792-3

8   Wehrmeister FC, Restrepo-Mendez MC, Franca GVA, Victora CG, Barros AJD. Summary indices for monitoring universal coverage in maternal and child health care. Bull World Health Organ. 2016;94:903-12. Medline:27994283 doi:10.2471/BLT.16.173138

9   Bryce J, Arnold F, Blanc A, Hancioglu A, Newby H, Requejo J, et al; CHERG Working Group on Improving Coverage Measurement. Measuring coverage in MNCH: new findings, new strategies, and recommendations for action. PLoS Med. 2013;10:e1001423. Medline:23667340 doi:10.1371/journal.pmed.1001423

10   Every Woman Every Child 2015 – The Global Strategy for Women's, Children's and Adolescents' Health 2016-2030 – New York 2015. Available: http://globalstrategy.everywomaneverychild.org/. Accessed: 1 August 2017.

11   World Health Organization. Every Newborn Action Plan. 2014. Geneva; World Health Organization: 2014.

12   Countdown to. 2015. A decade of tracking progress for maternal newborn and child survival: the 2015 report. New York; UNICEF: 2015.

13   UNICEF. Progress for Children Beyond Averages: Learning from the MDGs. New York; UNICEF: 2015.

14   UNICEF. Is Every Child Counted? Status of data for children in the SDGs. New York; UNICEF: 2015.

15   United Nations. Global strategy for women's and children's health. New York; United Nations: 2010.

16   Campbell OM, Graham WJ. Lancet Maternal Survival Series steering group. Strategies for reducing maternal mortality: getting on with what works. Lancet. 2006;368:1284-99. Medline:17027735 doi:10.1016/S0140-6736(06)69381-1

17   Global Health Group. Where women go to deliver: overview of the project and review of preliminary findings. San Francisco, California: University of California at San Francisco, Global Health Sciences; 2014.

18   World Health Organization. Consultation on improving measurement of the quality of maternal, newborn and child care in health facilities. Geneva; World Health Organization: 2014.

19   Austin A, Langer A, Salam RA, Lassi ZS, Das JK, Bhutta ZA. Approaches to improve the quality of maternal and newborn health care: an overview of the evidence. Reprod Health. 2014;11 Suppl 2:S1. Medline:25209614 doi:10.1186/1742-4755-11-S2-S1

20   van den Broek NR, Graham WJ. Quality of care for maternal and newborn health: the neglected agenda. BJOG. 2009;116:18-21. Medline:19740165 doi:10.1111/j.1471-0528.2009.02333.x

21   Souza JP, Gulmezoglu AM, Vogel J, Carroli G, Lumbiganon P, Quereshi Z, et al. Moving beyond essential interventions for reduction of maternal mortality (the WHO Multicountry Survey on Maternal and Newborn Health): a crosssectional study. Lancet. 2013;381:1747-55. Medline:23683641 doi:10.1016/S0140-6736(13)60686-8

22   Requejo JH, Newby H, Bryce J. Measuring Coverage in MNCH: Challenges and Opportunities in the Selection of Coverage Indicators for Global Monitoring. PLoS Med. 2013;10:e1001416. Medline:23667336 doi:10.1371/journal.pmed.1001416

23   Moran AC, Kerber K, Sitrin D, Guenther T, Morrissey CS, Newby H, et al. Measuring coverage in MNCH: indicators for global tracking of newborn care. PLoS Med. 2013;10:e1001415. Medline:23667335 doi:10.1371/journal.pmed.1001415

24 Hodgins S, D'Agostino A. The quality–coverage gap in antenatal care: toward better measurement of effective coverage. Glob Health Sci Pract. 2014;2:173-81. Medline:25276575 doi:10.9745/GHSP-D-13-00176

25 UNICEF. Statistics and monitoring: Multiple Indicator Cluster Surveys. Available: http://mics.unicef.org/surveys. Accessed: 1 August 2017.

26 The DHS Program. Demographic and Health Surveys. Available: https://dhsprogram.com/

27 Victora CG, Fenn B, Bryce J, Kirkwood BR. Co-coverage of preventive interventions and implications for child-survival strategies: evidence from national surveys. Lancet. 2005;366:1460-6. Medline:16243091 doi:10.1016/S0140-6736(05)67599-X

28 World Health Organization. ICM, FIGO. Making pregnancy safer: the critical role of the skilled attendant. Geneva; World Health Organization: 2004.

29 Abou-Zahr CL, Wardlaw TM. (2003). Antenatal care in developing countries: promises achievements and missed opportunities. An analysis of trends levels and differentials 1990-2001. Available: http://apps.who.int/iris/bitstream/10665/42784/1/9241590947.pdf. Accessed: 1 August 2017.

30 Marchant T, Tilley-Gyado RD, Tessema T, Singh K, Gautham M, Umar N, et al. Adding content to contacts: measurement of high quality contacts for maternal and newborn health in Ethiopia, north east Nigeria, and Uttar Pradesh, India. PLoS One. 2015;10:e0126840. Medline:26000829 doi:10.1371/journal.pone.0126840

31 Rani M, Bonu S, Harvey S. Differentials in the quality of antenatal care in India. Int J Qual Health Care. 2008;20:62-71. Medline:18024998 doi:10.1093/intqhc/mzm052

32 Carvajal-Aguirre L, Mehra V, Amouzou A, Khan SM, Vaz V, Guenther T, et al. Does health facility service environment matter for the receipt of essential newborn care? Linking health facility and household survey data in Malawi. J Glob Health. 2017;2:020509. doi:10.7189/jogh.07.020501

33 O'Neill K, Takane M, Sheffel A, Abou-Zahr C, Boerma T. Monitoring service delivery for universal health coverage: the Service Availability and Readiness Assessment. Bull World Health Organ. 2013;91:923-31. Medline:24347731 doi:10.2471/BLT.12.116798

Does health facility service environment matter for the receipt of essential newborn care? Linking health facility and household survey data in Malawi

Liliana Carvajal–Aguirre[1], Vrinda Mehra[1], Agbessi Amouzou[2], Shane M Khan[1], Lara Vaz[3], Tanya Guenther[3], Maggie Kalino[4], Nabila Zaka[5]

[1] Data and Analytics, Data Research and Policy, UNICEF, New York, New York, USA
[2] Department of International Health, Johns Hopkins School of Public Health, Baltimore, Maryland, USA
[3] Department of Global Health, Save the Children, Washington DC, USA
[4] National Statistical Office, Malawi
[5] Program Division, UNICEF, New York, New York, USA

Background Health facility service environment is an important factor for newborns survival and well–being in general and in particular in high mortality settings such as Malawi where despite high coverage of essential interventions, neonatal mortality remains high. The aim of this study is to assess whether the quality of the health service environment at birth is associated with quality of care received by the newborn.

Methods We used data from the Malawi Millennium Development Goals Endline household survey conducted as part of MICS survey program and Service Provision Assessment Survey carried out in 2014. The analysis is based on 6218 facility births that occurred during the past 2 years. Descriptive statistics, bivariate and multivariate random effect models are used to assess the association of health facility service readiness score for normal deliveries and newborn care with newborns receiving appropriate newborn care, defined for this analysis as receiving 5 out of 6 recommended interventions during the first 2 days after birth.

Results Newborns in districts with top facility service readiness score have 1.5 higher odds of receiving appropriate newborn care (adjusted odds ratio (aOR) = 1.52, 95% confidence interval CI = 1.19–1.95, $P = 0.001$), as compared to newborns in districts with a lower facility score after adjusting for potential confounders. Newborns in the Northern region were two times more likely to receive 5 newborn care interventions as compared to newborns in the Southern region (aOR = 2.06, 95% CI = 1.50–2.83, $P < 0.001$). Living in urban or rural areas did not have an impact on receiving appropriate newborn care.

Conclusions There is need to increase the level of service readiness across all facilities, so that all newborns irrespective of the health facility, district or region of delivery are able to receive all recommended essential interventions. Investments in health systems in Malawi should concentrate on increasing training and availability of health staff in facilities that offer normal delivery and newborn care services at all levels in the country.

Recent evidence estimates that care around the time of birth including having a skilled attendant at birth, emergency obstetric care, immediate care for newborns, and newborn resuscitation could prevent 1.5 million maternal and newborn deaths and stillbirths by 2025 [1]. The days and weeks around childbirth and immediate postnatal period – are the most vulnerable for both mothers and newborns. Most maternal and infant deaths occur during this time [2]. Care during the time of labour, child birth and early, postnatal care (PNC), presents a unique opportunity to set both mothers and babies on a good start. Postnatal care also provides the delivery platform for care of the newborn, including the promotion of preventive practices and detection of any complications. Care of the normal newborn includes early initiation of (exclusive) breastfeeding, prevention of hypothermia, clean postnatal care practices and appropriate cord care [3]. Close observation for 24 hours and at least three additional postnatal contacts is recommended for all mothers and newborns to establish good caregiving practices and detect any life–threatening conditions [4]. However, for improved effectiveness, newborn care interventions in the postnatal period should be delivered as a package. Every Newborn Action Plan launched in 2014 to end preventable newborn deaths envisages each country to ensure 90% of all births receive quality care improve PNC coverage at least by 20% by 2020 and 90% by 2030. PNC is also a key indicator for EWEC monitoring framework which will facilitate monitoring of SDG targets by 2030 [3].

Addressing newborns' health is a priority in Malawi as in many countries in sub–Saharan Africa. In 2015, newborns in Malawi accounted for 34% of all under–5 deaths, an increase from 2000 when newborns accounted for 20% of under–five deaths [5]. This increase in proportion of newborn deaths in overall under–five deaths speaks about the effect of immunization and reduction of diarrhoea and pneumonia related mortality. Malawi is one the few counties in sub–Saharan Africa which has reached the MDG goal 4 by reducing under–five deaths by 63% between 1990 and 2015. During the same period, the country also reduced its maternal mortality ratio by over one–third (34%) and witnessed a substantial increase in the rate of institutional deliveries; from 55% in 2000 to 91% in 2016 [6]. However, between 1990 and 2015, neonatal deaths have declined by only 36% (6). Additionally, recent data shows wide regional variations with regards to perinatal mortality rate. In 2016, the Central region had a perinatal mortality rate of 42 per 1000 pregnancies compared to 29 per 1000 in the Southern region [7]. The slower decline in newborn mortality relative to under–5 mortality in Malawi calls for a redoubling of efforts, including attention to premature babies and care for small and sick babies [8].

In Malawi, health care services are provided by three agencies; Government through the Ministry of Health (MoH) provides about 60%; the Christian Health Association of Malawi (CHAM) is responsible for about 39% plus a small contribution from the private–for profit health sector [9]. Attention to newborn health intensified after 2005 as the Government of Malawi integrated newborn survival and implemented the Essential Health Package and developed a multi–year national initiative (2005–2015), the 'Road Map' for Accelerating Reduction of Maternal and Newborn Mortality and Morbidity in Malawi [10]. Malawi Newborn Action Plan was developed and launched in 2015 and the country recently committed to WHO–UNICEF's network for Improving Quality of Care for Maternal, Newborn and Child Health. Ministry of Health engaged NSO to conduct partner resource mapping exercise and results showed variations in terms of support on MNCH interventions including newborns. There was more concentration mostly on maternal issue than new born issues leading to verticalization in the implementation on newborn care either by partners or districts. As identified by health authorities in the country, challenges in Malawi remain both acute and complex with projections on human resources. To ensure adequate staffing at health facilities, in 2012 the Government implemented an "Emergency Human Resource" program for re–engagement and redeployment of staff [11]. This has not been implemented fully and the health sector strategic plan 2 (2017–2022) is carrying on this work. Still, at current output levels, it will take many years to come anywhere near the numbers of health staff needed to provide minimum standards of service delivery [12].

The quality and availability of health services that are within reach to mothers and newborns, the service environment, plays a major role in the provision of good care. The relationship between health services and population outcomes is an important area of public health research that requires bringing together data on health outcomes and the relevant health service environment [13]. However, as newborn health is relatively new on the global agenda, data on the service environment for this vulnerable group is still scarce [14]. Malawi presents a great opportunity to explore the convergence of complementary data on health facilities and population–based data on this topic as it is one of the few countries with census facility data and household survey data within a range of close years readily and publicly available for analysis.

An important additional consideration in many low–income settings is the distance to health facilities, particularly in rural areas as roads may not be optimal and vehicles for transport are rarely available.

Distance to delivery care and the level of care provided are important determinants of facility delivery [15] and thus of the well–being of mothers and babies. Recent studies in sub–Saharan Africa show a significant variation in receiving postnatal care. Across communities in Nigeria and Uganda [16] studies have found that distance to health facilities as well as socio economic factors are important determinants for accessing services [17,18]. Recent geospatial analysis have also identified that targeted interventions at the district level are essential to strengthen maternal health programmes [19,20]. This study investigates if living in a district with health facilities that are ready to provide a high level of normal delivery and newborn care is associated with receiving a package of essential newborn care interventions during the first two days after birth.

METHODS

Data

Two main sources of data have been used for this analysis: the Malawi MDG Endline Survey 2014 – MES conducted as part of the UNICEF supported MICS survey program [21] which is a population–based household survey representative at the national and district level, and the Malawi Service Provision Assessment 2013–2014 – MSPA 2014 [22], which is based on a census of health facilities in the country. To determine population densities across districts, we used census data from the Malawi 2008 census as 2013–14 projections were not available at the time of the analysis [23].

Population based data

The Malawi MDG Endline Survey (MES) was carried out in 2013–14 by Malawi National Statistical Office as part of the global Multiple Indicator Cluster Survey (MICS) programme. Technical support was provided by the United Nations Children's Fund (UNICEF). The sample for the MES 2014 was designed to provide estimates for a large number of indicators at the national level; for urban and rural areas; the three regions (Northern Region, Central Region and Southern Region); and the 27 districts of Malawi excluding the island of Likoma due to logistical challenges. The sample was stratified by district with the aim of obtaining representative estimates at each district level. Within each district, the sample was further stratified by urban–rural, before a two stage cluster sampling was implemented. Within each stratum, a specified number of census enumeration areas were selected systematically with probability proportional to size [21]. All the information obtained from respondents remains strictly confidential and anonymous. Although GPS coordinates of each sample cluster was collected, this information was not collected of respondents' household.

In the MES 2014, a total of 24 230 women aged 15–49 years were interviewed between November 2013 and April 2014. Of the interviewed women, 31% had a live birth in the past two years, for a total of 7490 reported live births. Of these, 89% were born in health facilities (6661 live births). In the survey, women were asked questions about interventions related to maternal and newborn care that mothers and their newborns received immediately after birth and in the following few weeks. These questions include a number of critical interventions such as thermal care, feeding practices like early initiation of breastfeeding, weighing of the baby and more that are recommended to occur during the postnatal period to ensure the well–being of the baby [2]. Of the 6661 facility–based births in the last two years reported in the household survey, 6218 had complete data on all variables of newborn care and were included in the analysis.

Health facility data

The Malawi Service Provision Assessment MSPA 2014 was implemented by the Malawi Ministry of Health. ICF International provided technical assistance through the MEASURE DHS program, which is funded by USAID and is de-signed to assist countries in collecting data to monitor and evaluate population, health, and nutrition programmes [22]. The MSPA 2014 is considered a census of facilities in the country as it covers all of Malawi's health facilities including public and semi–public facilities of all levels, CHAM as well as major private facilities [22]. The survey assesses whether components considered essential for quality service delivery are present and functioning [22]. Data also includes precise location using GPS of all facilities in the country.

Of the 977 health facilities in Malawi, 528 (54%) were recorded as providing normal delivery and newborn care services and were included in the study. For this analysis, data from the MSPA 2014 facility and providers data sets were used. These modules collected information on basic emergency and neonatal services in key domains including: staff and training, equipment, and key medicines and commodities relevant during delivery and to provide care for the newborn. Variables about health facility services were ascertained through observation and health facility staff interviews, in the facility and providers data set of the MSPA 2014 [22]. No missing data was observed for the variables included from the MSPA 2014 facility and provider data sets in this analysis.

Definition of outcome and exposure

Outcome: Appropriate newborn care

In 2013, WHO released the Postnatal Care for Mother and Newborn guidelines which provided a list of recommendations for the care of the mother and newborn in the postnatal period [2]. The specific recommendations for the newborn included assessment of the baby, exclusive breastfeeding, cord care and thermal care interventions. We recognize that the scope of newborn care in the postnatal period is broad and encompasses a range of interventions. But, for the purposes of this analysis, appropriate newborn care is defined as co–coverage of essential interventions received by the newborn in the period immediately after birth and up to 2 days after birth for which data was available in the Malawi MES 2014 survey. Thus, a newborn was considered to have received appropriate newborn care if he/she received 5 out of 6 of the following interventions: 1) being weighed after birth, 2) being put to the breast during the first hour after birth, 3) not having received pre–lacteal feeds, 4) being wiped/dried after birth, 5) being bathed not before 6 hours after birth, 6) having received a postnatal check within 2 days following birth. The interventions for immediate care for newborns selected in this analysis were also consistent with the recommendations in the Every Newborn Action Plan (ENAP), which at its onset provided evidence of the effectiveness of these interventions for improving newborn survival [1]. The "appropriate newborn care" score was calculated using equal weights for each of the six components (Table S1a in **Online Supplementary Document**). The present analysis focused only on normal newborns and did not include premature, sick babies requiring additional interventions.

Exposure: Facility level readiness score

The quality of delivery and newborn care services offered in health facilities are characterized by calculating the service readiness score for "normal delivery and newborn care" based on the Service Availability and Readiness Assessment (SARA)."– Reference Manual [24]. The score includes three domains: 1) staff and training: having guidelines for integrated management of pregnancy and childbirth (IMPAC) and having staff trained in IMPAC. IMPAC was selected as the Malawi service provision assessment reports on IMPAC as the guidelines for facilities offering normal delivery service [22], 2) equipment and commodities (observed and functioning) and 3) medication and supplies availability. A total of 20 tracer indicators were included in the construction of the score (Table S1b in **Online Supplementary Document**), covering the 19 SARA tracer indicators plus having an infant scale given its relevance to the outcome under investigation. Facility specific scores ranged from 19 to 100. These scores were then aggregated at the district level using weighted average and the final scores were not stratified by the type of facility. To account for facility utilization, district level scores were weighed by the number of outpatient clients in each facility. District level service readiness scores ranged from 56 to 80 with a mean of 67.1. For ease of interpretation, these were then categorized into terciles based on their mean value: bottom (55.7–62), middle (62–70) and top (70–79.5) (**Figure 1**).

Method of analysis

To investigate the association between appropriate newborn care for newborns and district average facility service readiness score, the two data sources were

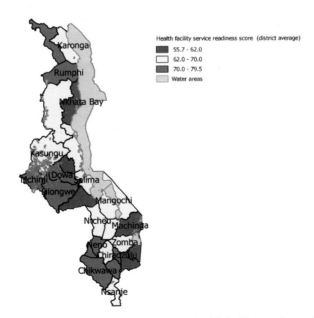

Figure 1. *District level 'normal delivery and newborn care' health facility service readiness score.*

linked using the administrative boundary linking method. This approach consists of linking the two data sets at a level at which both are representative [25]. Thus, following this method, facility data were aggregated at the district level and then merged with the individual level household survey data set for subsequent analysis. Recent analysis linked health facility and household survey using this same method for the analysis of availability of improved water and sanitation in the childbirth environment in 58 countries [26]. The study undertook an ecological type of analysis where facility births in a particular district were assigned their respective district average health facility score. Thus, each of the 6218 facility births from the individual data set included in the analysis was assigned a district average health facility score value according to their district location.

Bivariate regression analyses of potential confounders related to household, mother, delivery and infant (Table S1a in **Online Supplementary Document**) were analysed for association with the primary outcome of appropriate newborn care. Variables found to be significant in the bivariate analysis were selected for inclusion in the final model. A random effect multiple logistic model was used to assess the association between the variables of interest. This implies that levels of 'appropriate newborn care' in neighbouring districts are unrelated after adjusting for other variables in the model. This modelling technique was used given the structure of the data and to account for the effects of clustering. All variables kept in the model were checked for multicollinearity by assessing variance inflation factor. Analysis was conducted in Stata 14.0 [27] and maps were produced in QGIS desktop 2.14.0. [28].

Ethical approvals

All data are publicly available and therefore no ethics approval was required for this analysis. Ethical approval for data collection was the responsibility of data collectors.

RESULTS

Descriptive analysis

Table S2 in **Online Supplementary Document** presents the distribution of health facilities with service–readiness score (70 or above) in the top category in each domain. This descriptive analysis reveals that 52% of the facilities in urban areas have a service readiness score of 70 or higher, in contrast to rural areas where only 32% of the facilities recorded high scores. The results are further disaggregated by regions and districts. The domain with the lowest performance is staff and training. Across districts, there is a wide range in the proportion of facilities with a high score on this domain (range: 0–55%; mean 21.7%). For the equipment and supplies domain, the range is 25.2 to 77.6% (mean 46.7%) of facilities with scores in the top category. For the medicines and commodities domain, the range is 20.0 to 81.8% (mean 54.5%) with score 70 or higher. Across all districts, 35.3% of facilities (range 16.8 to 66.8%) have a service readiness score of 70% or higher. **Figure 1** presents the mean district health facility score.

At the individual level, of the 6218 facility births, 37% were in districts in which the average facility service readiness score was above 70%. Of all newborns included in the analysis, 88% were located in rural areas and 12% in urban areas, 14% were born to mothers younger than 20 years old, for 82% their mothers had either no education (11%) or only primary education (71%). Of the 6218 births, 86% were delivered in public health facilities (**Table 1**).

Bivariate analysis

Analysis of essential newborn care interventions across regions found that the Southern region presents lower coverage of newborns receiving all 6 newborn care interventions (37.1% CI = 34.4–39.9) (Table S3 in **Online Supplementary Document**). The interventions with significant differences in coverage across regions are: early initiation of breastfeeding, newborns being bathed 6 hours after birth or later and newborns receiving essential newborn care visit within 2 days. In terms of the combined 'appropriate newborn care' variable, in the Northern region nearly 90% (89.5% CI = 85.5–92.6) of the newborns received at least 5 newborn care interventions followed by Central (87.7%, CI = 85.8–89.4, $P < 0.001$) and Southern regions (81.4%, CI = 79.4–83.3, $P < 0.001$). Coverage of all 6 of the essential newborn interventions is considerably lower across all regions. While half of all newborns (49.5%) received all 6 interventions in the Central region, coverage was recorded at 41.1% in the Northern region and 37.1% in Southern region. These unadjusted distributions take account of the complex survey design but do not consider clustering, therefore should be interpreted with caution. **Figure 2** presents coverage of the appropriate newborn care interventions measured at the district level.

The crude analysis using simple logistic regression, presented in **Table 1**, shows a positive association between appropriate newborn care and service readiness facility score of 70 and above (OR = 1.60, 95% CI = 1.25–2.03, $P<0.001$). Other

Table 1. *Distribution of study population characteristics – live births in facilities in the past 2 years and crude associations with outcome (N = 6218)*

INDICATORS	TOTAL N (%)	PREVALENCE >5 5 NEWBORN CARE IN- TERVENTIONS (%)	UNADJUSTED OR (95% CI)	P
Health facility readiness score (district average):				<0.001
Bottom (55.7–62)	2117 (34)	1714 .0)	1	
Middle (62–70)	1813 (29)	1570 (86.6)	1.52 (1.21–1.91)	<0.001
Top (70–79.5)	2288 (37)	1994 (87.2)	1.60 (1.25–2.03)	<0.001
Place of residence:				
Urban	745 (12)	663 (88.9)	1	
Rural	5473 (88)	4615 (84.3)	0.67 (0.50–0.90)	<0.001
Region:				
Southern	3018 (48)	2457(81)	1	
Central	2467 (40)	2165 (87.7)	1.63 (1.32–2.02)	<0.001
Northern	733 (12)	656 (89.5)	1.95 (1.32–2.90)	<0.001
Mother's age at birth (years):				
<20	850 (14)	707 3.3)	1	
20–34	4617 (74)	3841 (85.1)	1.14 (0.85–.152)	0.374
35–49	852 (14)	729 (85.6)	1.18 (0.84–1.68)	0.329
Mother's education:				
None	664 (11)	542 1.6)	1	
Primary	4387 (71)	3722 (84.8)	1.27 (0.97–1.65)	0.080
Secondary or higher	1168 (19)	1014 (86.9)	1.49 (1.05–2.12)	0.025
Household wealth index:				
Poorest	1464 (24)	1203 .2)	1	
Second	1389 (22)	1176 (84.7)	1.19 (0.91–1.58)	0.200
Middle	1290 (21)	1093 (84.7)	1.20 (0.88–1.64)	0.240
Fourth	1059 (17)	911 (86.1)	1.34 (0.96–1.86)	0.081
Richest	1017 (16)	894 (87.9)	1.58 (1.12–2.22)	0.008
Type of health facility:				
Public health facility	5348 (86)	4563 (85.3)	1	
Private health facility	194 (3)	157 (81.1)	0.74 (0.43–1.26)	0.271
CHAM Mission	676 (11)	558 (82.5)	0.81 (0.60–1.09)	0.171
Type of delivery:				
Vaginal delivery	5032 (81)	5032 (85.3)	1	
C-Section	245 (4)	244 (76.3)	0.55 (0.39-0.79)	0.001
Parity (number of children):				
1 child	1466 (24)	1216 2.9)	1	
2-3 children	2293 (37)	1966 (85.7)	1.24 (0.96–1.60)	0.101
4–5 children	1483 (24)	1292 (87.1)	1.39 (1.08–1.79)	0.011
6+ children	975 (16)	804 (82.4)	0.96 (0.71–1.30)	0.809
Baby size:				
Not very small	6008 (97)	5107 (85.0)	1	
Very small	210 (3)	171 (81.2)	0.76 (0.49–1.18)	0.224
Density of facilities with score above 70%:				
Below mean	3820 (61)	3215 .2)	1	
Above mean	2398 (39)	2062 (86.0)	1.15 (0.95–1.40)	0.148

CHAM – Christian Health Association of Malawi, CI – confidence interval, OR – odds ratio

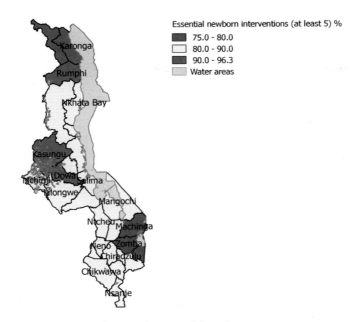

Figure 2. *Coverage of appropriate essential newborn care.*

variables found to be associated with appropriate newborn care are: residence, region, mother's education (secondary or higher), household wealth (fifth quintile), delivery by c–section and parity (having 4–5 children). For instance, newborns in the Northern and Central region of the country (as compared to newborns in the Southern part), newborns whose mothers have secondary or higher education (as compared to mothers with no education), newborns in households in the highest wealth quintile (as compared to the lowest wealth quintile) had higher likelihood of receiving appropriate newborn care in the postnatal period. On the other hand, newborns in rural areas, and newborns who were born by c–section had lower likelihood of receiving at least 5 newborn care interventions immediately after birth. There was no evidence of significant association between appropriate newborn care and mother's age at birth, type of health facility, baby size at birth or density of facilities with high score.

Multivariate analysis

The final model testing the association between receipt of appropriate newborn care and health facility service readiness score was adjusted for region, residence, household wealth, mother's education, type of delivery and baby's size at birth and residence. The results of the fully adjusted random effect logistic model are presented in **Table 2**.

The analysis reveals that newborns in districts with a facility score in the top category have 52% increased odds of receiving appropriate newborn care (OR = 1.52, 95% CI 1.19–1.95, P = 0.001), compared to newborns in districts with a facility score in the bottom category. Co–variates with a statistically significant positive association with newborns receiving at least 5 newborn care interventions are: region, household wealth, mother's education. Newborns residing in the Northern region are two times more likely to receive 5 essential newborn care interventions as compared to newborns in the Southern region (OR = 2.06, 95%CI 1.50–2.83, P < 0.001); the odds for newborns living in the Central region are increased by 1.5 as compared to newborns in the Southern region (OR:1.53, 95% CI 1.20–1.95, P = 0.001), having a mother with secondary or higher education increases the odds of better essential newborn care by 1.4 (OR = 1.40, 95% CI 1.05–1.86, P = 0.023) and by 1.37 if living in a household in

Table 2. *Association between appropriate PNC and district level health facility score for "normal delivery and newborn care" – random effect logistic model (N = 6218)*

VARIABLE	CATEGORIES	ADJUSTED OR (95%CI)	P
Health Facility Readiness Score	Bottom	1	
	Medium	1.29 (0.98–1.69)	0.067
	Top	1.52 (1.19–1.95)	0.001
Region	Southern	1	
	Central	1.53 (1.20–1.95)	0.001
	Northern	2.06 (1.50–2.83)	<0.001
C–Section	No	1	
	Yes	0.55 (0.42–0.73)	<0.001
Baby size at birth	Other	1	
	Very small	0.60 (0.43–0.84)	0.003
Household Wealth Index	Poorest	1	
	Second	1.20 (0.98–1.47)	0.070
	Middle	1.22 (0.99–1.50)	0.057
	Fourth	1.26 (1.01–1.59)	0.044
	Richest	1.37 (1.02–1.84)	0.036
Mother's education	None	1	
	Primary	1.21 (0.87–1.50)	0.091
	Secondary	1.40 (1.05–1.86)	0.023
Place of residence	Urban	1	
	Rural	0.84 (0.63–1.13)	0.254
Random effect variance (σ)		0.195	0.003
ICC (ρ)		0.011	

OR – odds ratio, CI – confidence interval, ICC – intra–cluster correlation coefficient the highest wealth quintile (OR = 1.37, 95% CI = 1.02–1.84, P = 0.036). On the other hand, newborns delivered by c–section (OR = 0.55, 95% CI 0.42–0.73, P < 0.001) and very small babies (OR = 0.60, 95% CI 0.43–0.84, P = 0.003) have lower odds of receiving the type of essential newborn care analyzed in this study. This may be due to the fact that the postnatal care protocol for c–section and low birth weight babies is different [29]. Unexpectedly, even though residing in rural areas showed a significant effect in the crude analysis, once the model was fully adjusted this effect was lost (OR = 0.84, 95% confidence interval 0.63–1.13, P = 0.254).

The cluster measures calculated in the model are the random effect variance (sigma = 0.195), which measures the in–between cluster variation and the intra–cluster correlation coefficient ICC (ρ = 0.011). These results give an indication of clustering within districts given that the values are not zero. The random effect variance is significant (P < 0.003). In other words, the result of the test of the null hypothesis of no within–district clustering provides strong evidence of within–district clustering in the model. Thus, it can be assumed that districts contributed to explain the variance in receiving appropriate newborn care.

DISCUSSION

This analysis investigated whether health facility service readiness score for normal delivery and newborn care at the district level is associated with receiving appropriate newborn care in the postnatal period in Malawi. The results indicate that newborns in districts with average facility service readiness score in the top category (score or 70% or higher) have 52% increased odds to receive appropriate newborn care than those in districts with lower facility score. The role of location is highlighted in the results as newborn in the Northern region have 2 times increased odds to receive appropriate newborn care as compared to newborns in the Southern region. As recent research has identified, addressing geographic and quality barriers is crucial to enhance service utilization and to lower maternal and perinatal mortality [30].

As reported in MSPA 2014 report, coverage of essential newborn care interventions is particularly high across health facilities in Malawi [22]. However, geographic location plays a role in the observed level of coverage disparity and health service environment. The level of health facility readiness to provide normal delivery and newborn care varies across the country (score range 56 to 80%) and only 35% of facilities across the country have a readiness score higher than 70%. A particular concern is that staff and training, which is a key domain of the health facility service readiness score is the lowest across the country. For instance, very few facilities in the Southern region have a score higher than 70% on the staff and training domain.

There are important limitations in this analysis that should be considered when interpreting the results. The measure of appropriate newborn care is based on a sub–set of recommended interventions for normal newborns for which data was available in the MES 2014 survey. Further, data on newborn care interventions is based on mother's recall of care provided to the newborn soon after birth. As with other measures based on mother's recall, this could have led to differential recall bias and may not entirely reflect the level of quality of care in facilities [31,32]. This is particularly the case for interventions that occur during the postpartum period as it is an extremely intense moment for mothers. Some mothers may not be aware of what is going on with their newborn given factors related to the dynamics of labour and delivery such as tiredness and soreness after labour, medical complications, or just the excitement of receiving their new child into the world.

Another limitation is the unavailability of GPS data at the cluster level which did not allow assessment of location within districts and distance to facilities. As the 2014 MES survey did not collect GPS data, the smallest level of aggregation possible was the district level. Districts have a number of facilities that provide different level of services. An average of the facility score at the district level may be an oversimplification of the reality. In addition, since districts are the lowest common level of geographic aggregation between the two data sets used in the analysis, further investigation of the effect of clustering at a lowest level of data collection (enumeration areas/clusters) was not possible and therefore would be a great choice for further research. To link the population and health facility data, a number of important assumptions were made. For instance, mean district health facility service readiness scores have been assigned to districts where the respondent resided at time of interview. However, this is a considerable limitation as with the available data it cannot be determined if a woman delivered in her own district or in a health facility outside of her district.

Given that this is a cross–sectional study, a cause–effect relationship cannot be established. It was also not possible to adjust for other potential confounding factors in the final model not available in the MES 2014. For instance, distance to health facility, motivation or awareness of mothers and health staff of essential newborn care procedures, availability of roads and transportation to access health facility, family support, the quality of the actual services received, women's autonomy, etc. A major confounder which could not be assessed in this study is the presence of a strong component of community–based maternal and newborn care in Malawi. For example: Ministry of Health revised the 2 week training on Community Based maternal and new born care to a 6–day training to increase coverage and improve access of these services. This process has so far covered almost 50% of the districts in the country. Supervision and mentorship tools have also been developed to support and strengthen implementation at district level [33].

Despite these limitations, the study provides evidence that the geographic proximity to facilities that provide optimal delivery and newborn care services can have an impact on the number of essential services received by the newborn. The main strengths of this analysis are the linking of health facility data with household survey data that allowed for joint analysis of health service environment and coverage indicators. Analysing these two sources of data also allowed for the inclusion of confounders at the individual, household and facility level. An important aspect of the analysis was that it looked into the quality of health facilities by analysing 3 main aspects important for normal deliveries and newborn care: staff and training, medicines and commodities as well as equipment and supplies. Previous quantitative studies have linked facility data and household data from DHS [15,34]. This methodology has a strong bearing on quality of care measurements which can use measures of essential newborn care interventions in household surveys as predictors of facility readiness.

CONCLUSION

The analysis reveals that in Malawi, newborns in districts with higher health facility service readiness score have increased odds of receiving a more complete set of essential newborn care interventions compared to those residing in districts with a lower facility score. These variations in readiness among geographical areas require a focused programming in order to address newborn care problems and achieve the targets that were set in the Every Newborn Action Plan. Therefore, it is imperative to increase the level of service readiness across all facilities, so that newborns regardless of the place and type of facility delivery receive all recommended essential interventions.

Staff availability and training emerged as an issue across all the districts in the country that can negatively affect the services received by newborns. Our study results suggest that given limited resources, priority should be given to high volume facilities in the poorly performing districts in the southern and northern regions. The essential newborn care interventions assessed in this study can for the most part be implemented with basic equipment available in most facilities and thus improvement strategies will need to address facility staff knowledge and motivation and other barriers including inadequate staffing levels. Strengthening of supervision, provision of simple job aids/checklists around essential newborn care, and ensuring adequate staffing for delivery and newborn care should be explored. In February 2017, the Malawi Ministry of Health joined eight other countries in launching a network for improving quality of care for maternal, newborn and child health and established a Quality of Care Management Directorate focussed on improving quality of care. Results of this study can help guide priority setting around what are the critical factors for the provision of quality services particularly in a context of a high neonatal mortality setting as Malawi [33]. Similarly, tracking of progress from mapping exercise and human resource development plan should be given attention as it will be critical for improvements in newborn care service delivery.

Over the last decade, the Government of Malawi has undertaken major initiatives to strengthen maternal and newborn care and improve staffing levels at health facilities. Getting performance reports and results from implementation of the current tools and instruments following the revised new born care guidelines will be a necessary as the Ministry looks forward for future domestic and international investments in health systems in Malawi. Additionally, it is critical to continue to analyse available data to generate evidence that will lead to the development of evidence based and focused programming for newborn care to the required standards in all parts of the country.

Acknowledgements: The authors are grateful to the following researchers for their inputs and guidance: Melissa Newman (LSHTM) for guidance throughout the development of the initial version of this analysis; Clara R. Burgert–Brucker, Wenjuan Wang, Tanya Marchant, Maria Muniz, Rocco Panciera and Maria Clara Restrepo–Mendez for support and guidance during the development of the various pieces of the analysis and for providing relevant inputs. The authors also thank Mr. Norman Lufesi (National Statistical Office of Malawi) and Mr. Humpfreys Nsona (Ministry of Health of Malawi) for their contributions in regards to the health policy in the country.

Disclaimer: The findings and conclusions in this report are those of the authors and do not necessarily represent the official position of the respective organizations.

Funding: None.

Authorship declaration: LCA conceptualized the original idea, conducted data analysis and produced the first draft. VM provided support on data analysis interpretation of results and drafting of manuscript. AA, VM, SMK provided overall guidance in interpretation of results. MK, LV, TG, NZ provided inputs regarding specific health program in country.

MK provided specific information about health policies in country. All authors reviewed the drafts and agreed on the final version.

Competing interests: *All authors have completed the ICMJE uniform disclosure form at http://www.icmje.org/coi_disclosure.pdf (available upon request from the corresponding author) and declare no conflict of interest.*

References

1 Bhutta ZA, Das JK, Bahl R, Lawn JE, Salam RA, Paul VK, et al. Can available interventions end preventable deaths in mothers, newborn babies, and stillbirths, and at what cost? Lancet. 2014;384:347-70. Medline:24853604 doi:10.1016/S0140-6736(14)60792-3

2 World Health Organization. Postnatal care of the mother and newborn. Geneva: World Health Organization; 2013.

3 World Health Organization. UNICEF. Every Newborn: An action plan to end preventable newborn deaths. Geneva: World Health Organisation; 2014. Available: http://www.everynewborn.org/every-newborn-action-plan/. Accessed: 13 October 2017.

4 World Health Organization. WHO recommendations on postnatal care for mother and newborn. Geneva: World Health Organization; 2013.

5 UNICEF. Committing to child survival: a promise renewed - progress report 2015. New York: UNICEF; 2015.

6 United Nations Inter-agency Group for Child Mortality Estimation. Levels and trends in child mortality: Report 2015. New York: UNICEF; 2015. Available: http://www.child-mortality.org/files_v20/download/IGME%20Report%202015_9_3%20LR%20Web.pdf. Accessed: 13 October 2017.

7 National Statistical Office (NSO) [Malawi] and ICF. Malawi Demographic and Health Survey 2015-16. Zomba, Malawi, and Rockville, Maryland, USA: NSO and ICF; 2017.

8 Kanyuka M, Ndawala J, Mleme T, Chisesa L, Makwemba M, Amouzou A, et al. Malawi and Millennium Development Goal 4: a Countdown to 2015 country case study. Lancet Glob Health. 2016;4:e201-14. Medline:26805586 doi:10.1016/S2214-109X(15)00294-6

9 USAID U. UNICEF, CHAI, Save the Children. Malawi Emergency Obstetric and Newborn Care Needs Assessment, 2014. Available: https://www.healthynewbornnetwork.org/hnn-content/uploads/Malawi-EmONC-Report-June-2015_FINAL.pdf. Accessed: 13 October 2017.

10 Zimba E, Kachale F, Waltensperger KZ, Blencowe H, Colbourn T, George J, et al. Newborn survival in Malawi: a decade of change and future implications. Health Policy Plan. 2012;27 Suppl 3:iii88-103. Medline:22692419 doi:10.1093/heapol/czs043

11 Republic of Malawi, Ministry of Health. Road Map for accelerating the reduction of maternal and neonatal mortality and morbidity in Malawi. Malawi: Ministry of Health; 2012. Available: https://www.healthynewbornnetwork.org/hnn-content/uploads/Malawi-Roadmap-for-Reducing-MN-mortality-2012.pdf. Accessed: 13 October 2017.

12 Republic of Malawi, Ministry of Health. Guidelines for the management of task shifting to health surveillance assistants in Malawi. Malawi: Ministry of Health; 2014.

13 Skiles MP, Burgert CR, Curtis SL, Spencer J. Geographically linking population and facility surveys: methodological considerations. Popul Health Metr. 2013;11:14. Medline:23926907 doi:10.1186/1478-7954-11-14

14 Moxon SG, Ruysen H, Kerber KJ, Amouzou A, Fournier S, Grove J, et al. Count every newborn; a measurement improvement roadmap for coverage data. BMC Pregnancy Childbirth. 2015;15 Suppl 2:S8. Medline:26391444 doi:10.1186/1471-2393-15-S2-S8

15 Lohela TJ, Campbell OM, Gabrysch S. Distance to care, facility delivery and early neonatal mortality in Malawi and Zambia. PLoS One. 2012;7:e52110. Medline:23300599 doi:10.1371/journal.pone.0052110

16 Ononokpono DN, Odimegwu CO, Imasiku EN, Adedini SA. Does it really matter where women live? A multilevel analysis of the determinants of postnatal care in Nigeria. Matern Child Health J. 2014;18:950-9. Medline:23812800 doi:10.1007/s10995-013-1323-9

17 Ugboaja JO, Nwosu OB, Igwegbe AO. OBI-Nwosu AL. Barriers to postnatal care and exclusive breastfeeding among urban women in southeastern Nigeria. Niger Med J. 2013;54:45-50. Medline:23661899 doi:10.4103/0300-1652.108895

18 Izudi J, Amongin D. Use of early postnatal care among postpartum women in Eastern Uganda. Int J Gynaecol Obstet. 2015;129:161-4. Medline:25661323 doi:10.1016/j.ijgo.2014.11.017

19 Amoako Johnson F. A geospatial analysis of the impacts of maternity care fee payment policies on the uptake of skilled birth care in Ghana. BMC Pregnancy Childbirth. 2016;16:41. Medline:26925575 doi:10.1186/s12884-016-0833-z

20 Burgert-Brucker CR, Yourkavitch J, Assaf S, Delgado S. Geographic variation in key indicators of maternal and child health across 27 countries in Sub-Saharan Africa. Rockville, Maryland, USA: ICF International; 2015.

21 Malawi NSO. Malawi MDG Endline Survey 2014. Zomba, Malawi: National Statistical Office; 2015.

22 Malawi MoH II. Malawi Service Provision Assessment (MSPA) 2013-14. Lilongwe, Malawi, and Rockville, Maryland, USA: MoH and ICF International; 2014.

23 Malawi NSO. Population and Housing Census. Malawi: National Stastical Office; 2008. Available: http://www.nsomalawi.mw/images/stories/data_on_line/demography/census_2008/Main%20Report/Census%20Main%20Report.pdf. Accessed: 13 October 2017.

24 World Health Organization. Service Availability and Readiness Assessment (SARA): an annual monitoring system for service delivery. Geneva: World Health Organization; 2015.

25 Do M, Micah A, Brondi L, Campbell H, Marchant T, Eisele T, et al. Linking household and facility data for better coverage measures in reproductive, maternal, newborn, and child health care: systematic review. J Glob Health. 2016;6:020501. Medline:27606060 doi:10.7189/jogh.06.020501

26 Gon G, Restrepo-Mendez MC, Campbell OM, Barros AJ, Woodd S, Benova L, et al. Who delivers without water? A multi-country analysis of water and sanitation in the childbirth environment. PLoS One. 2016;11:e0160572. Medline:27532291 doi:10.1371/journal.pone.0160572

27 Statacorp. Stata Statistical Software: Release 14, College Station, TX: Stata Corp LP; 2015.

28 QGIS. Free and Open Source Geographic Information System 2016.

29 Blanc AK, Warren C, McCarthy KJ, Kimani J, Ndwiga C. RamaRao S. Assessing the validity of indicators of the quality of maternal and newborn health care in Kenya. J Glob Health. 2016;6:010405. Medline:27231541 doi:10.7189/jogh.06.010405

30 Gabrysch S, Cousens S, Cox J, Campbell OM. The influence of distance and level of care on delivery place in rural Zambia: a study of linked national data in a Geographic Information System. PLoS Med. 2011;8:e1000394. Medline:21283606 doi:10.1371/journal.pmed.1000394

31 Stanton CK, Rawlins B, Drake M, Dos Anjos M, Cantor D, Chongo L, et al. Measuring coverage in MNCH: testing the validity of women's self-report of key maternal and newborn health interventions during the peripartum period in Mozambique. PLoS One. 2013;8:e60694. Medline:23667427 doi:10.1371/journal.pone.0060694

32 Carvajal-Velez L, Amouzou A, Perin J, Abdoulaye M, Tarekegn H, Akinyemi A, et al. Diarrhea management in children under five in sub-Saharan Africa: does the source of care matter? A Countdown analysis. BMC Public Health. 2016;16:830. Medline:27538438 doi:10.1186/s12889-016-3475-1

33 Kalino, Maggie (National Statistical Office, Malawi). Conversation with: Humphreys Nsona (Integrated Management of Childhood Illnesses Unit, Ministry of Health, Malawi). 2017 August 10.

34 Gabrysch S, Civitelli G, Edmond KM, Mathai M, Ali M, Bhutta ZA, et al. New signal functions to measure the ability of health facilities to provide routine and emergency newborn care. PLoS Med. 2012;9:e1001340. Medline:23152724 doi:10.1371/journal.pmed.1001340

Assessment of health facility capacity to provide newborn care in Bangladesh, Haiti, Malawi, Senegal, and Tanzania

Rebecca Winter[1], Jennifer Yourkavitch[2], Wenjuan Wang[3], Lindsay Mallick[4]

[1] Department of Health, The District of Columbia, Washington DC, USA
[2] ICF, Rockville, Maryland, USA
[3] The DHS Program, ICF, Rockville, Maryland, USA
[4] The DHS Program, Avenir Health, Glastonbury, Connecticut, USA

Background Despite the importance of health facility capacity to provide comprehensive care, the most widely used indicators for global monitoring of maternal and child health remain contact measures which assess women's use of services only and not the capacity of health facilities to provide those services; there is a gap in monitoring health facilities' capacity to provide newborn care services in low and middle income countries.

Methods In this study we demonstrate a measurable framework for assessing health facility capacity to provide newborn care using open access, nationally–representative Service Provision Assessment (SPA) data from the Demographic Health Surveys Program. In particular, we examine whether key newborn–related services are available at the facility (ie, service availability, measured by the availability of basic emergency obstetric care (BEmOC) signal functions, newborn signal functions, and routine perinatal services), and whether the facility has the equipment, medications, training and knowledge necessary to provide those services (ie, service readiness, measured by general facility requirements, equipment, medicines and commodities, and guidelines and staffing) in five countries with high levels of neonatal mortality and recent SPA data: Bangladesh, Haiti, Malawi, Senegal, and Tanzania.

Findings In each country, we find that key services and commodities needed for comprehensive delivery and newborn care are missing from a large percentage of facilities with delivery services. Of three domains of service availability examined, scores for routine care availability are highest, while scores for newborn signal function availability are lowest. Of four domains of service readiness examined, scores for general requirements and equipment are highest, while scores for guidelines and staffing are lowest.

Conclusions Both service availability and readiness tend to be highest in hospitals and facilities in urban areas, pointing to substantial equity gaps in the availability of essential newborn care services for rural areas and for people accessing lower–level facilities. Together, the low levels of both service availability and readiness across the five countries reinforce the vital importance of monitoring health facility capacity to provide care. In order to save newborn lives and improve equity in child survival, not only does women's use of services need to increase, but facility capacity to provide those services must also be enhanced.

Sustainable Development Target 3.2 aims to end the preventable death of newborns and children under age 5, with specific goals to reduce newborn deaths to less than 12 deaths per 1000 live births, and under–five deaths to less than 25 deaths per 1000 live births in all countries by 2030 [1]. Recent gains in child survival have been concentrated in the post–neonatal period, with slower gains made in survival during the first month of life [2]. As a result, the percentage of under–five deaths occurring in the first month of life has increased from 38 percent in 2000 to 45 percent in 2015 [3,4]. To continue making gains in child survival, it is essential to ensure that all newborns receive the care they need to survive.

Mothers are advised to give birth in health facilities in order to protect both their own and their infants' health [5,6]. Interventions during labor and birth, including those addressing obstetric complications, are known to have the greatest impact on neonatal survival, followed by appropriate care for small or ill newborns [7]. Specific interventions that have an impact on neonatal mortality include umbilical cord antiseptics, neonatal resuscitation, hypothermia for hypoxic ischaemic encephalopathy, topical emollient therapy, hypothermia prevention for preterm infants, Kangaroo Mother Care in preterm infants, oral and injectable antibiotics for pneumonia, and antibiotics for sepsis [7]. While evidence from a systematic review and meta–analysis suggests that delivering in a facility reduces the overall risk of neonatal mortality in low– and middle–income countries [6], not all studies have found facility delivery to be protective for newborn survival [8–10]. In fact, several recent studies using household survey data have found no evidence that the scale–up of facility deliveries or skilled birth attendance has been associated with reductions in neonatal mortality [10–12]. The provision of newborn care in the immediate and early postnatal period is particularly dependent on health facility infrastructure, capacity, and resources [13], and delivering in a facility that is ill–equipped to provide newborn care may not protect the infant. It is critical to ensure an optimal standard of care for mothers and newborns in health facilities, yet there is a gap in monitoring the quality of newborn care [14]. This study focuses on one specific aspect of quality of care: health facility capacity to provide newborn care, which is measured with service availability and service readiness to provide newborn care services. Service availability refers to the physical presence of essential newborn care services. Service readiness refers to the presence of essential infrastructure, functioning equipment, supplies, medicines that are in–stock and non–expired, trained staff, and current guidelines to provide the services. Both are prerequisite to providing good–quality services [15].

Despite agreement on the key packages and health interventions needed to protect and save newborn lives, there is little consensus on which are the key indicators needed to assess health facilities' capacity to provide newborn care [16]. The basic and comprehensive emergency obstetric care (EmOC) signal functions – shortlists of life–saving services first introduced in 1997 by the United Nations – are widely used to assess the functionality of health facility delivery care. But these functions focus primarily on provisions to treat the main causes of maternal mortality. With the exception of one recently added signal function on newborn resuscitation (introduced in 2009), the EmOC signal functions do not gauge facility readiness to provide essential newborn care [17]. Work has been under way to develop metrics for measuring facility provision of newborn care [15,16,18]. In 2008, Save the Children's Saving Newborn Lives program (SNL) convened a Newborn Indicators Technical Working Group (TWG) composed of evaluation and measurement experts, researchers, UN agencies, non–governmental organizations and donors. This group collaborated to construct a list of survey–based indicators to assess whether a facility is able to address the three leading causes of newborn death: intrapartum causes (eg, birth asphyxia), preterm birth, and infection. The evidence–based list of newborn care service indicators that they developed includes measures of service availability, equipment and supplies, documentation, staff training, supervision, and additional optional indicators [17]. Gabrysch and colleagues (2012) also proposed a set of obstetric and newborn signal functions that includes four areas: general health facility requirements, routine care for all mothers and babies, basic emergency care for mothers and babies with complications, and comprehensive emergency care functions [15]. Finally, the WHO Service Availability and Readiness Assessment (SARA) includes numerous indicators on newborn care [18]. In this study we combined indicators from these three sources to generate metrics to assess the availability and readiness of labor and delivery and immediate postnatal care provided at health facilities, in light of their impact on newborn morbidity and mortality.

The USAID–funded Service Provision Assessment (SPA) survey, implemented by the Demographic Health Surveys (DHS) Program, collects nationally–representative information about health facilities' service delivery, providing a key resource for assessing the extent to which facilities can provide comprehensive newborn care. In this study, we examined facility capacity to provide newborn care among facilities that offer delivery services in Bangladesh, Haiti, Malawi, Senegal, and Tanzania, five countries with high levels of neonatal mortality and recent SPA data. As of 2015, the neonatal mortality rates in the five countries ranged from 19 deaths per 1000 live births in Tanzania to 25 deaths per 1000 live births in Haiti, according to the UN Inter–agency Group for Child Mortality. For Senegal, Malawi, and Bangladesh, the rates were 21, 22, and 23 deaths per 1000 live births, respectively [19]. This study is the first comparative presentation of facility capacity to provide newborn care in multiple countries, using a measurable framework that could inform future studies. The manuscript originated from an earlier analysis carried out by the same authors [20] with a narrowed scope on key findings regarding newborn care service availability and readiness.

METHODS

Data

Study countries were selected according to two criteria. We focused the initial selection on the 25 USAID maternal and child health (MCH) priority countries (for a listing of the countries, see [21]). These countries account for more than 66% of global maternal and child deaths and are the focus of USAID programmatic efforts to scale up high–impact interventions and strengthen health systems [21]. We then restricted the analysis to countries with a SPA survey conducted within the last five years (ie, since 2011) with data available as of May 2016. Three of the five surveys included in the study are nationally representative sample surveys, while two (Haiti 2013 and Malawi 2013–14) are a census of all health facilities in the country (**Table 1**). The study was restricted to facilities that offer delivery services. Sample weights were applied throughout the study so that indicator estimates are representative of each country's actual mix of facilities, rather than the sample's mix of facilities. All five surveys produced indicators that are representative at the national level by facility type, managing authority, and geographic region.

SPA surveys provide information on the availability and readiness of health services. Specifically, the SPA surveys collect data on facility infrastructure (running water, electricity, privacy, etc.), the availability of resources (equipment, supplies, and medicines) and supportive processes and systems (client records, supervision, staff training, etc.) related to antenatal care, delivery care, and newborn care services (For more information on SPA surveys, see [22]).

Table 1. *Description of SPA surveys included in the study*

Country/y	Number of facilities*	Unweighted number of facilities with delivery services	Weighted number of facilities with delivery services	Sample or census
Bangladesh 2014	1548	586	280	sample
Haiti 2013	905	389	389	census
Malawi 2013–14	977	528	528	census
Senegal 2014†	363	282	279	sample
Tanzania 2014–15	1188	951	905	sample

*For all SPA surveys, the facility weights are normalized to have an equal unweighted and weighted total number of facilities.

†The Senegal 2014 SPA is part of the Senegal Continuous Survey project, which is designed to have five annual rounds of both DHS and SPA data collection, with the last round in 2017. This study uses the most recent available year of data, 2014. This survey included a subsample of health huts (case de santé). However, the methodology used to select health huts was different and their probability of selection was dependent on that of the health posts with which they were affiliated. Health huts are excluded from the current study.

SPA surveys include four standardized data collection instruments—the Facility Inventory Questionnaire, the Provider Interview Questionnaire, Observation Protocol, and Client Exit Interview—which provide general and service–specific information on the availability and quality of health services. This study relied primarily on the Facility Inventory Questionnaire, which collects information on health facilities' infrastructure, supplies, medicines, staffing, training, and procedures, as well as on the availability of specific delivery and newborn services, through interviews with the person most knowledgeable about delivery services in the facility. The study also drew upon the Provider Interview Questionnaire, which collects information on the experience, qualifications, and perceptions of the service delivery environment among health care workers who provide selected services.

Measurement of readiness

Our analysis focused on 38 tracer indicators to assess facilities' capacity to provide newborn care. In order to have this capacity, a facility must (1) offer key newborn–related services, and (2) have on–site the technology, equipment, medicine, training, and knowledge required to provide those services. Thus, we assessed two dimensions of facilities' capacity to provide newborn care: service availability and service readiness. Service availability captures the reported availability of essential newborn care services at the facility, while service readiness captures the facility's observed capacity to provide those services [23]. We assessed three domains of service availability: the availability of basic emergency obstetric care (BEmOC) signal functions, newborn signal functions, and routine perinatal practices; and four domains of service readiness: general facility requirements, equipment, medicines and commodities, and guidelines and staffing. Table S1 in **Online Supplementary Document** presents the seven domains, lists and defines the indicators, and notes their relevance to newborn health.

The 38 newborn care indicators were drawn primarily from a list of indicators suggested by the SNL TWG, and supplemented with additional WHO SARA indicators of "basic obstetric and newborn care" [18], and with Gabrysch and colleagues' [15] proposed obstetric and newborn signal function indicators. The study did not include prevention of mother to child transmission of HIV indicators since the burden of HIV varies substantially across the study countries and HIV is not a common cause of newborn death; it becomes more relevant for the post–neonatal period [24]. Several other suggested indicators (eg, referral services for lower–level facilities) are not available in the SPA surveys, along with information on these items: resuscitation table, towel for drying the baby, or up–to–date delivery register.

In accordance with the WHO SARA approach, we computed composite indicators to assess overall newborn care service availability and readiness in the facilities. We weighted the indicators within each domain of service availability and service readiness equally to produce a domain score, and weighted each domain equally to produce a summary score for service availability and for service readiness. This simple additive scale is easily replicable.

We examined newborn care service availability and readiness nationally, as well by type of facility (hospital, health center, dispensary/clinic), managing authority (public vs private/other), urban–rural location, and region (see Section B in **Online Supplementary Document**). For managing authority, the private/other category included NGOs, Mission or religious–run health facilities, and parastatal facilities. For region, the 14 regions presented in Senegal's 2014 SPA final report were aggregated into six geographic zones to have sufficient sample size in each geographic area [25].For additional detail, refer to Tables S2a–S6g in the **Online Supplementary Document** that show the individual components that comprise the seven dimensions of newborn care service availability and readiness disaggregated by facility characteristics, separately for each country.

For the three countries with sampled health facilities, we presented confidence intervals around coverage point estimates (Stata v. 14), accounting for the SPA complex sample design. For the two countries that used censuses of all formal health facilities, confidence intervals are not needed, since the point estimates describe the full population of formal health facilities.

RESULTS

Profile of facilities with delivery services

Table 2 shows the percent distribution of facilities offering delivery services by facility characteristics and country. In all five countries, the majority of facilities with delivery services were in rural areas—ranging from 61% in Haiti to 85% in Tanzania and Malawi. In Bangladesh and Haiti there was a fairly even distribution of hospitals, health centers, and dispensaries or clinics. In both countries, hospitals constituted roughly one–quarter of facilities with delivery services. In Senegal and Tanzania the vast majority of facilities with delivery services were either dispensaries or clinics (89% and 83%, respectively). Malawi stands out as the only country where the majority of facilities with delivery services were health centers (78%). Between 50% and 90% of the facilities were public. The managing authorities included within "private or other" varied by country, and included private, parastatal, NGO, for profit, and religious–affiliated facilities. Haiti had the largest share of private or other facilities with delivery services (50%). In Haiti these were a mix of NGO/private not for profit, private for profit, and Mission or faith–based facilities.

Overall service availability and readiness

Figure 1 shows national scores for each domain of availability and readiness, as well as national summary scores for service availability and service readiness. All scores range from 0 to 100 and indicate the average percentage of component tracer items that are available within the domain.

Table 2. *Percent distribution of facilities with delivery services by facility characteristics, Bangladesh, Haiti, Malawi, Senegal, Tanzania*

	BANGLADESH		HAITI		MALAWI		SENEGAL		TANZANIA	
	%	N	%	N	%	N	%	N	%	N
Facility type:										
Hospital	26.1	73	24.1	94	18.0	95	4.0	11	4.8	44
Health Center	35.2	99	42.9	167	78.5	414	7.3	20	12.1	110
Dispensary/Clinic	38.7	109	33.0	128	3.5	19	88.7	248	83.1	751
Urban–rural:										
Urban	29.3	82	38.8	151	14.8	78	25.9	72	14.6	132
Rural	70.7	198	61.2	238	85.2	450	74.1	207	85.4	773
Managing authority:										
Public	79.8	224	50.0	195	65.7	347	89.8	251	83.6	756
Private or other	20.2	57	49.8	194	34.3	181	10.2	29	16.4	149
Total	**100.0**	**280**	**100.0**	**389**	**100.0**	**528**	**100.0**	**279**	**100.0**	**905**

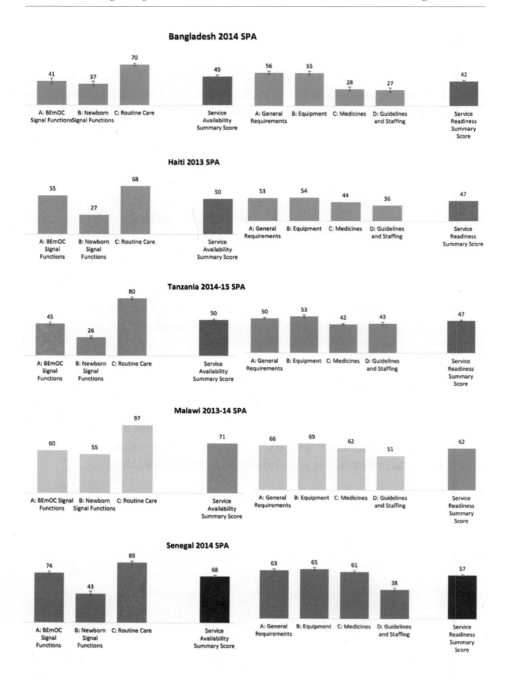

Figure 1. National service availability and service readiness summary scores, Bangladesh, Haiti, Tanzania, Malawi, Senegal. Confidence intervals are not shown for Haiti or Malawi, since those surveys were a census of all formal health facilities.

In all countries, of the three domains of service availability, scores for routine care availability were highest and scores for newborn signal function availability were lowest. Routine care scores ranged from about 70 in Bangladesh and Haiti to 97 in Malawi. This domain assessed the availability of three services: routine use of a partograph at the facility to monitor and manage labor, routine early initiation of breastfeeding, and routine thermal care, including drying and wrapping. While early initiation of breastfeeding and routine thermal care were nearly universal in each country, routine use of the partograph was less prevalent (see Tables S2a–S6g in the **Online Supplementary Document**).

Scores for the newborn signal function domain ranged from 26 and 27 in Tanzania and Haiti, respectively, to 55 in Malawi. Coverage of each of the three services included in the domain–corticosteroids in preterm labor, KMC for premature/very small babies, and neonatal resuscitation—was low, with the availability of corticosteroids in preterm labor scoring lowest (see Tables S2a–S6g in the **Online Supplementary Document**).

Scores for the third domain of service availability, the BEmOC signal functions, ranged from 41 in Haiti to 74 in Senegal. Of the six BEmOC functions, parenteral administration of anticonvulsants was least available in facilities, while parenteral administration of uterotonic drugs was most available (see Tables S2a–S6g in the **Online Supplementary Document**). Overall, the summary scores for newborn care service availability ranged from 49 in Bangladesh to 71 in Malawi.

Coverage patterns for the four domains of service readiness were consistent across the countries. Of the four domains, scores for guidelines and staffing were lowest, followed by scores for medicines. Guidelines and staffing scores ranged from 27 in Bangladesh to 51 in Malawi. This domain included six indicators of newborn–care related staff training, three indicators on the presence of key guidelines, and one indicator of supervision. Nearly all indicators in the domain scored poorly, with the exception of staff supervision (see Tables S2a–S6g in the **Online Supplementary Document).**

Scores in the medicines domain were also low, ranging from 28 in Bangladesh to about 60 in Malawi and Senegal. Of eight essential medicines in the domain, five were unavailable in more than half of facilities with delivery services in Bangladesh, Haiti, and Tanzania. These five medicines were chlorhexidine for cord cleaning, magnesium sulfate, hydrocortisone, injectable antibiotic, and antibiotic eye ointment for the newborn (see Tables S2a–S6g in the **Online Supplementary Document).**

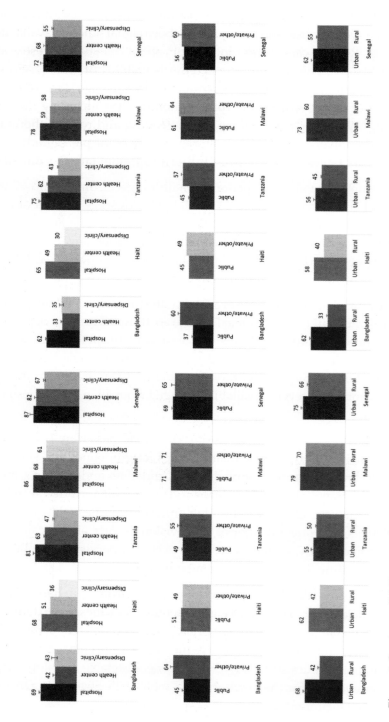

Figure 2. Service availability (panels on left) and service readiness (panels on right) summary scores by facility characteristics, Bangladesh, Haiti, Tanzania, Malawi, Senegal. Confidence intervals are not shown for Haiti or Malawi, since those surveys were a census of all formal health facilities.

Within each country, scores for the general requirements and equipment domains were higher, and were similar to each other. General requirements scores ranged from 50 in Tanzania to 66 in Malawi. This domain included five indicators: the availability of emergency transport, 24/7 skilled birth attendance, improved sanitation, an improved water source, and electricity. Of these, 24/7 skilled birth attendance was least prevalent, followed by emergency transport and improved sanitation (see Tables S2a–S6g in the **Online Supplementary Document).**

Equipment scores ranged from 53 in Tanzania to 69 in Malawi. The domain included 13 indicators, including sterilization equipment, delivery bed, examination light, delivery pack, suction apparatus, manual vacuum extractor, vacuum aspirator or D&C kit, partograph, disposable latex gloves, newborn back and mask, infant scale, blood pressure apparatus, and handwashing soap and running water or hand disinfectant. Of these, facility coverage of manual vacuum extractors and vacuum aspirator or D&C kits tended to be lowest, followed by newborn bag and masks and sterilization equipment (see Tables S2a–S6g in the **Online Supplementary Document).** Overall, the summary scores for newborn care service readiness ranged from 42 in Bangladesh to 62 in Malawi.

Figure 2 presents differentials in the composite service availability and service readiness scores side by side. The patterns in service availability and service readiness are strikingly similar across countries. Scores for both service availability and service readiness tended to be highest in hospitals and in urban areas. There was less difference in scores between public and private facilities, except for Bangladesh and Tanzania, where private facilities scored notably higher for both service availability and service readiness. To see the individual components that comprise the seven dimensions of newborn care service availability and readiness disaggregated by facility characteristics, see Tables S2a–S6g in the **Online Supplementary Document.**

DISCUSSION

Where you are born strongly affects your chance of survival [26]. Previous studies have found that access to delivery care alone is not enough to reduce early neonatal mortality rates [8]. It is essential that the facility where the birth occurs be equipped to provide key life–saving services for the newborn. Our study is the first study to examine the capacity of facilities to provide newborn care in five countries with high neonatal mortality. In all five countries, key services, commodities, and medicines needed for comprehensive delivery and newborn care were missing from a large proportion of the facilities that offer delivery services. This is important not only because it indicates a likelihood of poor quality of care, or possibly no care, but also because widespread perceptions of services of poor quality can deter women from seeking any care at a facility [27].

Of the five countries assessed, Malawi had the highest scores for both service availability and service readiness. Service availability scores in Malawi varied by domain, with the lowest scores being for BEmOC signal functions and newborn signal functions. Service readiness domain scores were generally consistent, at around 60. However, a need for improvement remains for all domains except routine care. Hospitals scored the highest for service availability and service readiness, while health centers scored much lower. Because health centers constitute nearly 80% of the facilities that provide delivery services, and they have the potential to serve more people than hospitals, further investment in the availability and readiness of their newborn care services is greatly needed. Urban facilities generally scored higher than rural facilities, and there was only a slight difference between public and private facility scores. Most facilities are located in rural areas (85%), and investments to increase the scores of those facilities in Malawi could have a significant impact on the population. Our findings are consistent with a study by Zimba and colleagues (2012) that found most facilities had staffing and supply shortages and lacked three or more signal functions [28].

Senegal's newborn care quality scores were nearly as high as those in Malawi, at 68 points for service availability and 57 points for service readiness. Senegal's highest score was for routine care (89); its lowest scores were for guidelines and staffing (38) and the availability of newborn signal functions (43). Compared with the other countries, disparities are markedly less drastic in Senegal. There was little difference between public and private facilities in service availability and readiness, and on average the differences between urban and rural facilities are smaller than for other countries except Malawi. Still, health posts—which constitute nearly 90% of all facilities that offer delivery services and 100% of the "dispensaries and clinics" category–scored substantially lower than hospitals. Investments to increase the scores of health posts could have a significant impact on population health.

Bangladesh showed impressive reductions in neonatal mortality between 1990 and 2015, with the NMR declining steadily and incrementally from 63 deaths per 1000 live births in 1990 to 23 deaths per 1000 live births in 2015 [19]. Despite this improvement, we found that the country had relatively low scores for newborn care service capacity, with scores below 50 for both service availability and service readiness. Its highest score was for routine care (70) and its lowest was for the availability of medicines (28). Of the five countries, Bangladesh also showed the widest gaps in coverage across subgroups: hospitals generally had much higher scores than health centers or dispensaries/clinics; private facilities had higher scores than public facilities, and urban facilities had higher scores than rural facilities, suggesting geographic and economic inequities in access to high–quality newborn care. These findings are consistent with other studies that reported inadequate quality of obstetric care in the country and marked urban–rural gaps in quality [29]. Bangladesh has been a global leader in priori-tizing newborn survival and care [30], and its policy efforts have been highly successful, as evidenced by the reductions in NMR. The relatively low quality scores could be explained by the country's newborn care policy emphasis on community health workers and home and community–based interventions [30]. That emphasis makes sense given that 62% of women in Bangladesh deliver at home, according to the 2014 Bangladesh DHS [31]. However, given that the remaining 38% of women deliver in health facilities, concentrated efforts to improve the quality of newborn care in health facilities are urgently needed, and could lead to further reductions in neonatal mortality.

Tanzania also scored around 50 for overall service availability and service read-iness, with its highest score attained for routine care (80) and its lowest score for newborn signal functions (26). Hospitals, which constitute just 5% of the country's health facilities with delivery services, had higher scores than health centers or dispensaries/clinics; private facilities had higher scores than public facilities; and urban facilities had higher scores than rural facilities, suggesting both geographic and economic inequities. While Tanzania made impressive gains in child survival between 2000 and 2015, improvements in neonatal survival were far slower [32]. Afnan–Holme and colleagues (2015) reported important differences in funding and implementation strategies among child, maternal, and newborn health policies in Tanzania that could have contributed to these different trajectories [32]. Child survival began receiving consistent policy attention in the mid–1980s, while attention to maternal health came later, in the mid–1990s, and attention to newborn care even later, in 2005. While Tanzania's child survival policy strategy has focused primarily on implement-ing high–impact interventions at the first level of the health system, maternal health interventions have often been targeted at higher levels of the health system [32]. Newborn care policies are just now rapidly scaling up in Tanzania [32]. These policies should target newborn care readiness at all facility levels, with an emphasis on first level facilities where readiness is currently lowest, and where more than 30% of women deliver [33].

Haiti scored around 50 for both service availability and service readiness, with a highest score of 68 for routine care and a lowest score of 27 for newborn signal functions. Overall in Haiti, public and private facilities scored similarly, but hospitals scored higher than health centers and dispensaries/clinics, and urban facilities scored higher than rural facilities, signaling geographic inequities and probable barriers to access. These findings are consistent with those of Wang and colleagues (2014), who also found that lower–level facilities in Haiti—and specifically health centers without beds and dispensaries—are poorly prepared to provide delivery services. In Haiti, health centers without beds and dispensaries lack a government mandate to provide delivery services [34], yet these facilities constitute half of all facilities that report offering delivery care [35]. Facilities that lack an official mandate may not receive necessary support from the government. Since lower–level facilities are often the only option in rural areas, the government should formally include them as providers of delivery care and equip them with the medicines, commodities, personnel, and training necessary to provide high–quality delivery and newborn care [35].

The study has several limitations. Our choice of countries was limited by the availability of SPA surveys. With data from SPA surveys, we cannot assess all aspects of the quality of newborn care. In this study we focused on two measurable dimensions of quality: service availability and service readiness. These two dimensions are necessary—but not sufficient—components of providing high–quality newborn care. While the indicators used to measure service availability and readiness were suggested by global experts in the field, there is a lack of evidence on a few indicators (eg, recent staff training in neonatal resuscitation, use of corticosteroids in preterm labor) about their association with newborn health outcomes. Furthermore, the service availability and readiness scores we created include 38 tracer indicators and condense a great deal of information that needs to be "unpacked" for clear interpretation and program purposes. However, we believe the scores provided a valid way to summarize a large amount of related information. The strength of our study is our multifaceted analysis, through which we sought to expose the current status of two components of newborn care quality from different angles.

We conclude that facility capacity to provide newborn care is lacking in five countries with a high burden of neonatal mortality. Of the seven domains of service availability and service readiness studied, routine care consistently scored highest, while newborn signal functions and guidelines and staffing tended to score lowest. The results point to persistent inequality in access to high–quality newborn care between urban and rural areas and between hospitals and the more commonly used health centers and dispensaries/clinics.

Health system initiatives to improve facility capacity are needed in each of the five countries. All facilities that offer delivery services must have trained staff available around–the–clock and be equipped with the essential supplies, medicines, and commodities needed to care for the mother–newborn dyad during labor, delivery, and the immediate postnatal period.

Disclaimers: *The views expressed are those of the authors and do not necessarily reflect the views of USAID or the United States Government.*

Funding: *This study was carried out with support provided by the United States Agency for International Development (USAID) through The DHS Program.*

Authorship contributions: *RW: research concept, developing analysis plan, data analysis, interpretation, and writing and revising the manuscript. JY: literature review, writing and reviewing the manuscript, WW: research concept, developing analysis plan, data analysis, interpretation, writing and revising the manuscript. LM: Data analysis and reviewing the manuscript. All authors have read and approved the final manuscript.*

Competing interests: *The authors have completed the Unified Competing Interest form at www.icmje.org/coi_disclosure.pdf (available on request from the corresponding author) and declare no competing interests.*

References

1 United Nations. Sustainable Development Goal 3: Ensure healthy lives and promote well-being for all at all ages. 2016. Available: https://sustainabledevelopment.un.org/sdg3. Accessed: 1 August 2017.

2 UNICEF, WHO, World Bank, UN-DESA Population Division. Levels and trends in child mortality 20152015. Available: http://www.childmortality.org/files_v20/download/IGME%20report%202015%20child%20mortality%20final.pdf. Accessed: 1 August 2017.

3 Liu L, Johnson HL, Cousens S, Perin J, Scott S, Lawn JE, et al. Global, regional, and national causes of child mortality: an updated systematic analysis for 2010 with time trends since 2000. Lancet. 2012;379:2151-61. Medline:22579125 doi:10.1016/S0140-6736(12)60560-1

4 WHO. Global Health Observatory visualizations: Child mortality causes of child mortality. 2015. Available: http://apps.who.int/gho/data/view.wrapper.CHILDCODv?lang=en. Accessed: 1 August 2017.

5 Exavery A, Kante AM, Njozi M, Tani K, Doctor HV, Hingora A, et al. Access to institutional delivery care and reasons for home delivery in three districts of Tanzania. Int J Equity Health. 2014;13:48. Medline:24934657 doi:10.1186/1475-9276-13-48

6 Tura G, Fantahun M, Worku A. The effect of health facility delivery on neonatal mortality: systematic review and meta-analysis. BMC Pregnancy Childbirth. 2013;13:18. Medline:23339515 doi:10.1186/1471-2393-13-18

7 Bhutta ZA, Das JK, Bahl R, Lawn JE, Salam RA, Paul VK, et al. Can available interventions end preventable deaths in mothers, newborn babies, and stillbirths, and at what cost? Lancet. 2014;384:347-70. Medline:24853604 doi:10.1016/S0140-6736(14)60792-3

8 Lohela TJ, Campbell OMR, Gabrysch S. Distance to care facility delivery and early neonatal mortality in Malawi and Zambia. PLoS One. 2012;7:e52110. Medline:23300599 doi:10.1371/journal.pone.0052110

9 Moyer CA, Dako-Gyeke P, Adanu RM. Facility-based delivery and maternal and early neonatal mortality in sub-Saharan Africa: a regional review of the literature. Afr J Reprod Health. 2013;17:30-43. Medline:24069765

10 Winter R, Pullum T, Florey L, Hodgins S. Impact of scale-up of maternal and delivery care on reductions in neonatal mortality in USAID MCH priority countries, 2000-2010. Rockville, Maryland, USA: ICF International; 2014.

11 Singh SK, Kaur R, Gupta M, Kumar R. Impact of National Rural Health Mission on perinatal mortality in rural India. Indian Pediatr. 2012;49:136-8. Medline:21992866 doi:10.1007/s13312-012-0022-8

12 Nathan R, Mwanyangala MA. Survival of neonates in rural Southern Tanzania: does place of delivery or continuum of care matter? BMC Pregnancy Childbirth. 2012;12:18. Medline:22439592 doi:10.1186/1471-2393-12-18

13 Dickson KE, Simen-Kapeu A, Kinney MV, Huicho L, Vesel L, Lackritz E, et al. Every Newborn: health-systems bottlenecks and strategies to accelerate scale-up in countries. 2014;384:438-54.

14 Rubayet S, Shahidullah M, Hossain A, Corbett E, Moran AC, Mannan I, et al. Newborn survival in Bangladesh: a decade of change and future implications. Health Policy Plan. 2012;27 Suppl 3:iii40-56. Medline:22692415 doi:10.1093/heapol/czs044

15 WHO. Service Availability and Readiness Assessment (SARA): An annual monitoring system for service delivery Reference Manual2015 May 1, 2016. Available: http://www.who.int/healthinfo/systems/SARA_Reference_Manual_Chapter3.pdf?ua=1. Accessed: 1 August 2017.

16 Gabrysch S, Civitelli G, Edmond KM, Mathai M, Ali M, Bhutta ZA, et al. New Signal Functions to Measure the Ability of Health Facilities to Provide Routine and Emergency Newborn Care. PloS Med. 2012;9:e1001340.

17 WHO. UNFPA, UNICF, AMDD. Monitoring emergency obstetric care: a handbook. Geneva, Switzerland: WHO; 2009.

18 Newborn Indicators Technical Working Group. Newborn Services Rapid Health Facility Assessment. 2012. Available: http://www.healthynewbornnetwork.org/hnn-content/uploads/Newborn-Services-Rapid-HFA_HNN_25June2012.pdf. Accessed: 1 August 2017.

19 UN Inter-agency Group for Child Mortality Estimation. Bangladesh Mortality rate, neonatal (per 1000 live births). 2015. Available: http://data.worldbank.org/indicator/SH.DYN.NMRT?end=2015&locations=BD&start=1990&view=chart&year_high_desc=false. Accessed: 1 August 2017.

20 Winter R, Yourkavitch J, Mallick L, Wang W. Levels and trends in newborn care service availability and readiness in Bangladesh, Haiti, Malawi, Senegal, and Tanzania. Rockville, Maryland, USA: ICF International; 2016.

21 USAID. Maternal and Child Health Priority Countries. 2017. Available: https://www.usaid.gov/what-we-do/global-health/maternal-and-child-health/priority-countries. Accessed: 1 August 2017.

22 USAID. SPA Overview. n.d. Available: http://dhsprogram.com/What-We-Do/Survey-Types/SPA.cfm. Accessed: 1 August 2017.

23 WHO. Service Availability and Readiness Assessment (SARA): Indicators and questionnaire. 2016. Available: http://www.who.int/healthinfo/systems/sara_indicators_questionnaire/en/. Accessed: 1 August 2017.

24   Naniche D, Bardaji A, Lahuerta M, Berenguera A, Mandomando I, Sanz S, et al. Impact of maternal human immunodeficiency virus infection on birth outcomes and infant survival in rural Mozambique. Am J Trop Med Hyg. 2009;80:870-6. Medline:19407140

25   Agence Nationale de la Statistique et de la Démographie - ANSD/Sénégal. ICF International. Sénégal Enquęte Continue sur la Prestation des Services de Soins de Santé (ECPSS) 2014. Rockville, Maryland, USA: ANSD/Sénégal and ICF International; 2015.

26   Lawn JE, Blencowe H, Darmstadt GL, Bhutta ZA. Beyond newborn survival: the world you are born into determines your risk of disability-free survival. Pediatr Res. 2013;74 Suppl 1:1-3. Medline:24240732 doi:10.1038/pr.2013.202

27   Darmstadt GL, Kinney MV, Chopra M, Cousens S, Kak L, Paul VK, et al. Who has been caring for the baby? Lancet. 2014;384:174-884;384:174-88. Medline:24853603 doi:10.1016/S0140-6736(14)60458-X

28   Zimba E, Kinney MV, Kachale F, Waltensperger KZ, Blencowe H, Colbourn T, et al. Newborn survival in Malawi: a decade of change and future implications. Health Policy Plan. 2012;27 Suppl 3:iii88-103. Medline:22692419 doi:10.1093/heapol/czs043

29   Anwar I, Kalim N, Koblinsky M. Quality of obstetric care in public-sector facilities and constraints to implementing emergency obstetric care services: evidence from high-and low-performing districts of Bangladesh. J Health Popul Nutr. 2009;27:139-55. Medline:19489412 doi:10.3329/jhpn.v27i2.3327

30   Shiffman J, Sultana S. Generating political priority for neonatal mortality reduction in Bangladesh. Am J Public Health. 2013;103:623-31. Medline:23237181 doi:10.2105/AJPH.2012.300919

31   Research NIoP. Training - NIPORT/Bangladesh, Mitra, Associates, ICF International. Bangladesh Demographic and Health Survey 2014. Dhaka, Bangladesh: NIPORT, Mitra and Associates, and ICF International; 2016.

32   Afnan-Holmes H, Magoma M, John T, Levira F, Msemo G, Armstrong CE, et al. Tanzania's Countdown to 2015: an analysis of two decades of progress and gaps for reproductive, maternal, newborn, and child health, to inform priorities for post-2015. Lancet Glob Health. 2015;3:e396-e409. Medline:26087986 doi:10.1016/S2214-109X(15)00059-5

33   Ministry of Health CD, Gender, Elderly, Children - MoHCDGEC/Tanzania Mainland, Ministry of Health - MoH/Zanzibar, National Bureau of Statistics - NBS/Tanzania, Office of Chief Government Statistician - OCGS/Zanzibar, ICF. Tanzania Demographic and Health Survey and Malaria Indicator Survey 2015-2016. Dar es Salaam, Tanzania: MoHCDGEC, MoH, NBS, OCGS, and ICF; 2016.

34   Ministere de la Santé Publique et de la Population (MSPP). Représentation du Systeme de Santé. Port-au-Prince, Haiti: 2000.

35   Wang W, Winter R, Mallick L, Florey L, Burgert-Brucker C, Carter E. The relationship between the health service environment and service utilization: linking population data to health facilities data in Haiti and Malawi. Rockville, Maryland, USA: ICF International; 2015.

SECTION 3

Methodological analysis: Improving measurement of maternal and newborn care interventions

"Every Newborn-BIRTH" protocol: observational study validating indicators for coverage and quality of maternal and newborn health care in Bangladesh, Nepal and Tanzania

Louise T Day[*,1], Harriet Ruysen[*,1], Vladimir S Gordeev[1], Georgia R Gore-Langton[1], Dorothy Boggs[1], Simon Cousens[1], Sarah G Moxon[1], Hannah Blencowe[1], Angela Baschieri[1], Ahmed Ehsanur Rahman[2], Tazeen Tahsina[2], Sojib Bin Zaman[2], Tanvir Hossain[2], Qazi Sadeq-ur Rahman[2], Shafiqul Ameen[2], Shams El Arifeen[2], Ashish KC[3], Shree Krishna Shrestha[4], Naresh P KC[5], Dela Singh[4], Anjani Kumar Jha[6], Bijay Jha[6], Nisha Rana[3], Omkar Basnet[7], Elisha Joshi[8], Asmita Paudel[10], Parashu Ram Shrestha[5], Deepak Jha[5], Ram Chandra Bastola[9], Jagat Jeevan Ghimire[6], Rajendra Paudel[10], Nahya Salim[11], Donat Shamba[12], Karim Manji[11], Josephine Shabani[12], Kizito Shirima[12], Namala Mkopi[11], Mwifadhi Mrisho[12], Fatuma Manzi[12], Jennie Jaribu[12], Edward Kija[11], Evelyne Assenga[11], Rodrick Kisenge[11], Andrea Pembe[11], Claudia Hanson[13], Godfrey Mbaruku[12†], Honorati Masanja[12], Agbessi Amouzou[14], Tariq Azim[15], Debra Jackson[16], Theopista John Kabuteni[17], Matthews Mathai[18], Jean-Pierre Monet[19], Allisyn Moran[20], Pavani Ram[21], Barbara Rawlins[22], Johan Ivar Sæbø[23], Florina Serbanescu[24], Lara ME Vaz[25], Nabila Zaka[16], Joy E Lawn[1]

[1] Maternal, Adolescent, Reproductive & Child Health (MARCH) Centre, London School of Hygiene & Tropical Medicine (LSHTM), London, UK
[2] Maternal and Child Health Division, International Centre for Diarrhoeal Disease Research, Bangladesh (iccdr, b), Dhaka, Bangladesh
[3] Department of Women's and Children's Health, Uppsala University, Uppsala, Sweden
[4] Pokhara Academy of Health Science, Pokhara Ranipauwa, Nepal
[5] Department of Health Services, Ministry of Health, Kathmandu, Nepal
[6] Nepal Health Research Council, Kathmandu, Nepal
[7] Golden Community, Kathmandu, Nepal
[8] LifeLine Nepal, Kathmandu, Nepal
[9] Matri Shishu Miteri Hospital, Pokhara, Nepal
[10] Kanti Children's Hospital, Kathmandu, Nepal
[11] Department of Paediatrics and Child Health, Muhimbili University of Health and Allied Sciences, Dar Es Salaam, Tanzania
[12] Department of Health Systems, Impact Evaluation and Policy, Ifakara Health Institute, Dar es Salaam, Tanzania
[13] Public Health Sciences – Global Health – Health Systems and Policy, Karolinska Institutet, Stockholm, Sweden
[14] Institute for International Programs, Department of International Health, Johns Hopkins University, Baltimore, Maryland, USA
[15] MEASURE Evaluation, University of North Carolina, North Carolina, USA
[16] Knowledge Management & Implementation Research Unit, Health Section, UNICEF, New York, USA
[17] Family and Reproductive Health WHO Tanzania
[18] Centre for Maternal and Newborn Health, Liverpool School of Tropical Medicine, Liverpool, UK
[19] Department for Sexual and Reproductive Health, UNFPA, New York, USA
[20] Department of Maternal, Newborn, Child and Adolescent Health, World Health Organization, Geneva, Switzerland
[21] Office of Health, Infectious Disease and Nutrition, Bureau for Global Health, United States Agency for International Development, Washington, DC, USA
[22] Jhpiego Baltimore, Baltimore, MD, USA
[23] Department for Informatics, University of Oslo, Oslo, Norway
[24] Division of Reproductive Health, Centres for Disease Control and Prevention (CDC), Atlanta, Georgia, USA
[25] Department of Global Health, Save the Children, Washington DC, USA

Background To achieve Sustainable Development Goals and Universal Health Coverage, programmatic data are essential. The *Every Newborn* Action Plan, agreed by all United Nations member states and >80 development partners, includes an ambitious Measurement Improvement Roadmap. Quality of care at birth is prioritised by both *Every Newborn* and Ending Preventable Maternal Mortality strategies, hence metrics need to advance from health service contact alone, to content of care. As facility births increase, monitoring using routine facility data in DHIS2 has potential, yet validation research has mainly focussed on maternal recall surveys. The *Every Newborn* –Birth Indicators Research Tracking in Hospitals (EN-BIRTH) study aims to validate selected newborn and maternal indicators for routine tracking of coverage and quality of facility-based care for use at district, national and global levels.

Methods EN-BIRTH is an observational study including >20 000 facility births in three countries (Tanzania, Bangladesh and Nepal) to validate selected indicators. Direct clinical observation will be compared with facility register data and a pre-discharge maternal recall survey for indicators including: uterotonic administration, immediate newborn care, neonatal resuscitation and Kangaroo mother care. Indicators including neonatal infection management and antenatal corticosteroid administration, which cannot be easily observed, will be validated using inpatient records. Trained clinical observers in Labour/Delivery ward, Operation theatre, and Kangaroo mother care ward/areas will collect data using a tablet-based customised data capturing application. Sensitivity will be calculated for numerators of all indicators and specificity for those numerators with adequate information. Other objectives include comparison of denominator options (ie, true target population or surrogates) and quality of care analyses, especially regarding intervention timing. Barriers and enablers to routine recording and data usage will be assessed by data flow assessments, quantitative and qualitative analyses.

Conclusions To our knowledge, this is the first large, multi-country study validating facility-based routine data compared to direct observation for maternal and newborn care, designed to provide evidence to inform selection of a core list of indicators recommended for inclusion in national DHIS2. Availability and use of such data are fundamental to drive progress towards ending the annual 5.5 million preventable stillbirths, maternal and newborn deaths.

Valid data and measurement are central to achieving the Sustainable Development Goal (SDG) aspiration of "no-one left behind" [1]. In the United Nation's Global Strategy for Women's Children's and Adolescent's Health the ongoing imperative for the right to survive, is joined by a new focus on thriving, with wider transformation [2]. Progress for survival has been slowest for the 5.5 million deaths of women and babies around the time of birth each year, including an estimated 2.5 million newborns dying in the first 28 days of life, 2.6 million babies stillborn and 303 000 maternal deaths [3-5]. Most of these deaths happen to the poorest families in the poorest countries, and most are preventable [6]. Opportunity exists to save an estimated 3 million lives per year by improving quality of care at birth and care of small and sick newborns [7,8]. Based on this evidence, the *Every Newborn* Action Plan (ENAP) was launched in 2014 and endorsed by all member states in a World Health Assembly resolution [9]. The plan outlines 2030 country targets of 12 or fewer newborn deaths per 1000 live births and 12 or fewer stillbirths per 1000 total births. *Every Newborn* is closely aligned with the World Health Organization (WHO) Strategy for Ending Preventable Maternal Mortality (EPMM) [10] since both include a priority for quality of care at birth alongside the Quality, Equity, Dignity movement led by WHO, UNICEF and UNFPA in 11 countries, aiming to halve facility deaths by 2020 [11].

Accurate data are essential to drive progress towards these targets. However, at the dawn of the SDG era, most deaths around the time of birth still occur in settings with the least data on coverage and quality of care – the "inverse data law" [12]. One of five strategic objectives of *Every Newborn* is to transform measurement and use of data to track coverage and quality of care [8,9,13]. A top priority has been to develop and implement a time-limited plan to ensure required core indicators are validated and feasible to measure at scale. In support, WHO and the London School of Hygiene & Tropical Medicine (LSHTM) have coordinated an ambitious Measurement Improvement Roadmap which reviews specific measurement gaps and provides a multi-year, multi-partner pathway to define specific indicators, test validity if needed, develop tools, and promote use of data by 2020 [14-16].

Ten core indicators were prioritised as part of the *Every Newborn* multi-country consultation process including those for impact, coverage and input (**Figure 1**) [9,16,17]. This protocol relates to the coverage indicators shown in the middle of **Figure 1**. Indicators of coverage of care for all women and newborns are shaded amber, because whilst definitions are clear, content and quality of care data requires improvement. The greatest metrics gap is core coverage indicators for specific, high impact interventions, shown in red in **Figure 1**. The combination of core indicators for *Every Newborn* and EPMM is illustrated in **Figure 2** and approximately half of these indicators are the same [10]. Validating the highest priority indicators, highlighted in red in **Figure 2**, is the topic of this research: all women to receive uterotonics and newborns with complications to receive neonatal resuscitation, Kangaroo mother care (KMC), treatment for possible serious infections and maternal antenatal corticosteroids (ACS)[16]. The assumed need for these interventions, likely coverage and expected prevalence is shown in the Appendix S2, Table S1 in **Online Supplementary Document**.

Current Status		Core Indicators	Additional indicators
Definitions clear – but quantity and consistency of data lacking	*Impact*	1. Maternal mortality ratio*	
		2. Stillbirth rate*	Intrapartum stillbirth rate
		3. Neonatal mortality rate*	Low birth weight rate
			Preterm birth rate
			Small for gestational age
			Neonatal morbidity rates
			Disability after neonatal conditions
Contact point definitions clear but data on content of care are lacking	*Coverage:* Care for All Mothers and Newborns	4. Skilled attendant at birth*	Antenatal Care*
		5. Early postnatal care for mothers and babies*	
		6. Essential newborn care (tracer is early breastfeeding)	Exclusive breastfeeding up to 6 months*
Gaps in coverage definitions, and requiring validation and feasibility testing for HMIS use	*Coverage:* Complications and Extra Care	7. Neonatal resuscitation	Caesarean section rate
		8. Kangaroo mother care	
		9. Treatment of serious neonatal infections	
		10. Antenatal corticosteroid use	Chlorhexidine cord cleansing
	Input: Service Delivery Packages for Quality of Care	Emergency Obstetric Care	
		Care of Small and Sick Newborns	
		Every Mother Every Newborn Quality Initiative with measurable norms and standards	
	Input: Counting	Birth Registration	Death registration, cause of death

Figure 1. *Every Newborn Action Plan core and additional indicators. Shaded – not currently routinely tracked at global level. Bold red – indicator requiring additional testing to inform consistent measurement. Asterisk – also SDG core or complementary indicator. Indicators disaggregated by equity such as urban/rural, income, and education. Adapted from references [9,16,17].*

	Ending Preventable Maternal Mortality (Phase 1)	Every Newborn	
IMPACT	1.Maternal mortality ratio Maternal cause of death with ICD-MM	1.Maternal mortality ratio	
		2.Stillbirth rate + intrapartum stillbirth rate	
		3.Neonatal mortality rate	
	4.Adolescent birth rate		
COVERAGE Care for all women and newborns	5.Antenatal visits – four or more		
	6.Skilled birth attendance	6.Skilled birth attendance	
	7.Institutional Delivery		
	8.Early postnatal care	8.Early postnatal care	
	9.Met need for family planning		
	10.Uterotonic immediately after birth		
		11.Immediate newborn care (tracer immediate breastfeeding)	
COVERAGE Care for all women and newborns with complications	12.Caesarean section rate	12.Caesarean section rate	FOCUS OF EN-BIRTH STUDY
		13.Newborn resuscitation	
		14.Kangaroo mother care	
		15.Treatment of serious newborn infection	
		Antenatal corticosteroid use	
INPUTS Counting	Maternal death registration	Birth registration, death registration, cause of death	
Availability of services and care	Availability of functional EmONC facilities	EmONC + service readiness for newborns (including small and sick newborns)	
	Respectful maternity care	Quality of Care- measurable norms and standards	

Figure 2. *Combined priority indicator table for relevant plans: Ending Preventable Maternal Mortality and Every Newborn [10]. Highlighted in red with box is the priority for measurement improvement and the focus of this research.*

Coverage is defined as the number of individuals receiving an intervention or service (numerator), from among the population in need of the intervention or service (denominator). To date the main source of coverage and impact data in high-burden countries has been intermittent household surveys, including:

Demographic Health Survey (DHS) and Multiple Indicator Cluster Survey (MICS) [18,19]. Currently monitored coverage indicators, including antenatal care, skilled birth attendance and postnatal care, mainly measure contact points with health care services but additional indicators are required to capture effective content of care [16,20,21]. Quality of care measurement requires definitions of characteristics for both provision (eg, safety, effectiveness, timeliness, equity, completeness) and experience of care (eg, client satisfaction) [22,23]. Household survey data accuracy depends first on the woman's interpretation of what took place at the time and second on recalling and reporting this understanding up to five years after the event. Evidence suggests that household surveys do not always accurately capture either numerator or denominator for some treatment interventions, such as pneumonia in young children [24] and events during labour [25]. In addition, since measurement of newborns with complications occur only for a subset of births (3%-15%, see Appendix S2, Table S1 in the **Online Supplementary Document**), the sample size required is higher than possible in most national DHS. Consequently, not all desired maternal and newborn intervention coverage indicators specifically relating to content and quality of care, can be captured through household surveys [16,26].

Globally more than 75% of babies are now born in facilities, and local count data from routine registers is increasingly available [27]. Whilst health-facility data can be used to track coverage more frequently than surveys, previous studies have demonstrated mixed data quality [28-30]. Health workers recording the care they deliver face many barriers in documentation [31,32]. Capturing denominators through routine data are also a major challenge. Firstly, for indicators regarding interventions for the whole population, disaggregated by equity criteria, facility births are not the "true" population denominators. Given the lack of specific and appropriate denominator data, a national health management information system (HMIS) typically use census-based data for deriving forecasts and key population calculations [28]. Secondly, the challenge is magnified if the "true" denominator for the intervention is based on clinical need, so targeted at a proportion of the total population eg, requiring treatment for possible serious bacterial infection. Measurement of the "true" denominator requires consistent and objective measure of clinical need. Yet clinical judgement and decision making, even using evidence based algorithms, is often still subjective [33,34]. Live births are often used as a proxy denominator when it is challenging to define and measure the "true" denominator. A benchmark "target coverage level" is required when proxy denominators are used, because 100% coverage is only a target for a "true" denominator. For example, the "true" denominator for Caesarean Section rate is "women in need for Caesarean section". Because this is challenging to define and measure, the proxy denominator per 100 live births is used, but benchmarking a "target Caesarean Section rate" has proved complex [35-39]. Large inequity within countries and over- and under-provision occurring in parallel [40] highlight the problem of constructing useful indicators to measure and compare met need for complications. Therefore, an important focus of this study will be to compare various denominator options and, if using a proxy denominator to consider benchmarking.

The hierarchy of data needs (**Figure 3**) illustrates scope and granularity of data use decreases at higher levels of the health system [41]. At the point of service delivery, data are needed for individual clinical decisions and to measure the client's perspective of care received. At facility level, aggregate data are collated to inform administrative and managerial decisions for planning and local quality improvement, mortality audit etc. At district level, data are required for planning (eg, human resources, equipment and drug availability). At national and global level, it is not possible or useful to collate all these data used at lower levels of the system. But it is crucial for accountability purposes to track a few core, standardised indicators to monitor SDGs and Universal Health Coverage at all levels – these "core indicators" are shown in the centre of the pyramid (**Figure 3**). WHO maintains a core list of 100 health indicators [42] and ENAP has prioritised 10 core indicators [9,16,17].

Improvements in civil and vital registration systems are enabling a more rapid transition to more timely denominator data on births and deaths. Data systems

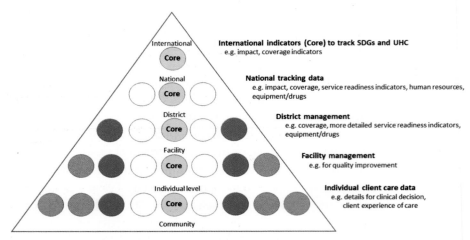

Figure 3. *Data collection and use by level of health system. Adapted from [41].*

are transitioning to increasing use of HMIS to collect, collate, analyse and report routine data from health facilities up to district and national level. This has potential to be cost-efficient and generate more frequent coverage measurements [16,27]. Electronic HMIS platforms are increasingly being applied, offering great potential to harmonize traditionally fragmented information streams [43]. One such platform, the District Health Information System, version 2 (DHIS2) [44] is now being successfully implemented in >50 countries with high mortality burdens. Infrastructure and software development advances are currently driving a transition from predominately paper-based to mixed recording systems, even at clinical data level, ie, electronic patient records will increasingly be the basis of HMIS data in low-middle income country (LMIC) contexts.

Testing indicator validity is critical to improve measurement and inform decision makers of the likely accuracy of coverage collected by household survey and/or routine facility data [20]. Comparison of the reported indicator to an external data source "gold standard" is recommended [45]. Previous validation studies have mainly focused on population-based intervention coverage indicators for use in household surveys [25,46-48]. Observational studies to determine accuracy of facility registers in high burden settings have typically focused on outcome indicators [29]. The EN-BIRTH study seeks to address current evidence gaps by testing validity of priority coverage indicators for newborn and maternal health, in facilities in three high burden country settings.

Aim

This paper is the protocol paper for the *Every Newborn*-Birth Indicators Research Tracking in Hospitals (EN-BIRTH) Study, which aims to test validity of selected newborn and maternal care health intervention indicators (coverage/quality aspects and/or safety) in facilities (Table 1). This study, as part of the *Every Newborn* Measurement Improvement Roadmap, and working closely with EPMM, aims to increase the evidence base to inform selection and use of maternal and newborn indicators in national HMIS (particularly DHIS2), and global tracking.

Research objectives

The research questions per objective, methods and analysis are detailed in Table 2.

Objective 1 – Numerators: To determine validity (accuracy) of both routine facility register and maternal recall surveys, compared to direct observation for selected maternal and newborn care interventions: uterotonics for 3rd stage labour, immediate breastfeeding, neonatal resuscitation, KMC; and, verification with patient case notes: neonatal infection management, and ACS administration (Table 1).

Objective 2 – Denominators: To compare different denominator options including proxies, and assess feasibility of their use in routine data platforms (Table 1), including:

- Target population requiring intervention (clinical need) in the facility ("true" denominator)
- Live births in the facility
- Total births (live births and stillbirths) in the facility
- Estimated population births (live or total): facility births *and* home births

Table 1. *EN-BIRTH study selected indicators to be assessed for validity*

INDICATOR	PLACE OF CARE	NUMERATOR	DENOMINATOR OPTIONS
Uterotonic use for 3rd stage of labour	Labour/Delivery ward, or operating Theatre	Number of women who received a uterotonic immediately after birth	- Per 100 live births (currently used denominator) - Per 100 total births
Immediate newborn care		Number of babies who breastfed immediately after birth as possible surrogate for immediate newborn care	Per 100 live births (currently used denominator)
		Number of newborns who had chlorhexidine applied to the cord stump after birth (*Bangladesh and Nepal only*)	
Newborn resuscitation		Number of newborns for whom resuscitation actions (Bag and Mask Ventilation) were initiated	**To be compared for all 4 denominators options:** - Target population requiring the specific intervention (eg, admitted to the facility with presumed infection or at risk of preterm birth as per WHO guideline) - Live births in the facility - Total births in the facility (including stillbirths) - Estimated births in the population (live or total)
Kangaroo mother care (KMC)	KMC ward/ area	Number of eligible (<2000g) newborns initiated on facility-based KMC	
Treatment of neonatal infection	Newborn or postnatal wards	Number of neonates (<28 days old) who received at least one dose of antibiotic injection*	
Antenatal corticosteroid (ACS) use	Labour/delivery ward or antenatal ward	All women giving birth in a facility who are 24-34 weeks and received at least one dose of ACS†	

*Specific exclusions apply to exclude other primary diagnoses eg, congenital abnormalities, preterm births <32 weeks or <1500g and neonatal encephalopathy.
†ACS focus is to track safety, test methods to include gestational age and relevant safety outcomes.

Table 2. *EN-BIRTH study summary of research questions, data collection and analysis by objective*

RESEARCH QUESTIONS	DATA COLLECTION METHOD	DATA ANALYSIS APPROACH
Objective 1 – Numerators		
- Do registers give a valid representation of observed maternal and newborn interventions? - Do maternal recall survey questions used in household surveys capture a valid representation of the observed maternal and newborn interventions? - What is the consistency between observers?	- Observation of clinical practice (or verification from inpatient records for neonatal infections and ACS) plus video film for neonatal resuscitation (Nepal only) - Maternal recall survey (all six indicators) - Extraction from routine data sources	- Sensitivity, positive predictive value - Specificity of numerator for those with all birth denominator or clearly measurable denominator - Inter-rater reliability (Cohen's Kappa)
Objective 2 – Denominators		
- How different are the coverage estimates when using alternative denominator options? - Which denominator options are feasible for use in each country HMIS?	Observation of clinical practice for measurement of "true" denominator Collection of hospital documentation for the denominator or alternative denominator options	- Descriptive statistics - Quantitative analysis with inflation factor for indicators with all-birth denominator
Objective 3 – Content and quality of care		
- What content of care are women and newborns observed to receive for each intervention, with focus on timing? - Which aspects of the content of care are already accurately recorded in registers? - Which aspects of the content of care are accurately recalled by women?	Observation of clinical practice (or verification from inpatient records for neonatal infections and ACS) plus video film for neonatal resuscitation (Nepal only) Maternal recall survey (all six indicators) Extraction from routine data sources	- Assessment of content/quality of care for specific aspects related to each intervention with emphasis on timing
Objective 4 – Barriers and enablers		
- Are some indicators recorded more completely than others? - Has routine recording changed during the time of the study? - What are the barriers and enablers to measurement of these indicators? - What are the barriers and enablers to perceived use of data regarding these indicators? - How can facility recording and flow of information into DHIS2 for these indicators be improved?	Quantitative – Register review for 12 months before and during study Qualitative FGD/IDI of study data collectors Qualitative FGD/IDI of health workers Qualitative FGD/IDI of other data users (policymakers etc) regarding data utility Process evaluation of data flow from patient level to DHIS2	- Quantitative comparison of registers applying data quality scores comparing before and after - Qualitative data for data collectors, health workers and data users - Process evaluation of data flow to DHIS2

FGD – focus group discussion, IDI – in-depth interview, DHIS2 – District Health Information System 2

Objective 3 – Content /quality of care: To evaluate different domains of coverage (eg, timing, completion rates, safety) for selected interventions (**Table 3**).

Objective 4 – Barriers and enablers: To evaluate barriers and enablers to routine recording of selected indicators, and to explore perceived utility of these data to improve decision-making, coverage and quality of care at all levels.

Table 3. *EN-BIRTH study – Examples of indicator quality of care research questions, particularly regarding timing*

INTERVENTION	RESEARCH QUESTION TO ANSWER USING OBSERVATION DATA
Uterotonic	Proportion of mothers who received oxytocin within recommended one minute after birth
Immediate breastfeeding	Proportion of babies whose breastfeeding was initiated within one hour of birth
Resuscitation	Proportion of non-breathing babies who had bag-and-mask initiated within one minute of birth
Kangaroo mother care	Proportion of babies receiving KMC, held in skin-to-skin position for 18 h or more, during the last 24 h
Neonatal infection	Proportion of cases with presumed sepsis, treated with antibiotics and for whom a blood culture result was available
Antenatal corticosteroids	Proportion of preterm labour cases who received antenatal corticosteroids according to WHO criteria for safety

METHODS

Study design

The EN-BIRTH study uses quantitative and qualitative methods across four objectives (**Table 2**). The validity of coverage indicators of selected maternal and newborn interventions as measured by routine facility registers and maternal recall surveys will be assessed by comparison with the "gold standard" of direct observation (**Figure 4**, panel A). Observation will be undertaken in three clinical settings (labour/delivery ward, operation theatre, and KMC ward/area) by trained clinical observers. Data will be extracted from facility registers and verification of inpatient records carried out for newborns who received antibiotics for presumed infection, and for women who received ACS. Interviews to capture maternal recall will be conducted prior to discharge with all women whose births and/or their newborn's care were observed or case notes were verified. In addition, barriers and enablers to recording of selected indicators in routine facility registers will be evaluated. Data flow into national HMIS platforms and perceived utility of data will be documented.

A

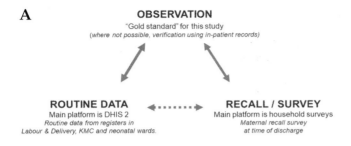

OBSERVATION
"Gold standard" for this study
(where not possible, verification using in-patient records)

ROUTINE DATA ◄┄┄┄► **RECALL / SURVEY**
Main platform is DHIS 2   Main platform is household surveys
Routine data from registers in   *Maternal recall survey*
Labour & Delivery, KMC and neonatal wards.   *at time of discharge*

B

OBSERVED INTERVENTION (GOLD STANDARD)

		Positive	Negative	
RECORD OF INTERVENTION	**Positive**	True positive (TP) Intervention occurred and recorded /reported*	False positive (FP) Intervention did not occur, but recorded /reported*	Total recorded /reported* as receiving intervention = TP + FP
	Negative	False negative (FN) Intervention occurred but not recorded/reported *	True negative (TN) Intervention did not occur and not recorded/reported*	Total recorded /reported* as not receiving intervention = FN + TN
		Total receiving the intervention TP + FN	Total not receiving the intervention FP +TN	Total observed cases TP+FN+FP+TN
		Sensitivity =TP/ (TP+FN) Those receiving the intervention who were recorded /reported* as receiving the intervention i.e. expressing the level of true positives recorded /reported*	Specificity =TN/ (FP +TN) Those who did not receive the intervention who were recorded / reported* as having received the intervention i.e. the chances of misreporting /recording an intervention that did not happen	

TERMS	DEFINITION
Accuracy	Closeness of a measured value to a standard value For EN-BIRTH study, closeness of register recorded or maternal recall survey compared to direct clinical observation
Validation	The process whereby the ability of health indicators to measure what they are supposed to measure is determined compared to a standard
Positive Predictive Value (PPV)	The probability that an intervention recorded/reported as received had been observed as received = TP/ (TP + FP)
Negative predictive value (NPV)	The probability that an intervention not recorded/reported had been observed as not received = TN/ (TN+FN)

Figure 4. *EN-BIRTH study validation and analysis approach.* **Panel A.** *Validation "gold standard" comparison to routine data (eg, HMIS/DHIS2) and to maternal recall survey data (eg, for household surveys).* **Panel B.** *Analysis for validation of sensitivity and specificity. Asterisk – recorded in facility L&D or KMC register / reported in maternal recall survey.*

Research questions were informed by consultation with many *Every Newborn* stakeholders [9,17] including WHO-led Measurement Improvement Road-map meeting [15] and EN-BIRTH Expert Advisory Group (listed as author group). More than 60 participants in an EN-BIRTH study design workshop [49] provided representation from country partners, national stakeholders, UN agencies, leading academic and professional experts in the field, governmental and non-governmental organisations, clinicians, program managers, other key experts and donors (see Appendix S1 in **Online Supplementary Document**) and contributed to development of the research protocol (**Box 1**).

Box 1. *Authorship teams for EN-BIRTH study*

EN-BIRTH LSHTM Team: Louise T Day, Harriet Ruysen, Vladimir S Gordeev, Georgia R Gore-Langton, Dorothy Boggs, Simon Cousens, Sarah G Moxon, Hannah Blencowe, Angela Baschieri.

EN-BIRTH Co-PI and country teams

Bangladesh: Ahmed Ehsanur Rahman, Tazeen Tahsina, Sojib Bin Zaman, Tanvir Hossain, Qazi Sadeq-ur Rahman, Shafiqul Ameen, Shams El Arifeen.

Nepal: Ashish KC, Shree Krishna Shrestha, Naresh P KC, Dela Singh, Anjani Kumar Jha, Bijay Jha, Nisha Rana, Omkar Basnet, Elisha Joshi, Asmita Paudel, Parashu Ram Shrestha, Deepak Jha, Ram Chandra Bastola, Jagat Jeevan Ghimire, Rajendra Paudel.

Tanzania: Nahya Salim, Donat Shamba, Karim Manji, Josephine Shabani, Kizito Shirima, Namala Mkopi, Mwifadhi Mrisho, Fatuma Manzi, Jennie Jaribu, Edward Kija, Evelyne Assenga, Rodrick Kisenge, Andrea Pembe, Claudia Hanson, Godfrey Mbaruku, Honorati Masanja.

Senior author/corresponding: Joy E Lawn

With the EN-BIRTH Expert Advisory group

Agbessi Amouzou, Tariq Azim, Debra Jackson, Theopista John Kabuteni, Matthews Mathai, Jean-Pierre Monet, Allisyn Moran, Pavani Ram, Barbara Rawlins, Johan Ivar Sæbø, Florina Serbanescu, Lara Vaz, Nabila Zaka.

On behalf of the EN-BIRTH study research design Windsor Workshop Invitees (not already names in above author groups)

AI Ayede, Simon Azariah, Anne-Marie Bergh, Elahi Chowdhury, Olive Cocoman, Patricia Coffey, Jai Das, Ashok Deorari, Mary Drake, Queen Dube, Suzanne Fournier, John Grove, Rima Jolivet, Amira Khan, Dyson Likomwa, James Litch, Goldy Mazia, Kate Milner, Indira Narayanan, Susan Niermeyer, Alfred Osoti, Sayed Rubayet, Joanna Schellenberg, Wilfred Senyoni, Gaurav Sharma, Kavita Singh, Nalini Singhal, Cally Tann, Steve Wall.

Study settings

Tanzania, Bangladesh and Nepal were chosen as LMIC's currently implementing the selected maternal and newborn interventions within Sub-Saharan Africa and Asia [50]. Within these countries, research centres of excellence with a strong track record in maternal and newborn health were selected: Ifakara Health Institute (IHI) and Muhimbili University of Health and Allied Sciences (MUHAS) in Tanzania, International Centre for Diarrhoeal Disease Research, Bangladesh (icddr,b); UNICEF-Nepal with Lifeline in Nepal. Criteria for selection of facilities were: providing the selected interventions in line with current WHO recommendations for improving quality of care; existing registers recording most interventions; and sufficient number of births to ensure sample size (except for ACS discussed under sample size section below).

Study populations

Inclusion / exclusion criteria for consenting women according to data collection methods (**Figure 5**) are:

- **Observation on labour and delivery, operating theatre:** All admitted women in active labour excluding those likely to deliver immediately. Women with a prior diagnosis of intrauterine death, were also excluded to avoid further maternal distress.
- **Observation KMC ward/area:** All in-born and out-born neonates admitted for KMC.
- **Verification from inpatient records for ACS administration:** All women being observed and reported to be <34 weeks' gestation at admission from Expected Date of Delivery (EDD).
- **Verification from inpatient records for neonatal infection cases:** All babies < 28 days old with a main diagnosis of infection (sepsis/meningitis) recorded in neonatal register or admission/discharge book. Babies will be excluded for major congenital abnormality, neonatal encephalopathy/severe asphyxia, <32 weeks' gestation and/or admission weight <1500 grammes.
- **Maternal recall survey:** All women whose birth and/or their newborn's KMC will be observed, or case notes verified for ACS or neonatal infection.
- **Routine register extraction:** All women whose birth and/or their newborn's KMC will be observed.

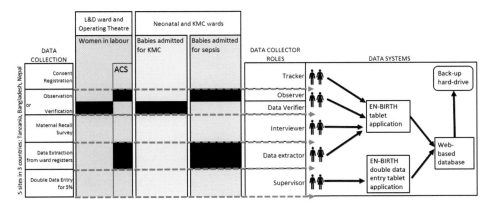

Figure 5. *EN-BIRTH study – overview of data flow in study sites. Data Collection – "ward registers" on one line. Data collector roles revised with "Data Verifier" added. Data Systems needed "web based database" (word database was missing). ACS – antenatal corticosteroids.*

Sample size

Sample size was based on planned analysis for validity in objective one, by assuming 50% sensitivity ±10% precision, 50% specificity ±10% precision, with $\alpha = 0.05$ and then applying the lowest previously published rates for neonatal resuscitation [51] and for KMC initiation [52,53]. Since formative data suggested >80% coverage for uterotonic administration, this indicator will be well-powered (see Appendix S2, Tables S2-3 in **Online Supplementary Document**). Hence minimal sample size is 4850 observations in each country, increased to 5390 observations to allow for a non-consent rate of 10% (**Table 4**). As expected prevalence of ACS is less than 0.5%, the resulting very large sample size was

Table 4. *EN-BIRTH study – national mortality rates, facility context and expected number of births and cases per indicator*

	Context	Facilities		Sample size			
Country	National mortality rates*	Name	Hospital type	Annual total births	Expected births in study	Uterotonic use†	Each for: resuscitation, Kangaroo mother care, neonatal infection management††
Tanzania	MMR = 398 /100 000 NMR = 22/1000 SBR = 22/1000	Muhimbili National Hospital, Dar es Salaam	National Referral & University Teaching	9773	5390	>4310	>106
		Temeke Regional Hospital, Dar es Salaam	Regional Referral	14 655	5390	>4310	>106
Subtotal					10780	>8620	>212
Bangladesh	MMR = 176/100 000 NMR = 21/1000 SBR = 25/1000	Maternal and Child Health Training Institute (MCHTI), Dhaka	Tertiary	4488	2695	>2150	>53
		Kushtia District Hospital	Secondary	2581	2695	>2,150	>53
Subtotal					5390	>4,310	>106
Nepal	MMR = 258 /100 000 NMR = 22/1000 SBR = 18/1000	Pokhara Academy of Health Sciences	Tertiary	9427	5390	>4310	>106
TOTAL all				40 924	21 560	>17 240	>424

*MMR – maternal mortality ratio per 100 000 live births [5]; NMR – neonatal mortality rate per 1000 live births [54]; SBR – stillbirth rate per 1000 total births [4].
†Prevalence/incidence based on references [51-53,55,56]. More details in Appendix S2 of **Online Supplementary Document**.

not feasible for this study [54,55]. The 5390 observations will be collected from three countries. In Tanzania and Nepal, each facility will observe this number of births, and in Bangladesh observations will take place in two facilities (**Table 4**) [4,5,56]. We anticipate a total >20 000 observed births aiming to capture at least 106 observations per intervention per country, except for ACS (**Table 4** and Appendix S2, Table S3 in **Online Supplementary Document**).

Tool development

A formative research phase was undertaken from July – December 2016 including: health facility assessments [57], register reviews, data flow assessments, and interviews/focus group discussions (FGDs) with women, caregivers, health workers and senior facility-level staff. The results helped ensure study sites could meet inclusion criteria, achieve required sample size and informed refinement of observer checklists and data collection processes. Maternal Recall survey tools were translated into local languages and back-translated.

Data collection software application

The development of a customised tablet-based software application (Android-based) for data collection and monitoring was undertaken by the icddr,b team supported by LSHTM (**Figure 5** and **Figure 6**) [58]. The software application has different permissions for various data collector cadres (observation, verification, maternal recall survey, and data extraction) and translated into local languages where relevant. Time-stamped data will be collected using this EN-BIRTH data collection software, stored locally on the tablet, and synchronised regularly to the local central secure database server.

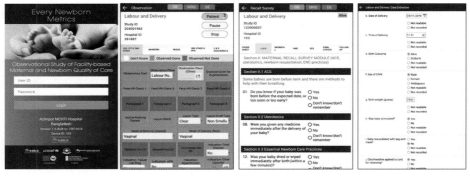

Figure 6. *EN-BIRTH study software data collection showing examples of the tablet application screen shots.*

Training of data collectors and supervisors

Data collector cadres include: tracker (responsible for consent, registration and assigning for observation/record verification and subsequent tracking); observer (direct observational data for assigned women and babies); interviewer (maternal recall survey interviews); data verifier/extractor (data from facility registers or case notes); and supervisor (responsible for all data collectors and quality assurance) (**Figure 5**). Observers with a clinical background (eg, nurses) will be recruited. Data collection staff will receive two weeks of training using classroom-based sessions, group activities and mock data collection within the health facility, detailed in the Data Collectors Training Handbook [58]. Observer training will include guidance on response to specific events, including managing maternal distress and when to pause data collection and assist in the care of the patient, if they perceive facility staff are responding inappropriately to a life-threatening situation. A minimum individual post-training assessment score of ≥80% is required before data collection can commence.

Procedures according to data collection method

Observation (Objectives 1, 2, and 3)

Informed written consent will be obtained prior to study registration and basic demographic data collected (**Figure 5**) by the tracker. Verbal consent will be obtained from the health workers. Observers working in Labour/Delivery ward, Operating theatre and KMC ward/areas will collect direct clinical observation data. These observers will not interact with participating pregnant women, her family members or attending health workers during observation (except to respond to a life-threatening event [58]).

Observations on Labour/Delivery ward will focus on specific aspects of: 1st, 2nd and 3rd stage of labour, postpartum haemorrhage, immediate newborn care and neonatal resuscitation. Multiple parameters will be recorded to assess content/quality of care, particularly related to intervention timing. KMC observations will focus on domains of initiation, position, feeding and other treatment administered. Mother and baby outcome at discharge from hospital will be documented [58].

Additionally in Nepal for neonatal resuscitation, observation video film recording and physiological assessment will be undertaken. Information regarding these additional processes will be provided separately to women and informed, signed consent taken [59]. Video cameras and pulse oximeters will be placed on resuscitation tables within Labour/Delivery ward and Operating theatres and research staff trained in this equipment operation and maintenance. A trained data collector will complete the observation checklist for resuscitation using the recorded video within 24 hours of birth [60,61]. If consent is subsequently withdrawn for video use, this data will be excluded, and the video deleted.

Verification using inpatient notes (Objectives 1, 2, and 3)

During the formative phase it was recognised that direct observation was not feasible for two of the selected interventions (neonatal infection and antenatal corticosteroids). For these interventions, data verifiers will use patient charts/ case notes, drug charts, laboratory reports and other relevant routine documentation to verify intervention and quality of care measurements. Supervisors will review/search for any missing or illegible documents before confirming data not readable/ not recorded [58].

Maternal Recall Survey (Objectives 1, 2, and 3)

Data collectors will interview mothers whose baby's birth or treatment is observed and/or verified prior to discharge from postnatal or KMC ward/areas The software programming of the structured questionnaires will automatically skip certain questions to minimise any risk of further emotional trauma if the mother has experienced a stillborn or neonatal death [58]. For multiple births the interview will be completed only for first-born babies. Consent will be repeated before this interview in recognition that the mother may have been in labour when she first consented to participation in this research. Consent will also be taken for repeat maternal recall surveys at different intervals after discharge, if funded for follow-up.

Routine register data extraction (Objectives 1, 2 and 3)

Data extractors will use routine labour/delivery registers, KMC registers and neonatal ward registers to extract participant data recorded by facility staff. If data are illegible or cannot be found, supervisors will review/search for these documents, before documenting data not readable/not recorded [58].

Assess barriers and enablers (Objective 4)

Mixed methods will be used to identify barriers and enablers to routine data recording and use of selected indicators (Table 1). Completeness and quality of existing documentation in routine registers (labour/delivery, KMC and/or neonatal) for 12 months prior to the study will be evaluated. In Bangladesh and Nepal, 100% of cases in these registers will be extracted. In the Tanzanian facilities, with a high number of births, a 20% sample randomly selected will be used for labour/delivery cases with 100% for KMC and neonatal infection cases.

Qualitative data collection tools for FGD, in-depth and key informant interviews will be informed by the MEASURE Evaluation Performance of Routine Information System Management (PRISM) conceptual framework and tools [62], including constructs for Technical, Organizational and Behavioural factors. Data will be collected from study data collectors and facility health workers. Data flow assessments will provide information on movement of data from registers, into DHIS2 and up to national level. Additionally, perceptions regarding indicators which are considered most valuable and most feasible to collect will be explored through interviews with policy makers and technical managers of DHIS2.

Data quality monitoring

The EN-BIRTH data collection software includes skip rules, and consistency checks as well as pre-defined value ranges for some variables. Progress will be monitored by an online data dashboard, providing real-time summary tables per site, including data capture cascade for selected coverage indicators at each step; registration, consent, observation/ verification, maternal recall survey and register data extraction. A traffic light system will indicate overall progress for each indicator using pre-defined thresholds. Bi-weekly all-site calls will provide an opportunity for country teams to review and discuss progress using these data dashboards, in addition to promoting collaborative quality improvement initiatives between countries and sites.

As part of the quality assurance process, for approximately 5% of cases in each site, simultaneous supervisor observation and duplicate data verification and extraction will also be conducted using EN-BIRTH data collection software. The supervisor data will be regarded as the standard, stored in a separate database, and variability between individual data collectors estimated by calculating inter-rater reliability using Cohen's kappa (κ) coefficient. Minimum agreement levels of $\geq$71% for observation and $\geq$91% for data extraction/case verification will be used [63].

Data management

EN-BIRTH tablet data will be synchronised, and uploaded to an in-country central server, regularly backed-up. Raw data will be encrypted, and access restricted to country data manager who will anonymise data before data sets are pooled. Server maintenance, data management, and cleaning will be coordinated according to agreed protocols including logical and completeness checks. A unified variable code book will contain description of variable names and answer options. Qualitative data will be digitally recorded, transcribed, and translated into English. All data will be stored on password-protected computers.

Analysis plan

Analyses will be coordinated, using a standard approach, both combining sites, and with site-specific and/or country-specific analyses. An overview of research objectives, main research questions and data analysis approach are summarised in **Table 2**. Quantitative analyses will be undertaken with Stata 15 (*Stata Statistical Software: Release 15*).

Objective 1 – Numerator

The "gold standard" used for comparison will be direct observation of selected interventions by research observer, except for neonatal infection and ACS, where in-patient note verification will be used. Data extracted from facility routine register records and data collected during maternal recall survey will be compared with this "gold standard" separately (**Figure 4**, panel A). Accuracy of each individual coverage indicator will be assessed by constructing two-by-two tables to analyse the sensitivity and positive-predictive value of routine data (**Figure 4**, panel B). Specificity of routine data will be assessed for those indicators with true negatives and confidence intervals will be computed. "Area Under the Curve" previously used for coverage indicators validation will be used for indicators with true negatives [25,46-48,64].

Objective 2 – Denominators

Various denominator options (**Table 1**) will be compared using descriptive statistics to assess variation in estimated coverage and undertake analyses to guide benchmarking. Information on denominators will come from the EN-BIRTH data set, facility total birth data collected from facility reports, and population birth data from estimates based on census or survey and fertility rates, as used in DHIS2. For indicators with a whole population denominator (ie, uterotonics, breastfeeding) or a clearly measurable "true" denominator regarding clinical need (eg, KMC – birth weight <2000g), the inflation factor will be used. Inflation factor is the ratio of estimated routine recording-based prevalence to true (observed) population-based prevalence. It represents the magnitude of over- or under-estimation in the study setting relative to true population-based prevalence.

Objective 3 – Content/quality of care

Multiple recorded parameters will be analysed to assess measurement related to content/quality of care, particularly regarding timing of interventions and in relation to WHO Guideline recommendations (Table 3).

Objective 4 – Barriers and enablers

To assess barriers and enablers to indicator data recording and use, mixed methods will be used based on a framework adapted from PRISM [62] and considering other tools [65]. Quantitative analysis of routine register data collected prior to and during the study will address two research questions: (1) Are some indicators recorded more completely than others? (2) Has routine recording changed during the study time? Qualitative data from FGDs, in-depth and key informant interviews will be analysed using QSR International's NVivo 12 qualitative software (NVivo qualitative data analysis Software; QSR International Pty Ltd Version 12.1, 2018). Predetermined codes will be applied by two independent researchers, data managed into units of information covering broad categories with grouping of relevant emerging themes of importance.

DISCUSSION

EN-BIRTH is the first large study to assess validity of newborn and maternal care indicators in routine data systems, doing so at very large scale (>20 000 observed births) across three countries with a high-burden of mortality. Previous maternal and newborn indicator validation studies have focused on testing the validity of women's self-report method, used in population-based household surveys [25,46-48,64]. Validation of facility registers have focussed on outcome measures [29]. The EN-BIRTH study seeks to validate both routine registers and maternal recall at discharge for coverage indicators of high impact interventions. The novel software developed for this research allows detailed and precise recording of events around the time of birth, and particularly the timing of interventions. There are many studies examining quality of care at birth [66,67], and this research is not repeating that, but is focused on accuracy of routine reporting of care.

This research responds to calls from country and programme leaders for guidance on indicators for maternal and newborn services, tracking progress towards meeting national targets and Universal Health Coverage [9,17,68]. The high reporting load for many countries with multiple programmes, donors, and indicators, may result in the so-called data rich, information poor (DRIP) syndrome [69]. In addition to high reporting burden on the system, the individual midwives and doctors are responsible for recording data in multiple registers and patient records, sometimes at the expense of providing respectful quality care for women and babies. Hence a shorter list of evidence-based, indicators is required for national tracking, taking in to account validity and utility in low-resource, high-burden settings. The results of this study will inform recommendations for indicators appropriate for uptake within HMIS, and may also identify some that are not appropriate for use at higher levels of the health system (Figure 3). This research will also help inform improved capture and quality of data in HMIS, and especially DHIS2.

During the MDG-era, population-level surveys were the most common data source in high-burden countries, but studies consistently demonstrate challenges with maternal recall data, especially regarding details of clinical interventions [24,25,46,47,64]. For data that require medical knowledge and especially events that women may not have closely witnessed (eg, neonatal resuscitation), we expect poor maternal recall, which may reflect the lack of information given to families experiencing complications. Given continued reliance on household surveys for demographic and health data in many remote or unstable settings, we anticipate the main value of our maternal recall survey validation findings will be to contribute to the understanding of which indicators are not suitable for use in household surveys. We anticipate that if the woman does not know about the intervention at discharge from hospital, then recall later will not be useful.

A strength of this study design is the rigorous assessment of validity at scale, of facility routine data by comparison with direct observation, defined here as the "gold standard". Another strength is a specific focus on the denominator challenge. In an era of Universal Health Coverage, with discussions surrounding scale-up of more complex care for targeted populations, the science of denominator measurement, use of proxies, and selection of benchmarks will be increasingly important. This challenge applies to denominator measurement for maternal and newborn complications (as well as other large burden conditions, notably non-communicable diseases). This study, however, is not designed to validate the denominator based on subjective assessment of clinical need (eg, requiring neonatal resuscitation). Hence, we will only be able to measure true negatives, calculate specificity, and undertake analysis of "area under the curve" for interventions with a total population or clearly defined denominator [25,46-48,64].

This research also offers a unique opportunity to examine quality of care data from >20 000 births and assess to what extent we can accurately capture specific components including content and timing of selected interventions. Although multiple specific aspects of care may be measured locally to drive quality of care improvement at facility level, here we will focus on quality of care indicators that may be useful at district or national levels of the health system. Timing of interventions is a critical marker of quality of care, since delays are a matter of life or death: a woman may die in hours, a baby in minutes. Moreover, the sequence of interventions is complex and even concurrent (eg, how often is the correct dose of uterotonic given <1 minute after birth to prevent a woman bleeding from postpartum haemorrhage; How soon is bag-and-mask ventilation initiated for a baby who is not breathing; How many hours each day is a baby kept in KMC position). The time-stamped design of EN-BIRTH data collection software will permit analysis of such sequences.

Whilst direct observation is considered the "gold standard", data collectors might miss interventions, with concurrent actions at birth, especially in an emergency. We will limit potential recording bias by using observers with health backgrounds who are familiar with the procedures under observation [70-72]. EN-BIRTH data will also be directly on the tablet software to allow fast data capture. The study also presents several ethical challenges including the dilemma of observing a life-threatening situation without appropriate response from facility staff, and gaining informed consent during labour [58]. The clinically trained observers will have underlying familiarity of hospital environments, experience to uphold study protocols correctly [70] and experience in maintaining participant confidentiality. Training and processes will be put in place to take account of professional and legal duty of care.

The "Hawthorne effect" describes the phenomenon when a research participant's behavior is altered as a consequence of being studied or observed, and can be a source of bias in observational research [73]. Within this study, it is possible that clinical observers' presence will influence health workers to change their approach to care and routine register data. However, there is some evidence to suggest that sustained contact with participants (as with this study) may mitigate altered behaviors in health care settings [74]. To assess this bias, we will analyze changes in register data completeness and quality before and during the study.

Although the EN-BIRTH study is not powered to validate an ACS administration indicator, this will be included. Current WHO guidelines provide strong recommendation for the provision of a single course of ACS for any woman at risk of imminent preterm birth (24-34 weeks of gestation) provided the following criteria are met: 1) accurate assessment of gestational age; 2) no evidence of maternal infection; 3) preterm birth is considered imminent; 4) available adequate childbirth and newborn care services [75]. EN-BIRTH study sites were assessed in accordance with these WHO guidelines. The Antenatal Corticosteroid Trial (ACT) evaluated use of ACS at lower levels of the health system, with half of study births in home settings and care often provided by traditional birth attendants [76]. ACT reported an adverse outcome risk particularly in cases where ACS administration was after 34 weeks and outlines important challenges for measurement of gestational age, and assessment of maternal infection. This demonstrated need for robust data and further evidence in such settings, along with the imperative of ensuring safety and effectiveness, make measurement of ACS coverage and outcomes essential. Therefore, the EN-BIRTH study ACS analysis will focus on assessing relevant documentation to report the current ACS administration practice, compared with WHO safety criteria [75].

Given the importance of the neonatal period in terms of risk and prevention of long-term adverse child development outcomes, we plan a five-year follow-up for EN-BIRTH study recruited children who received basic neonatal interventions [77]. The *Every Newborn* – Simplified Measurement Integrating Longitudinal Neurodevelopment & Growth (EN-SMILING) aims to detect child development outcomes as early as possible for referral to services, and to improve routine measurement of child development outcomes in programme settings.

The EN-BIRTH study is richer through active involvement of experts and policymakers from the EN-BIRTH Expert Advisory Group, *Every Newborn* implementation community, EPMM, UN Agencies including WHO, UNICEF and UNFPA as well as many partners and donors. In further support of this goal, each of the three countries have National Advisory Committees who will actively participate in the research process and support uptake of findings. Results will also be published in peer reviewed journals and disseminated with all relevant audiences. Following EN-BIRTH study validity testing, an important next step will be to evaluate feasibility of a short-list of indicators at different levels of the health system.

Most of the 5.5 million deaths around the time of birth [3] still occur in settings with the least data. Household surveys remain a key data source in the poorest countries, and *Every Newborn* is also involved in a multi-site study, EN-INDEPTH, to assess and improve these data [78]. Data improvement is fundamental for monitoring more rapid progress towards meeting global and national mortality targets, and in achieving Universal Health Coverage for all women and newborns [15]. With ongoing investment in electronic data platforms (including DHIS2) and increasing country demand for evidence-based indicators, we anticipate that these results will advance availability and use of data to change coverage, quality and equity, to help end preventable maternal and newborn mortality, as well as stillbirths.

Acknowledgements: We credit the inspiration of the late Godfrey Mbaruku. Many thanks to Claudia DaSilva, Fion Hay, Alegria Perez, Sadie Sareen, Adeline Herman, Veronica Ulay, Mohammad Raisul Islam and Ziaul Haque Shaikh, Susheel Karki and Bhula Rai for their administrative support. We thank Sabrina Jabeen, Tamatun Islam Tanha, Goutom Banik and Md Moshiur Rahman for their support in providing training to data collectors in the Bangladesh sites. We would also like to thank Ann Blanc, Liliana Carvajal, Doris Chou, Kim Dickson, Tanya Marchant, Claire-Helene Mershon, Natalie Roos, Anna Seale, Theresa Shaver, Deborah Sitrin, Kate Somers, and Cindy Stanton for sharing relevant technical inputs and expertise.

We *acknowledge the National Advisory Groups:* **Tanzania:** *Muhammad Bakari Kambi, Georgina Msemo, Asia Husein, Talhiya Yahya, Claud Kumalija, Eliakim Eliud, Mary Azayo, Onest Kimaro.* **Bangladesh:** *Mohammad Shahidullah, Khaleda Islam, Md Jahurul Islam (joining the EN-BIRTH Expert Advisory Group in 2018).* **Nepal:** *Tara Pokharel, Uwe Ewald.*

Finally, *and most importantly we thank the women, their families, the health workers and the hundreds of data collectors involved in the EN-BIRTH study.*

Ethics and consent to participate: *This study was granted ethical approval by institutional review boards in all operating counties including the London School of Hygiene & Tropical Medicine (Appendix S3 of* **Online Supplementary Document***).*

Availability of data and material: *All collaborating partners have signed data sharing and transfer agreements.*

Funding: *The Children's Investment Fund Foundation (CIFF) are the main funder of this research which is administered via The London School of Hygiene & Tropical Medicine. The Swedish Research Council specifically funded the Nepal site through UNICEF and Lifeline Nepal. The main funding for the Windsor research design workshop was provided by CIFF and in addition, the United States Agency for International Development, Saving Newborn Lives/Save the Children, WHO and Bill & Melinda Gates Foundation through the United States Fund for UNICEF funded many participants' travel and accommodation for attendance.*

Authorship contributions: *The study was conceptualized by JEL in 2014, and the initial protocol was coordinated by HR with JEL during 2016, with inputs from SC, SM, HB, the EN-BIRTH advisory group (names listed above), and during a multi-stakeholder Windsor research design workshop (names listed above). From mid-2016 VSG, GGL, DB and AB, with LTD joining in 2017. GGL and HR led inputs to observation checklists and led development of training materials with country coordinators (Bangladesh, TT and AER, Nepal, NR, Tanzania, NS). DB led development of the maternal recall survey and coordinated the health facility assessments. Each of the three country research teams input to all the data collection tools and review processes. The iccdr,b team from Bangladesh (notably AER, TT, TH, QSR, SA and SBZ) led the development of the software application, data dashboards and database development with VSG and the LSHTM team. iccdr,b (AER) also led the development of the verification form for infection case management and the data variable dictionary. The IHI and MUHAS in Tanzania hosted the study implementation workshop, input to data collection tools and training materials and are leading work on objective 4 (barriers and enablers for data collection and use). The Nepal team input to data collection tools and training materials, and led on use of video filming. The manuscript was drafted by HR, JEL and LTD with further review of the analysis sections by VSG and SC, in addition to major inputs particularly from GM, AER and TT. All authors reviewed and helped to revise the manuscript.*

Competing interests: *The authors completed the Unified Competing Interest form at www.icmje.org/coi_disclosure.pdf (available upon request from the corresponding author), and declare no conflicts of interest.*

Additional material
Online Supplementary Document

References

1 United Nations. Sustainable Development Goals. 2016. Available: http://www.un.org/sustainabledevelopment/health/. Accessed: 5 April 2018.

2 United Nations. Global Strategy for Women's, Children's and Adolescents' Health, 2016-2030. New York: United Nations; 2015.

3 UN IGME. Levels and Trends in Child Mortality Report 2018. Estimates developed by United Nations inter-agency group for child mortality estimation (UN IGME). New York: United Nations Children's Fund: 2018.

4 Blencowe H, Cousens S, Jassir FB, Say L, Chou D, Mathers C, et al. National, regional, and worldwide estimates of stillbirth rates in 2015, with trends from 2000: a systematic analysis. Lancet Glob Health. 2016;4:e98-108. Medline:26795602 doi:10.1016/S2214-109X(15)00275-2

5 World Health Organization, UNFPA, World Bank Group, United Nations Population Division. Trends in maternal mortality: 1990 to 2015: estimates by WHO, UNICEF, UNFPA, World Bank Group and the United Nations Population Division. Available: http://www.who.int/reproductivehealth/publications/monitoring/maternal-mortality-2015/en/. Accessed: 4 December 2018.

6 Liu L, Oza S, Hogan D, Chu Y, Perin J, Zhu J, et al. Global, regional, and national causes of under-5 mortality in 2000-15: an updated systematic analysis with implications

for the Sustainable Development Goals. Lancet. 2016;388:3027-35. Medline:27839855 doi:10.1016/S0140-6736(16)31593-8

7   Darmstadt GL, Kinney MV, Chopra M, Cousens S, Kak L, Paul VK, et al. Who has been caring for the baby? Lancet. 2014;384:174-88. Medline:24853603 doi:10.1016/S0140-6736(14)60458-X

8   Lawn JE, Blencowe H, Oza S, You D, Lee AC, Waiswa P, et al. *Every Newborn*: progress, priorities, and potential beyond survival. Lancet. 2014;384:189-205. Medline:24853593 doi:10.1016/S0140-6736(14)60496-7

9   World Health Organization. *Every Newborn*: An action plan to end preventable deaths (ENAP). 2014 ISBN 9789241507448.

10   World Health Organization. Strategies towards ending preventable maternal mortality (EPMM). 2015 ISBN 9241508485.

11   World Health Organization. What is the Quality of Care Network? 2017. Available: http://www.who.int/maternal_child_adolescent/topics/quality-of-care/network/en/. Accessed: 19 December 2017.

12   Lawn JE, Cousens S, Zupan J. 4 million neonatal deaths: when? Where? Why? Lancet. 2005;365:891-900. Medline:15752534 doi:10.1016/S0140-6736(05)71048-5

13   Dickson KE, Simen-Kapeu A, Kinney MV, Huicho L, Vesel L, Lackritz E, et al. *Every Newborn*: health-systems bottlenecks and strategies to accelerate scale-up in countries. Lancet. 2014;384:438-54. Medline:24853600 doi:10.1016/S0140-6736(14)60582-1

14   World Health Organization. UNICEF, LSHTM. *Every Newborn* Metrics Report Cards. 2016. Available: https://www.healthynewbornnetwork.org/resource/enap-metrics-cards. Accessed: 21 July 2017.

15   World Health Organization. WHO technical consultation on newborn health indicators: *Every Newborn* Action Plan metrics, Ferney Voltaire, France, 3-5 December 2014. 2015 Contract No.: ISBN: 9789241509381.

16   Moxon SG, Ruysen H, Kerber KJ, Amouzou A, Fournier S, Grove J, et al. Count *Every Newborn*; a measurement improvement roadmap for coverage data. BMC Pregnancy Childbirth. 2015;15:S8. Medline:26391444 doi:10.1186/1471-2393-15-S2-S8

17   Mason E, McDougall L, Lawn JE, Gupta A, Claeson M, Pillay Y, et al. From evidence to action to deliver a healthy start for the next generation. Lancet. 2014;384:455-67. Medline:24853599 doi:10.1016/S0140-6736(14)60750-9

18   Demographic and Health Surveys. The DHS program. 2017. Available: https://dhsprogram.com/. Accessed: 19 December 2017.

19   UNICEF. Multiple Indicator Cluster Surveys, 2017. Available: http://mics.unicef.org/. Accessed: 19 December 2017.

20   Munos MK, Stanton CK, Bryce J. Improving coverage measurement for reproductive, maternal, neonatal and child health: gaps and opportunities. J Glob Health. 2017;7:010801. Medline:28607675 doi:10.7189/jogh.07.010801

21   Marchant T, Tilley-Gyado RD, Tessema T, Singh K, Gautham M, Umar N, et al. Adding content to contacts: measurement of high quality contacts for maternal and newborn health in Ethiopia, North East Nigeria, and Uttar Pradesh, India. PLoS One. 2015;10:e0126840. Medline:26000829 doi:10.1371/journal.pone.0126840

22   World Health Organization. Standards for improving quality of maternal and newborn care in health facilities. Geneva. WHO; 2016.

23   Kruk ME, Gage AD, Arsenault C, Jordan K, Leslie HH, Roder-DeWan S, et al. High-quality health systems in the Sustainable Development Goals era: time for a revo-

lution. Lancet Glob Health. 2018;6:e1196-252. Medline:30196093 doi:10.1016/S2214-109X(18)30386-3

24 Campbell H, el Arifeen S, Hazir T, O'Kelly J, Bryce J, Rudan I, et al. Measuring coverage in MNCH: challenges in monitoring the proportion of young children with pneumonia who receive antibiotic treatment. PLoS Med. 2013;10:e1001421. Medline:23667338 doi:10.1371/journal.pmed.1001421

25 Stanton CK, Rawlins B, Drake M, dos Anjos M, Cantor D, Chongo L, et al. Measuring coverage in MNCH: Testing the validity of women's self-report of key maternal and newborn health Interventions during the peripartum period in Mozambique. PLoS One. 2013;8:e60694. Medline:23667427 doi:10.1371/journal.pone.0060694

26 Bryce J, Arnold F, Blanc A, Hancioglu A, Newby H, Requejo J, et al. Measuring coverage in MNCH: new findings, new strategies, and recommendations for action. PLoS Med. 2013;10:e1001423. Medline:23667340 doi:10.1371/journal.pmed.1001423

27 Maternal and Child Survival Program. What Data on Maternal and Newborn Health do National Health Management Information Systems include? A review of data elements for 24 low- and lower middle income countries. 2018 May 2018. Report No.

28 Maina I, Wanjala P, Soti D, Kipruto H, Droti B, Boerma T. Using health-facility data to assess subnational coverage of maternal and child health indicators, Kenya. Bull World Health Organ. 2017;95:683-94. Medline:29147041 doi:10.2471/BLT.17.194399

29 Broughton EI, Ikram AN, Sahak I. How accurate are medical record data in Afghanistan's maternal health facilities? An observational validity study. BMJ Open. 2013;3:e002554. Medline:23619087 doi:10.1136/bmjopen-2013-002554

30 Duffy S, Crangle M. Delivery room logbook–fact or fiction? Trop Doct. 2009;39:145-9. Medline:19535748 doi:10.1258/td.2009.080433

31 Chiba Y, Oguttu MA, Nakayama T. Quantitative and qualitative verification of data quality in the childbirth registers of two rural district hospitals in Western Kenya. Midwifery. 2012;28:329-39. Medline:21684639 doi:10.1016/j.midw.2011.05.005

32 Melberg A, Diallo AH, Storeng KT, Tylleskar T, Moland KM. Policy, paperwork and 'postographs': Global indicators and maternity care documentation in rural Burkina Faso. Soc Sci Med. 2018;215:28-35. Medline:30205276 doi:10.1016/j.socscimed.2018.09.001

33 Ronsmans C, Achadi E, Cohen S, Zazri A. Women's recall of obstetric complications in South Kalimantan, Indonesia. Stud Fam Plann. 1997;28:203-14. Medline:9322336 doi:10.2307/2137888

34 Wall SN, Lee AC, Niermeyer S, English M, Keenan WJ, Carlo W, et al. Neonatal resuscitation in low-resource settings: what, who, and how to overcome challenges to scale up? Int J Gynaecol Obstet. 2009;107 Suppl 1:S47-S64. Medline:19815203 doi:10.1016/j.ijgo.2009.07.013

35 Souza JP, Betran AP, Dumont A, de Mucio B, Gibbs Pickens CM, Deneux-Tharaux C, et al. A global reference for caesarean section rates (C-Model): a multicountry cross-sectional study. BJOG. 2016;123:427-36. Medline:26259689 doi:10.1111/1471-0528.13509

36 Ye J, Betrán AP, Guerrero Vela M, Souza JP, Zhang J. Searching for the optimal rate of medically necessary cesarean delivery. Birth. 2014;41:237-44. Medline:24720614 doi:10.1111/birt.12104

37 Vogel JP, Betrán AP, Vindevoghel N, Souza JP, Torloni MR, Zhang J, et al. Use of the Robson classification to assess caesarean section trends in 21 countries: a secondary analysis of two WHO multicountry surveys. Lancet Glob Health. 2015;3:e260-70. Medline:25866355 doi:10.1016/S2214-109X(15)70094-X

38 Betran AP, Torloni MR, Zhang JJ, Gulmezoglu AM. WHO Statement on Caesarean Section Rates. BJOG. 2016;123:667-70. Medline:26681211 doi:10.1111/1471-0528.13526

39 Ye J, Zhang J, Mikolajczyk R, Torloni M, Gülmezoglu A, Betran A. Association between rates of caesarean section and maternal and neonatal mortality in the 21st century: a worldwide population-based ecological study with longitudinal data. BJOG. 2016;123:745-53. Medline:26331389 doi:10.1111/1471-0528.13592

40 Boatin AA, Schlotheuber A, Betran AP, Moller AB, Barros AJD, Boerma T, et al. Within country inequalities in caesarean section rates: observational study of 72 low and middle income countries. BMJ. 2018;360:k55. Medline:29367432 doi:10.1136/bmj.k55

41 Heywood A, Rohde J. Using information for action - a manual for health workers at facility level. University of Western Cape/HISP/MSH/EQUITY Project.

42 World Health Organization. 2018 Global Reference List of 100 Core Health Indicators - plus health-related SDGs. 2018 World Health Organization 2018. Licence: CC BY-NC-SA 3.0 IGO.

43 Maternal & Child Survival Program. Health Management Information Systems Review - Survey on Data Availability in Electronic Systems for Maternal and Newborn Health Indicators in 24 USAID Priority Countries. 2016.

44 DHIS2. Oslo: Health Information Systems Programme. 2016. Available: https://www.dhis2.org/. Accessed: 25 January 2018.

45 Munos MK, Blanc AK, Carter ED, Eisele TP, Gesuale S, Katz J, et al. Validation studies for population-based intervention coverage indicators: design, analysis, and interpretation. J Glob Health. 2018;8:020804. Medline:30202519 doi:10.7189/jogh.08.020804

46 Blanc AK, Warren C, McCarthy KJ, Kimani J, Ndwiga C. RamaRao S. Assessing the validity of indicators of the quality of maternal and newborn health care in Kenya. J Glob Health. 2016;6:010405. Medline:27231541 doi:10.7189/jogh.06.010405

47 McCarthy KJ, Blanc AK, Warren CE, Kimani J, Mdawida B, Ndwidga C. Can surveys of women accurately track indicators of maternal and newborn care? A validity and reliability study in Kenya. J Glob Health. 2016;6:020502. Medline:27606061 doi:10.7189/jogh.06.020502

48 Blanc AK, Diaz C, McCarthy KJ, Berdichevsky K. Measuring progress in maternal and newborn health care in Mexico: validating indicators of health system contact and quality of care. BMC Pregnancy Childbirth. 2016;16:255. Medline:27577266 doi:10.1186/s12884-016-1047-0

49 The London School of Hygiene & Tropical Medicine. *Every Newborn* Action Plan Metrics Design Workshop for Facility-based Testing of Coverage Metrics, Windsor. 2016. Available: https://www.healthynewbornnetwork.org/hnn-content/uploads/ENAP-Metrics-Facility-based-Workshop-Report_April-2016_FINAL.pdf Accessed: 5 April 2018.

50 World Health Organization. Accountability for Women's and Children's Health Countries Oversight Platform. 2017. Available: http://www.who.int/woman_child_accountability/countries/en/. Accessed: 23 October 2017.

51 Lee AC, Cousens S, Wall SN, Niermeyer S, Darmstadt GL, Carlo WA, et al. Neonatal resuscitation and immediate newborn assessment and stimulation for the prevention of neonatal deaths: a systematic review, meta-analysis and Delphi estimation of mortality effect. BMC Public Health. 2011;11:S12. Medline:21501429 doi:10.1186/1471-2458-11-S3-S12

52 Oza S, Lawn JE, Hogan DR, Mathers C, Cousens SN. Neonatal cause-of-death estimates for the early and late neonatal periods for 194 countries: 2000–2013. Bull World Health Organ. 2015;93:19-28. Medline:25558104 doi:10.2471/BLT.14.139790

53 Vesel L, Bergh A-M, Kerber KJ, Valsangkar B, Mazia G, Moxon SG, et al. Kangaroo mother care: a multi-country analysis of health system bottlenecks and potential solutions. BMC Pregnancy Childbirth. 2015;15:S5. Medline:26391115 doi:10.1186/1471-2393-15-S2-S5

54 Blencowe H, Cousens S, Oestergaard MZ, Chou D, Moller A-B, Narwal R, et al. National, regional, and worldwide estimates of preterm birth rates in the year 2010 with time trends since 1990 for selected countries: a systematic analysis and implications. Lancet. 2012;379:2162-72. Medline:22682464 doi:10.1016/S0140-6736(12)60820-4

55 Vogel JP, Souza JP, Gülmezoglu AM, Mori R, Lumbiganon P, Qureshi Z, et al. Use of antenatal corticosteroids and tocolytic drugs in preterm births in 29 countries: an analysis of the WHO Multicountry Survey on Maternal and Newborn Health. Lancet. 2014;384:1869-77. Medline:25128271 doi:10.1016/S0140-6736(14)60580-8

56 World Health Organisation. World Health Statistics data visualization dashboard. 2015. Available: http://apps.who.int/gho/data/view.sdg.3-2-data-ctry. Accessed.

57 World Health Organisation. Monitoring emergency obstetric care: a handbook, 2009. Available: http://www.who.int/reproductivehealth/publications/monitoring/9789241547734/en/ Accessed: 31 August 2017.

58 EN-BIRTH Study at London School Hygiene and Tropical Medicine Data Compass. 2018. Available: https://doi.org/10.17037/DATA.00000955. Accessed: 4 December 2018.

59 Lindbäck C, Ashish K, Wrammert J, Vitrakoti R, Ewald U, Målqvist M. Poor adherence to neonatal resuscitation guidelines exposed; an observational study using camera surveillance at a tertiary hospital in Nepal. BMC Pediatr. 2014;14:233. Medline:25227941 doi:10.1186/1471-2431-14-233

60 Ashish KC, Målqvist M, Wrammert J, Verma S, Aryal DR, Clark R, et al. Implementing a simplified neonatal resuscitation protocol-helping babies breathe at birth (HBB)-at a tertiary level hospital in Nepal for an increased perinatal survival. BMC Pediatr. 2012;12:159. Medline:23039709

61 Ashish KC, Wrammert J, Clark RB, Ewald U, Vitrakoti R, Chaudhary P, et al. Reducing perinatal mortality in Nepal using helping babies breathe. Pediatrics. 2016;137:e20150117. Medline:27225317 doi:10.1542/peds.2015-0117

62 Aqil A, Lippeveld T, Hozumi D. PRISM framework: a paradigm shift for designing, strengthening and evaluating routine health information systems. Health Policy Plan. 2009;24:217-28. Medline:19304786 doi:10.1093/heapol/czp010

63 Gwet KL. Handbook of inter-rater reliability: The definitive guide to measuring the extent of agreement among raters: Advanced Analytics, LLC, Gaithersburg, Maryland, USA; 2014.

64 Liu L, Li M, Yang L, Ju L, Tan B, Walker N, et al. Measuring coverage in MNCH: A validation study linking population survey derived coverage to maternal, newborn, and child health care records in rural China. PLoS One. 2013;8:e60762. Medline:23667429 doi:10.1371/journal.pone.0060762

65 World Health Organization. Data quality review: a toolkit for facility data quality assessment. Module 2: Desk review of data quality. Geneva: WHO; 2017.

66 Tripathi V. A literature review of quantitative indicators to measure the quality of labor and delivery care. Int J Gynaecol Obstet. 2016;132:139-45. Medline:26686027 doi:10.1016/j.ijgo.2015.07.014

67 The Lancet Global Health Commission on High Quality Health Systems in the SDG Era. (in press). 2018. Available: https://www.hqsscommission.org/. Accessed: 11 April 2018.

68 Tunçalp Ö, Were W, MacLennan C, Oladapo O, Gülmezoglu A, Bahl R, et al. Quality of care for pregnant women and newborns—the WHO vision. BJOG. 2015;122:1045-9. Medline:25929823 doi:10.1111/1471-0528.13451

69 Goodwin S. Data rich, information poor (DRIP) syndrome: is there a treatment? Radiol Manage. 1996;18:45-9. Medline:10158370

70 Jackson D, McDonald G, Luck L, Waine M, Wilkes L. Some strategies to address the challenges of collecting observational data in a busy clinical environment. Collegian. 2016;23:47-52. Medline:27188039 doi:10.1016/j.colegn.2014.10.001

71 Rawlins B, Christenesen A, Bluestone J. Clinical Observer Learning Resource Package. 2013. Available: http://reprolineplus.org/resources/clinical-observer-learning-resource-package. Accessed: 9 December 2017.

72 Fry M, Curtis K, Considine J, Shaban RZ. Using observation to collect data in emergency research. Australas Emerg Nurs J. 2017;20:25-30. Medline:28169134 doi:10.1016/j.aenj.2017.01.001

73 McCambridge J, Witton J, Elbourne DR. Systematic review of the Hawthorne effect: new concepts are needed to study research participation effects. J Clin Epidemiol. 2014;67:267-77. Medline:24275499 doi:10.1016/j.jclinepi.2013.08.015

74 Paradis E, Sutkin G. Beyond a good story: from Hawthorne Effect to reactivity in health professions education research. Med Educ. 2017;51:31-9. Medline:27580703 doi:10.1111/medu.13122

75 World Health Organization. WHO Recommendations on Interventions to Improve Preterm Birth Outcomes. 2015. Available: http://apps.who.int/iris/bitstream/10665/183037/1/9789241508988_eng.pdf. Accessed: 4 Dec 2018.

76 Althabe F, Belizán JM, McClure EM, Hemingway-Foday J, Berrueta M, Mazzoni A, et al. A population-based, multifaceted strategy to implement antenatal corticosteroid treatment versus standard care for the reduction of neonatal mortality due to preterm birth in low-income and middle-income countries: the ACT cluster-randomised trial. Lancet. 2015;385:629-39. Medline:25458726 doi:10.1016/S0140-6736(14)61651-2

77 Lawn JE, Blencowe H, Darmstadt GL, Bhutta ZA. Beyond newborn survival: the world you are born into determines your risk of disability-free survival. Pediatr Res. 2013;74 Suppl 1:1-3. Medline:24240732 doi:10.1038/pr.2013.202

78 Baschieri A, Gordeev VS, Akuze J, Kwesiga D, Blencowe H, Cousens S, et al. "Every Newborn-INDEPTH" (EN-INDEPTH) study protocol for a randomised comparison of household survey modules for measuring stillbirths and neonatal deaths in five Health and Demographic Surveillance sites. J Glob Health. 2019;9:010901. doi:10.7189/jogh.09.010901

"Every Newborn-INDEPTH" (EN-INDEPTH) study protocol for a randomised comparison of household survey modules for measuring stillbirths and neonatal deaths in five Health and Demographic Surveillance sites

Angela Baschieri[1], Vladimir S Gordeev[1], Joseph Akuze[1,2,3], Doris Kwesiga[2,3], Hannah Blencowe[1], Simon Cousens[1], Peter Waiswa[2,3], Ane B Fisker[4,5,6], Sanne M Thysen[4,5,7], Amabelia Rodrigues[4], Gashaw A Biks[8], Solomon M Abebe[8], Kassahun A Gelaye[8], Mezgebu Y Mengistu[8], Bisrat M Geremew[8], Tadesse G Delele[8], Adane K Tesega[8], Temesgen A Yitayew[8], Simon Kasasa[2,9], Edward Galiwango[2,9], Davis Natukwatsa[2,9], Dan Kajungu[2,9], Yeetey AK Enuameh[10,11], Obed E Nettey[11], Francis Dzabeng[11], Seeba Amenga-Etego[11], Sam K Newton[10,11], Alexander A Manu[11], Charlotte Tawiah[11], Kwaku P Asante[11], Seth Owusu-Agyei[1,12,13], Nurul Alam[14], M M Haider[14], Sayed S Alam[14], Fred Arnold[15], Peter Byass[16], Trevor N Croft[15], Kobus Herbst[17], Sunita Kishor[18], Florina Serbanescu[19], Joy E Lawn[1]

---

[1] Maternal, Adolescent, Reproductive and Child Health (MARCH) Centre, London School of Hygiene &Tropical Medicine, London, United Kingdom

[2] School of Public Health, Makerere University, Kampala, Uganda

[3] INDEPTH Network Maternal, Newborn and Child Health Working Group Technical Secretariat

[4] Bandim Health Project, Bissau, Guinea-Bissau

[5] Research Center for Vitamins and Vaccines, Bandim Health Project, Statens Serum Institut, Copenhagen, Denmark

[6] OPEN, Odense Patient data Explorative Network, Odense University Hospital/Institute of Clinical Research, University of Southern Denmark, Odense, Denmark

[7] Center for Global Health, Department of Public Health, Aarhus University Denmark, Aarhus, Denmark

[8] Institute of Public Health, College of Medicine and Health Sciences, University of Gondar, Gondar, Ethiopia

[9] IgangaMayuge HDSS, Uganda

[10] Kwame Nkrumah University of Science and Technology, Kumasi, Ashanti, Ghana

[11] Kintampo Health Research Centre, Kintampo, Ghana

[12] University of Health and Allied Sciences, Kintampo Health Research Centre, Kintampo, Ghana

[13] Malaria Centre, London School of Hygiene &Tropical Medicine, London, United Kingdom

[14] Health Systems and Population Studies Division, icddr,b, Dhaka, Bangladesh

[15] ICF, Rockville, Maryland, USA

[16] Department of Epidemiology & Global Health, Umeå University, Umeå, Sweden

[17] Africa Health Research Institute, South Africa

[18] The DHS Program, ICF Rockville, Maryland, USA

[19] Centers for Disease Control and Prevention, Division of reproductive Health, USA

Background Under-five and maternal mortality were halved in the Millennium Development Goals (MDG) era, with slower reductions for 2.6 million neonatal deaths and 2.6 million stillbirths. The Every Newborn Action Plan aims to accelerate progress towards national targets, and includes an ambitious Measurement Improvement Roadmap. Population-based household surveys, notably Demographic and Health Surveys (DHS) and Multiple Indicator Cluster Surveys, are major sources of population-level data on child mortality in countries with weaker civil registration and vital statistics systems, where over two-thirds of global child deaths occur. To estimate neonatal/child mortality and pregnancy outcomes (stillbirths, miscarriages, birthweight, gestational age) the most common direct methods are: (1) the standard DHS-7 with Full Birth History with additional questions on pregnancy losses in the past 5 years (FBH⁺) or (2) a Full Pregnancy History (FPH). No direct comparison of these two methods has been undertaken, although descriptive analyses suggest that the FBH⁺ may underestimate mortality rates particularly for stillbirths.

Methods This is the protocol paper for the Every Newborn-INDEPTH study (IN-DEPTH Network, International Network for the Demographic Evaluation of Populations and their Health Every Newborn, Every Newborn Action Plan), aiming to undertake a randomised comparison of FBH⁺ and FPH to measure pregnancy outcomes in a household survey in five selected INDEPTH Network sites in Africa and South Asia (Bandim in urban and rural Guinea-Bissau; Dabat in Ethiopia; IgangaMayuge in Uganda; Kintampo in Ghana; Matlab in Bangladesh). The survey will reach >68 000 pregnancies to assess if there is ≥15% difference in stillbirth rates. Additional questions will capture birthweight, gestational age, birth/death certification, termination of pregnancy and fertility intentions. The World Bank's Survey Solutions platform will be tailored for data collection, including recording paradata to evaluate timing. A mixed methods assessment of barriers and enablers to reporting of pregnancy and adverse pregnancy outcomes will be undertaken.

Conclusions This large-scale study is the first randomised comparison of these two methods to capture pregnancy outcomes. Results are expected to inform the evidence base for survey methodology, especially in DHS, regarding capture of stillbirths and other outcomes, notably neonatal deaths, abortions (spontaneous and induced), birthweight and gestational age. In addition, this study will inform strategies to improve health and demographic surveillance capture of neonatal/child mortality and pregnancy outcomes.

Almost nine million women and children die each year, two-thirds during pregnancy and around the time of birth [1]. An estimated 2.6 million babies are stillborn (die in the last three months of pregnancy or during childbirth) [2], 2.6 million liveborn babies die within the first 28 days of life (neonatal deaths) [1], and 303 000 women die of pregnancy complications per year [3]. Whilst child and maternal mortality rates halved during the Millennium Development Goal era, slower progress has been made for preventing stillbirths and neonatal deaths [4]. To accelerate progress, the Every Newborn Action Plan

(Every Newborn) was launched in June 2014 [5], including national targets of 12 or fewer neonatal deaths per 1000 live births and 12 or fewer stillbirths per 1000 total births by 2030 [5,6]. Neonatal mortality is also a sub-target under the third Sustainable Development Goal (SDG 3). Both neonatal and stillbirth rates (SBR) are tracked in the United Nation's Global Strategy for Women's, Children's and Adolescent's Health 2016-2030 [6,7]. The countries needing the greatest acceleration to meet these targets are mainly in sub-Saharan Africa and South Asia, with both the highest risk of mortality and the lowest availability of data. To track SDG progress and inform investments towards the Every Newborn targets, data are essential on both coverage of interventions and impact.

In response, the World Health Organization (WHO) and the London School of Hygiene & Tropical Medicine (LSHTM) published an ambitious Every Newborn Measurement Improvement Roadmap. This Roadmap prioritises specific measurement gaps and provides a multi-year, multi-partner pathway to test validity of selected coverage indicators [8], develop tools (eg, improved birth and death registration, audit, minimum perinatal data set, gestational age and birthweight), and promote use of data by 2020 [5,9,10]. The roadmap includes improved measurement and classification of pregnancy outcomes including stillbirths, miscarriage, or termination of pregnancy (TOP) and neonatal deaths. Data on birthweight, gestational age and vital status at birth are critical for correct classification of these outcomes (**Figure 1**) [12].

Population-based household surveys are the major source of population-level data on child and neonatal mortality rates (NMR) in settings without high coverage Civil Registration and Vital Statistics (CRVS) systems, and will continue to be an important source of data in the SDG-era [13,14]. Surveys are also sources for adverse pregnancy outcome data including stillbirths, miscarriages, TOPs, and birthweight, and gestation age.

Birthweight data are collected in surveys from either health cards or maternal recall. Where this information is not available, surveys ask about 'maternal perceived size at birth', which has been used in the estimation of low birthweight rates from surveys [15]. Surveys have a high proportion of missing birthweight data and heaping of reported birthweights [15-17]. Gestational age data are not usually presented in the survey reports, although these data are collected in months in the reproductive calendar for live births and stillbirths, and in additional questions for non-live births (miscarriages and abortions), eg, "How many months pregnant were you when that pregnancy ended?". This answer relies on mother's recall of the length of her pregnancy. The usefulness and validity of these survey data on gestational age in months are not known. More information on gestational age is now increasingly available from health facilities, where the last menstrual period can be recorded by a clinician and

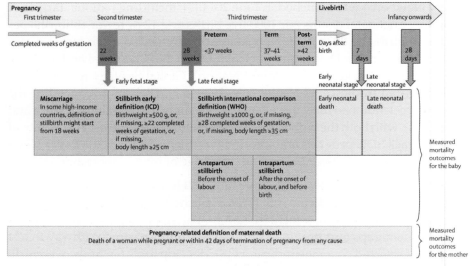

Figure 1. *Pregnancy outcomes and neonatal deaths with definitions for international comparison. From [11]. Pregnancy outcomes include miscarriage, stillbirth, termination of pregnancy, gestational age at birth and birthweight. This figure does not include induced termination of pregnancy which are defined as an induced termination of pregnancy by medical or surgical means and this definition be different in countries depending on their law and regulations.*

may be supplemented with an early ultrasound scan, fundal height during pregnancy, or clinical assessment of the newborn. Birth registration coverage is also assessed through household surveys, and these questions have not been assessed for feasibility or acceptability.

Although DHS collects data on abortions, most of these questions do not distinguish between induced abortions (TOP) or spontaneous abortions (miscarriages) and early/late fetal deaths or stillbirths [18]. This may contribute to undercounting of these different pregnancy outcomes. In some countries like Armenia and Nepal, the reproductive and health surveys go into more detail in collecting data on abortions, including the number of abortions and reasons why. A challenge with accurate capture of induced abortions is a reluctance to report, especially where they are illegal.

Currently, DHS use two alternative approaches to estimate NMR and SBR (**Figure 2**, panel A and panel B):

(1) *Standard DHS-7 core questionnaire Full Birth History (FBH⁺)*, with additional questions on pregnancies in the last five years resulting in a non-live birth used by a large majority of countries running DHS surveys;

(2) *Full Pregnancy History (FPH)*, used only in some countries in Eastern Europe and Central Asia, and more recently Afghanistan, Ghana, Nepal, the Philippines, South Africa, Vietnam.

The main difference between these two is that in FPH data are collected on all pregnancies in a woman's lifetime; whereas in the FBH⁺ data are collected on all live births in a woman's lifetime and on any pregnancies not resulting in a live birth only for the five years preceding the survey.

A

Survey Questions	Components
FBH+	Full history of all live births and questions on pregnancies in the last five years resulting in non-live births (including miscarriages, termination of pregnancy and stillbirths). Details of all pregnancies and pregnancy outcomes in the last five years entered in the reproductive calendar (calendar history). Used in reproduction module in DHS-7 model questionnaire.
FPH	Full history of all pregnancies and their outcomes (including live births, miscarriage, termination of pregnancy and stillbirths). Details of all pregnancies and outcomes in the last five years entered in the reproductive calendar (calendar history). Used in the reproduction module in some nationally adapted DHS questionnaires.

B

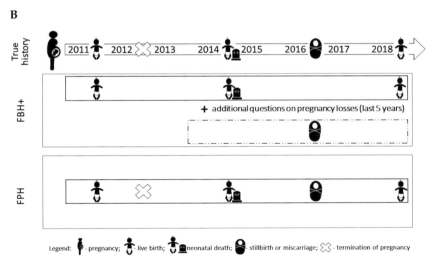

Figure 2. *Two DHS alternative approaches to estimate neonatal mortality rates and stillbirth rates.* **Panel A.** *Full Birth History (FBH⁺) and Full Pregnancy History (FPH) approaches used to collect pregnancy outcomes including stillbirth and neonatal death. DHS-6 and DHS-5 also collected similar information with a Full Birth History, but information on pregnancies not resulting in a live birth were collected in the reproductive calendar only. The new design of DHS-7 questionnaire has additional questions inserted in the questionnaire after the Full Birth History to capture this information.* **Panel B.** *Data capture by FBH⁺ and FPH methodologies.*

Few comparisons of these two methods are available and no rigorous evaluation has been undertaken. No studies have directly compared the performance of the two methods in estimating SBR, but an indirect comparison between two contemporaneous surveys in Ghana: (1) 2008 DHS (using the standard FBH+) and (2) 2007 Maternal Health Survey (using FPH) found SBR were 35% lower using the FBH+ but there was no difference in Early Neonatal Mortality Rates (ENMR) [19,20] (Appendix S1 in **Online Supplementary Document**). Another study in the Philippines compared two surveys, both using a FPH, found 34% higher SBR when the FPH was part of a short maternal health survey (SBR 12.5 per 1000 total births), compared to when it was administered as part of a full DHS (SBR 9.6 per 1000 total births) [21]. The difference observed may have been due to a shorter, more focused questionnaire in the maternal health survey and not by the question structure itself. Only one published study has made a direct (non-randomised) comparison between the two methods for ENMR, and found 2%-3% higher rates using the FPH [22].

Whilst it is plausible that a FPH may yield improved capture of adverse pregnancy outcomes, it may be more time consuming and hence, data are required to show evidence of better capture before recommending this as standard in the already long DHS core questionnaire. In addition, it is important to understand interview procedures and barriers and enablers to reporting pregnancies and adverse outcomes, which have been understudied. Data from Tanzania suggests that socio-economic and cultural factors affect the quality of information collected on adverse pregnancy outcomes [23]. An analysis of 39 DHS suggested that fieldwork procedures affect data quality, notably including sex of the interviewer; whether or not a translator was used; the timing of the interview; and how many call-backs an interviewer had to make [24]. Some studies have reported on the stigma for women after stillbirths, newborn deaths and abortions in developing country contexts [25-27].

Aim

This is the protocol paper for the **Every Newborn-INDEPTH** Network (EN-INDEPTH) study which is part of the Every Newborn Measurement Improvement Roadmap, and aims to improve household survey capture of stillbirths and neonatal deaths by assessing whether FPH leads to increased capture of selected pregnancy outcomes compared to the standard DHS-7 FBH+ (**Figure 2**, panel A and panel B). The study will investigate the performance of existing or modified survey questions regarding other important measures related to pregnancy related outcomes, including fertility intentions, TOP, birthweight, gestational age, and coverage of birth and death certification. In addition, the study will examine barriers and enablers to reporting of pregnancy and adverse pregnancy outcomes in surveys and through Health and Demographic Surveillance Systems (HDSS).

Research objectives

Research objectives, research questions and data analysis methods are summarised in **Table 1.**

Table 1. *EN-INDEPTH study summary of research questions and data analysis approach, according to the four study objectives.*

RESEARCH OBJECTIVE	RESEARCH QUESTION	DATA ANALYSIS APPROACH
Objective 1: Full Birth History (FBH+) approach vs Full Pregnancy History (FPH) approach		
To undertake a randomised comparison of the reproductive module used in the latest version of FBH+ vs a FPH module to examine the variation in capture of stillbirths and neonatal deaths.	Is the FPH method better at capturing stillbirths and neonatal deaths in the last five years than the FBH+?	Descriptive and bivariate analyses comparing the two methods including meta-analysis: SBR; and NMR.
	How long does it take to collect data using the FPH questionnaire? Does the length of data collection vary by context and/or fertility level?	Bivariate analyses of the FPH and FBH+ by the time spent answering the questionnaires, variation by context and maternal characteristics.
Objective 2: Pregnancy outcomes		
To evaluate the use of existing/modified survey questions to capture the fertility intentions and selected pregnancy outcomes (top, miscarriage, birthweight, gestational age), as well as birth and death certification.	What is the answerability and data quality by indicator?	Descriptive analyses of selected indicators, and assessment of data quality per indicator (eg, non-response, heaping, missingness).
	How long does it take to collect data regarding these indicators? Does the length of data collection vary by data collector context and/or fertility level?	Analyses of survey paradata to assess variation by data collector (eg, gender, education level and training), time of day, rural/urban location, and time needed to complete survey questions and sections, frequency of repeated corrections of answers to questions.
Objective 3: Survey vs HDSS data collection platforms		
To compare the capture of pregnancy outcomes in the survey to that in the routine HDSS data collection	How do outcomes reported in the EN-INDEPTH survey compare with HDSS data?	Assess level of agreement at population-level between survey and routine HDSS data over the same time period for several indicators: SBR, NMR, miscarriage, TOP, birthweight, GA.
		For individually linked data, compare capture of pregnancy outcomes between survey and HDSS and assess predictors of capture.

Table 1. *Continued*

RESEARCH OBJEC-TIVE	RESEARCH QUESTION	DATA ANALYSIS APPROACH
Objective 4: Barriers and enablers to reporting (adverse) pregnancy outcomes		
To identify barriers and enablers to the reporting of pregnancy and adverse pregnancy outcomes during the survey and HDSS data collection, and particularly if these differ for the two survey questionnaire methods (FBH⁺ and FPH).	What are barriers and enablers to reporting of pregnancies and pregnancy outcomes (geographic, socioeconomic, cultural, data collection methodologies, etc.) in HDSS and survey data collection?	Quantitative analyses. Qualitative analyses of FGDs or IDIs for:
	What are interviewers' perceptions (both HDSS and survey interviewers) of barriers and enablers to collect data on pregnancy losses in survey setting?	- survey interviewers
		- HDSS interviewers
		- supervisors
		- mothers who had a pregnancy in the past five years
	What are women's perceptions and barriers for reporting pregnancy losses?	A priori coding. Use of the grounded theory and identify emerging themes and outliers; relationships and theories.
	How can data collection process be improved to obtain better data on adverse pregnancy outcomes?	

FBH⁺ – Full Birth History⁺; FPH – Full Pregnancy History; SBR – stillbirth rates ; NMR – neonatal mortality rates; TOP – termination of pregnancy; HDSS – Health and Demographic Surveillance Systems; GA – gestation age; FGDs – focus group discussions ; IDIs – in-depth interviews

Objective 1. FBH⁺ vs FPH approach: To undertake a randomised comparison of the reproductive module used in the latest version of FBH⁺ vs a FPH module to examine the variation in capture of stillbirths and neonatal deaths.

Objective 2. Pregnancy outcomes: To evaluate the use of existing/modified survey questions to capture the fertility intentions and selected pregnancy outcomes (TOP, miscarriage, birthweight, gestational age), as well as birth and death certification.

Objective 3. Survey vs HDSS data collection platforms: To compare the capture of pregnancy outcomes in the survey to that in the routine HDSS data collection.

Objective 4. Barriers and enablers to reporting (adverse) pregnancy outcomes: To identify barriers and enablers to the reporting of pregnancy and adverse pregnancy outcomes during the survey and HDSS data collection, and particularly if these differ for the two survey questionnaire methods (FBH+ and FPH).

METHODS

Study design

This multi-site study will use a retrospective survey to compare two methods of recording pregnancy outcomes (FBH+ vs FPH methods), with random allocation at the individual woman level. Quantitative and qualitative data will be collected to answer four research objectives (**Table 1**).

Research protocol development was informed by wide consultation, including review by the research site teams and an Expert Advisory Group. 23 participants took part in a study design workshop in Kampala in mid-2016 [28]. In addition, in April 2017, a multi-site workshop was organised to agree on the data collection protocol in the five sites.

Study settings

The INDEPTH Network's HDSS is a network of research sites in 53 countries, established in 1998. Each site tracks vital events in a defined population on a continuous basis, but methods used vary [29]. Since some sites undertake pregnancy surveillance, the INDEPTH network provides an ideal platform for this multi-site retrospective population-based survey with a potential for linking with prospective HDSS data. The INDEPTH Network operates through Working Groups, one of which, the Maternal Newborn and Child Health (MNCH) working group [30], hosted by the Makerere University School of Public Health (MakSPH), Uganda, will coordinate this study, partnering with LSHTM.

A Request For Applications (RFA) was sent to all 53 HDSS sites in December 2015 by the INDEPTH Network secretariat. Fourteen proposals were received and reviewed by LSHTM, MakSPH and the INDEPTH Network secretariat [31]. The selection criteria were: HDSS total population of more than 30 000 people; annual SBR and NMR greater than 15 per 1000 total births; acceptable quality surveillance for pregnancy outcomes, including neonatal deaths and stillbirths; expertise on maternal and newborn health, and stillbirths among the HDSS team members and evidence of co-funding in the submitted estimated budgets. Five sites (Bandim, Dabat, IgangaMayuge, Kintampo, and Matlab) were selected (**Table 2** and **Figure 3**), all of which, as well as LSHTM, received ethical approval from local institutional review boards (Appendix S2 in **Online Supplementary Document**).

While all the selected HDSS sites undertake pregnancy surveillance, the quality of which is influenced by various factors including: frequency of surveillance rounds; the key informants ratio to population; gender; the method used to ask about pregnancy and pregnancy outcomes; the proportion of facility births; and linkage between HDSS and facility data. Cultural norms around pregnancy disclosure may also vary and affect the data collected (**Table 2**).

Table 2. *Expected sample size across the five INDEPTH sites*

CHARACTERIS-TICS	BANDIM	MATLAB	KINTAMPO	DABAT	IGANGAMA-YUGE	ACROSS THE FIVE SITES
Estimated number of total births over the five years captured within the HDSS	29 173	25 799	24 008	7031	11 489	97 499
Surveillance system	Bi-annual update rounds in the rural area and monthly updates in urban area. Update rounds includes registration of pregnancies	Two monthly update rounds including pregnancy testing and registration	Bi-annual update, from 2017 they have shifted to an annual update rounds	Bi-annual update rounds. Monthly updates of births and deaths from local guides.	Bi-annual update rounds. Monthly updates of births and deaths from local scouts.	
Sampling frame*	Women in HDSS site with recorded birth outcome in last 5 y. (all in urban site and 80% in rural site)	Women in HDSS site with recorded birth outcome in last 5 y. (all)	Women in HDSS site with recorded birth outcome in last 5 y. (random sample)	Women of reproductive age in HDSS site	Women of reproductive age in HDSS site	
Expected number of total births to be captured in survey	17 000	21 000	14 500	5700	9800	68 000

HDSS – Health and Demographic Surveillance Systems
*See Appendix S3 in **Online Supplementary Document** for details.

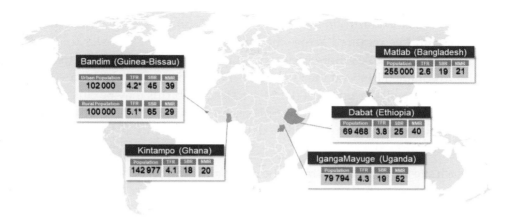

Figure 3. *Map showing the location of the EN-INDEPTH study HDSS sites. Total fertility rate (TFR) for women ages 15-49; neonatal mortality rate (NMR) per 1000 live births; stillbirth rate (SBR) per 1000 live births. More detailed information on study HDSS sites: Bandim (http://www. indepth-network.org/member-centres/bandim-hdss); Dabat (http://www.indepth-network.org/ member-centres/dabat-hdss); Iganga-Mayuge (http://www.indepth-network.org/member-centres/ igangamayuge); Kintampo (http://www.indepth-network.org/member-centres/kintampo-hdss); Matlab (http://www.indepth-network.org/member-centres/matlab-hdss). Asterisk: Bandim- children/ pregnancies only followed prospectively; TFR estimated by cumulative birth hazards (Nelson Ahlen) as observed for specific age bands between 2012-16 extrapolated to age span 15-50 years; SBR, NMR estimated among registered pregnancies ending in 2012-16.*

Sample size and data collection approach

Limited evidence from previous descriptive studies discussed above suggests a difference in SBR from 3 to 35% between a FBH+ and a FPH method [19,20]. A difference of at least 15% between the two methods could be sufficient to consider a major change in the DHS core questionnaire. Since this is the first direct comparisons of the two methodologies, we powered the randomized comparison to capture a 15% difference assuming that a difference less than 15% will not justify a change in survey methodology (see Appendix S1 in **Online Supplementary Document**).

Based on the recorded SBR and total births per HDSS over the last three years, the overall SBR for the final sample of births captured in the survey is expected to be around 28.4 per 1000 total births, if all women are surveyed. However, we needed to account for possible outmigration, unavailability of women at any visit, or non-consent. After adjusting for these factors, we expect the SBR for the FPH arm to be around 26.7 per 1000 total births (see Appendix S3, Table

S2.2 in **Online Supplementary Document** for details). Assuming a SBR of 26.7 per 1000 total births in the FPH arm, a total sample size of at least 68 000 births would be required across the five sites to have 80% power to detect a difference of 15% or more between the proportion of total births that are stillbirths in the FBH⁺ and the FPH at the 5% significance level (alpha = 0.05), including a small design effect (DEFF = 1.1), as stillbirths may be clustered in individual women. The lower the SBR captured in the FBH⁺ arm, the higher the sample size will be required to detect 15% difference between the two arms (see **Table 3**).

For each site the approach to reach the maximum number of births was agreed based on site-specific information on the level of migration, geographical accessibility, and assumed levels of non-response (either due to non-consent or inability to locate) and other factors. The numbers per site are shown in **Table 2** and details of the estimation are in Appendix S3, Table S2.2 in **Online Supplementary Document**. Three sites (ie, Matlab, Dabat and IgangaMayuge) will survey all women who have given birth in the last five years. Matlab has bi-monthly data collection with pregnancy testing for women who report having missed a menstrual period, and hence has reliable listings of total births, and will administer the EN-INDEPTH survey to eligible women (age 15-49) known to have had at least one birth (live birth or stillbirth) in the last five

Table 3. *Required sample size by stillbirth rate (SBR) for the household survey randomised comparison, assuming alpha = 0.05 and an expected 15% difference in SBR**

Assumed SBR in birth history group/ 1000 total births	Predicted SBR in pregnancy history group/ 1000 total births	Number of total births to achieve 80% power	Sample size - number of births required including design effect and non-response (15%)
23.00	26.45	63 604	80 459
23.20	26.70	62 348	68 583
24.00	27.60	60 886	77 021
25.00	28.75	58 386	73 858
26.00	29.90	56 078	70 939
27.00	31.05	53 942	68 237
28.00	32.20	51 958	65 727

*The Design effect (DEFF) is calculated as $DEFF = 1 + (r - 1) \times rho$, where r = average number of observations in a cluster and rho = correlation between pairs of observations selected at random from the same cluster). Assuming in a 5-year period women will experience on average a maximum of 2 births, and that as stillbirth is a rare outcome rho<0.1, a design effect of 1.1 is included. For Bandim, due to the challenge of reaching women in rural area, we can only account for a maximum of two visits to reach the interview, for this reason we have assumed a higher rate of non-response rate (30%).

years; Dabat and IgangaMayuge have bi-annual updates and do not have a specific system of pregnancy tracking and therefore, all women of reproductive age (15-49 years) in the HDSS site will be included. Bandim and Kintampo, will select a random sample of women residing in the HDSS known to have at least one birth in the last five years (**Table 2**).

Data collection software application

Currently, the DHS and Multiple Indicator Cluster Survey (MICS) surveys are administered either using a paper version of the questionnaire (PAPI) or computer assisted personal interviewing (CAPI) and the CSPro (Census and Survey Processing System) platform for entering the data entry or data capture. We elected to use Android-based tablet data collection as most of the selected HDSS sites had some experience with these. We compared several existing data collection platforms (ODK, CSPro, Qualtrics, Red Hat and Survey Solutions). We selected the Survey Solutions Computer Assisted Personal Interview and Computer Assisted Web Interviewing platform (Survey Solutions) developed by the World Bank [32], given its ability of linking questions to specific household members listed in the roster file; its flexible and user-friendly online interface for the questionnaire design; the ability to integrate validation rules; lack of user fees; the online tool for centralised survey administration and data management; data aggregation and reporting features; end-user technical support provided by the World Bank technical support team; as well as the Interviewer application available for Android devices.

The data will be entered on Android-based tablets using the Survey Solution platform, stored locally on the tablets, and synchronised regularly to the dedicated country's physical or virtual server. The platform has different user roles with varying level of permissions and functions: Interviewer (function – data collection), Supervisor (assigning and monitoring data collection by interviewers), Headquarters (overall survey and data management), and Observer (monitoring) (**Figure 4**). The platform's survey and data management component ('Survey Solutions Headquarters', HQ) provides a dashboard of the progress of data collection, including duration and speed of the interviews, Global Positioning System coordinates of the interviewer, as well as paradata. The paradata contains information about the process of collecting survey data and records all events with timestamps on a tablet during data collection (data entry, data correction, responsibility changes, etc.). This type of data can be used for analysis of time per interview and time per question and section, as well as changes in productivity over time for different interviewers and teams. These data can be used for live data quality control, data monitoring and interview progress evaluation.

Procedures

Informed consent and respondent identification

All participants will receive a verbal explanation of the study objective by a trained field assistant and an information sheet. An adapted version of the standard DHS consent form will be used (Appendix S4 in **Online Supplementary Document**). Both will be translated into local languages and written consent will be obtained from all study participants. Study participants will be informed of their right to refuse and/or withdraw at any point of time from the survey interviews, and at liberty to answer those questions they want to and will not be coerced in case they refuse. Information obtained will be viewed only by the researchers and anonymity will be guaranteed by using identification numbers. Separate written consent will be sought for women and interviewers participating in the qualitative aspects. We will follow fieldwork procedure as outlined in the DHS interviewer manual. Interviewers will make up to three attempts to find respondents.

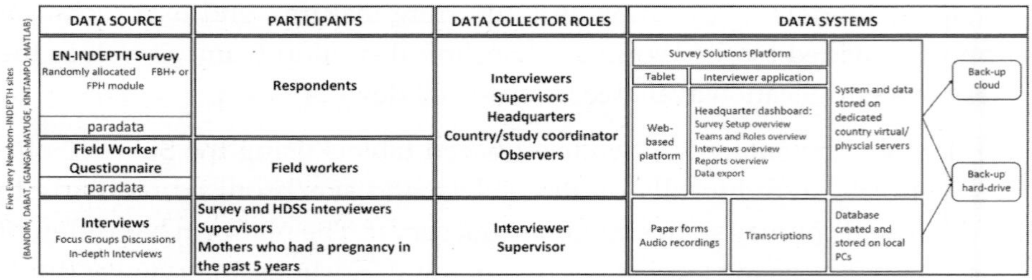

	DATA SOURCE	PARTICIPANTS	DATA COLLECTOR ROLES	DATA SYSTEMS				
Five Every Newborn-INDEPTH sites (BANDIM, DABAT, IGANGA-MAYUGE, KINTAMPO, MATLAB)	**EN-INDEPTH Survey** Randomly allocated FBH+ or FPH module	**Respondents**	Interviewers Supervisors Headquarters Country/study coordinator Observers	Survey Solutions Platform		System and data stored on dedicated country virtual/ physcial servers	Back-up cloud	
				Tablet	Interviewer application			
	paradata			Web-based platform	Headquarter dashboard: Survey Setup overview Teams and Roles overview Interviews overview Reports overview Data export			
	Field Worker Questionnaire	**Field workers**						
	paradata						Back-up hard-drive	
	Interviews Focus Groups Discussions In-depth Interviews	Survey and HDSS interviewers Supervisors Mothers who had a pregnancy in the past 5 years	Interviewer Supervisor	Paper forms Audio recordings	Transcriptions	Database created and stored on local PCs		

Figure 4. *EN-INDEPTH Data Collection and Flow.*

Randomisation and EN-INDEPTH survey

Women selected for the survey from all five sites will be randomised to receive either the reproduction questions from the DHS-7 women's questionnaire with a standard FBH+ or a FPH. Randomisation will be done automatically within the application-based questionnaire using an in-built random number generator.

Table 4 provides a summary of adaptations to the DHS-7 questionnaire sections to meet the study objectives including questions on gestational age, birth

Table 4. *Current standard DHS Phase 7 questionnaire sections and adaptations for this study*

SURVEY QUESTIONNAIRE WITH FBH+ OR FPH DETAILING ADAPTATIONS FROM STANDARD DHS PHASE 7 SECTION, WHERE APPLICABLE	
Section 1. Consent form and background of interview	The content of section 1 will be reduced to focus on key maternal background characteristics only.
Section 2. Reproduction	Standard FBH+ questions with pregnancy loss questions which include information on stillbirths, miscarriages and abortions. No adaptations made. Or randomly allocated to FPH from Nepal 2016 for the FPH and pregnancy losses questions – the detailed questions on abortion will only be administered in selected sites.
Section 4. Pregnancy and postnatal care	Section 4 will be administered with minor adaptations for all stillbirths and neonatal deaths, as well as for a sample of live births. Additional questions on gestational age (weeks), birth and death certification, and timing and characteristics of stillbirths will be added to test the feasibility of these questions in household surveys.
Section 8. Fertility preferences	Some questions on fertility intention to refine the measurement on unwanted pregnancy will be added. These questions have been developed and tested in a multi-country research study [33].
Section 9. Household characteristics	Questions on household socio-economic characteristics including household dwelling structure, flooring material, sanitation and toilet facility. These questions are adapted from the DHS household survey questionnaire.

FBH+ – full birth history +; FPH – full pregnancy history; DHS – Demographic and Health Surveys.

certification, characteristics of stillbirths and fertility intentions. The latest DHS questionnaire (DHS-7) will be used, with a shortened introduction section 1 of the DHS-7 women's questionnaire; section 2 on reproduction; section 4 on pregnancy, delivery and postnatal care; and an additional section 9 adapted on household characteristics. Section 8 on fertility intentions was optional and the Matlab site opted not to administer this as they have just recently completed the collection of similar data. Some specific country add-on modifications will be made to the questionnaire (eg, Bandim site will collect questions on vaccinations, and the IgangaMayuge site will collect data using the Dietary Diversity questionnaire in section 10). Apart from section 2, the questionnaires for the FBH+ and FPH arms will be identical. Section 2 in the FBH+ arm will contain the standard DHS-7 core reproduction questions. In the FPH arm, section 2 will contain the whole reproduction section from the Nepal 2016 DHS for sites willing to include detailed questions on abortion, and a reduced version without the detailed abortion questions for other sites. Appendix S5 in **Online Supplementary Document** gives full details of the questionnaires.

Local language translations of the questions already used by DHS will be used whenever available. Where not available, translations to local languages will be made by the site teams and checked using back translation.

Assessment of barriers and enablers to reporting of pregnancy and adverse pregnancy outcomes

For objective 4, a self-administered questionnaire adapted from DHS field-worker questionnaire, will assess demographic and other characteristics of the interviewers (Appendix S6 in **Online Supplementary Document**). A series of Focus Group Discussions (FGDs) will be held with HDSS and survey interviewers, as well as supervisors, to assess the barriers or enablers to collecting data on pregnancy and adverse pregnancy outcomes in the survey and HDSS. FGDs will be conducted with women who had at least one pregnancy in the past five years, focusing on perceptions, practices, barriers and enablers in the community. A minimum of six FGDs will be conducted in each site, each with approximately eight to ten participants. In-Depth Interviews (IDIs) will be undertaken in some sites with women who have experienced these adverse pregnancy outcomes, allowing for deeper exploration and triangulation of data.

Training of data collectors and supervisors

The EN-INDEPTH site teams with LSHTM and MakSPH jointly developed a training manual on the data collection procedures, adapting the standard DHS Interviewer's Manual [34], and tailored it to the specific country context and the HDSS site. Four additional manuals (data collection setup, Survey Solutions data management procedures, listing process, Survey Solutions Tester/Interviewer application) were developed adapting the World Bank Survey Solutions Manuals [35]. The training of data collectors and supervisors was led by the HDSS team with initial support from the core team for a minimum of two weeks in all HDSS sites. The training included at least one-week on the paper-based questionnaire and one to two weeks on tablet use, data collection using the Survey Solutions Tester application, as well as the Survey Solutions Interviewer application and interviewer field practice. Prior to data collection, additional trainings on survey management using Survey Solutions HQ were provided to supervisors and data analysists.

For the qualitative work, training manuals will be developed to guide the interviewers during the FGDs and IDIs to ensure comparability of interviews across sites. Additionally, a protocol will be developed to guide the interviewers on how to react in situations where the respondent gets distressed. After the initial two to three weeks training, all sites will initiate the pilot phase of data collection. The length of the data collection will vary by site depending on the fieldwork schedule and allocated sample size ranging between six to 12 months.

Data quality monitoring

Validations for value ranges were defined and programmed into the tablet application to avert predictable human errors. The skipping rules were programmed and additional rules were set to perform consistency checks. Warning messages were programmed to prompt to correct the input when values are outside the defined range, and to provide guidance as per the DHS manual. Data quality will be monitored using Survey Solutions platform's online data dashboard, providing real-time cumulative and detailed summary of ongoing surveys across teams and individual interviewers in each country. The platform allows Supervisors and Headquarters to validate collected data by Interviewer online and, if necessary, incomplete or erroneous questionnaires can be returned to the Interviewer for timely re-assignment and correction. In addition, bi-weekly reports will be sent to the LSHTM and MakSPH core teams by data analysts from all sites summarising the overall data collection progress. Regular all-site data monitoring calls will provide an opportunity for country teams to review and discuss progress in addition to promoting collaborative quality improvement initiatives between countries and sites.

Data management

Following synchronisation, data from tablets will be uploaded to the country's dedicated virtual or physical server with regular automatic back-up, with additional back-up on a separate server or external hard drive. The raw data will be stored in an encrypted format, accessed only by the country's data manager. The anonymization of the quantitative and qualitative data (removing any direct or indirect identifiers, including enumeration identifiers, geo-referenced data, transcripts and audio recording) will take place in-country before data sets are pooled into one multi-site data set (**Figure 4**).

Analysis by objective

The overview of research objectives, main research questions, and analytical approaches are summarised in **Table 1**. For all study objectives, the primarily analyses will be performed overall across countries (as pooled analyses), and comparative secondary analyses will be performed by site separately, whenever possible. Data will be cleaned according to an agreed protocol, including logical and completeness checks. Quantitative analyses will be undertaken with

Stata 15SE (Stata Statistical Software: Release 15. College Station, TX: StataCorp LLC). Qualitative analyses will be conducted using NVivo software (NVivo qualitative data analysis Software; QSR International Pty Ltd Version 12, 2018).

Objective 1

A population-level descriptive analysis will be conducted comparing SBR and NMR by FBH+ or FPH, and by maternal characteristics (age, parity, residence, and education status). Crude risk ratios with its 95% confidence interval will be computed for comparison of SBR and NMR between FBH+ and FPH overall and by study site using the meta-analysis methods with Random Effects. Regression models will be fitted to assess determinants of adverse pregnancy outcomes using Generalised Estimation Equations to adjust for clustering of stillbirths or neonatal deaths within the same woman, therefore taking into account design effect. We will use paradata to assess differences in average time taken to complete the FBH+ and FPH.

Objective 2

We will undertake descriptive analyses of selected indicators including fertility intentions, selected pregnancy outcomes (TOP, miscarriage, birthweight, gestational age), as well as birth and death registration. This will include estimates of frequency of reported TOP and miscarriage, coverage of reported birthweight, gestational age, birth and death certification, and of fertility intentions. The answerability of new/refined questions will be assessed by describing patterns of non-response and heaping, where appropriate. Variation in these indicators by pregnancy outcome, maternal or interviewer characteristics will be assessed. For gestational age, internal consistency in the survey will be assessed by comparing women's reporting of gestation in months compared to weeks, and reported maternal perception of the birth to be preterm. Survey paradata will also be analysed to assess time taken to complete and frequency of repeated corrections to relevant survey questions.

Objective 3

Women-level data from the survey will be individually matched with the routine HDSS surveillance data to establish matching rates for stillbirths and neonatal deaths. We will assess determinants of reporting or not reporting of these outcomes in the survey by women's and interviewers' characteristics and HDSS settings (geographic, socioeconomic, cultural, data collection methodologies, etc.). We will also assess levels of agreement between the survey and the routine HDSS data over the same time period at a population level for several indicators, such as SBR, NMR, miscarriage, TOP, birthweight, and gestational age. Predictors of disagreement (eg, length of recall, maternal education, etc.) will be examined. We recognize that neither HDSS nor survey data can be considered 'gold standard' and that the difference in measurement might be in both or either direction and variable by site.

Objective 4

For qualitative data, we will use a grounded theory approach for analysis, with an iterative process involving reading the text, detecting potential emerging themes and outliers, comparing themes and searching for relationships, as well as building theoretical models. A priori coding will be done, with a codebook listing potential codes developed before the analysis begins, to guide the process, and new codes identified from data included as analysis proceeds. Results will be presented with verbatim quotes from respondents. Reliability will be checked by multiple members of the team, two from each site, independently coding data.

DISCUSSION

The EN-INDEPTH is the first randomised comparison of two survey methods to capture pregnancy outcomes, the current DHS-7 FBH+ and FPH. This is a large-scale study (at least 68 000 births) based in five high-burden countries, including one site in South Asia and four sites across West and East Africa. The study is powered to be able to detect a 15% difference in the estimated SBR, but it is also expected to inform our understanding of survey capture of other pregnancy outcomes, notably neonatal deaths, birthweight, gestational age and abortions (spontaneous and induced). Even if the results show a convincing increase in capture of stillbirths or other pregnancy outcomes, a key operational question is whether the FPH takes longer. The software used for our study (Survey Solutions) allows recording of the paradata, including precise timing by section of the questionnaire. This study will, therefore, enable us to conduct more detailed analyses of time spent by question and section, as well as by the fertility context. Underreporting of pregnancy and adverse outcomes may be affected by socio-cultural barriers and survey data collection procedures, so the mixed methods assessment of barriers and enablers to reporting and recording will be valuable.

In addition to omission of events, household surveys are known to have important limitations in the measurement of stillbirths and neonatal deaths, including displacement of reported day of death and misclassification between stillbirths and neonatal deaths [36,37]. Distinguishing between stillbirths and neonatal deaths requires detection of signs of life at birth, notably assessment of heart rate. Recall by a mother in a survey requires her to know whether there were signs of life at birth and for her to report this. Differences in assessment at birth, perceptions of viability, availability of neonatal resuscitation and cultural and religious factors - all potentially have a role in whether a mother will report her baby's death as a stillbirth or an early neonatal death. This study will examine any differences between reporting of these outcomes in the survey compared to HDSS data, and explore women's perceptions of stillbirth and neonatal deaths, but will not have the ability to assess "true" stillbirths based on lack of accurate measures of heart rate at birth. Another important misclassification is between early fetal death and late fetal death/stillbirth with a threshold of 28 weeks, based on errors in gestational age measurement and reporting. Again, this study will not have "true" gestational age based on first trimester ultrasound.

Birthweight and gestational age measurements are important from individual, clinical and public health perspectives. From a clinical perspective, they are important to identify liveborn neonates at increased risk of mortality and morbidity, for example, those preterm (born at <37 completed weeks of gestation) or low birthweight (<2500g), to enable provision of extra care [12]. From a classification perspective, this information is critical to differentiate between miscarriages and stillbirths. Studies have shown that data on perceived size at birth recorded in surveys are not consistent with data recorded from health cards and that the quality of recalled birthweight data are variable [38]. In addition, little is known on community perceptions of the importance of birthweight and how this may influence reporting. This study seeks to provide further insights on how to obtain better birthweight data in surveys. Although a gestational age in months is collected in the five-year reproductive calendar in DHS surveys, concerns have been raised regarding the validity of these data. Whilst months are used to differentiate between miscarriages and stillbirths, they are currently not reported in most survey reports and are not used in the estimation of population-level measures, such as preterm birth. In this study, we will assess standard and modified questions that seek to capture gestational age, as well as the internal validity of the reporting of gestational age in months, in weeks, and reported maternal perception of the birth as preterm. In the Matlab site, where more accurate gestational age information is captured in the HDSS through early routine urinary pregnancy testing following a missed period, we will assess the validity of these questions by comparing the information captured in the EN-INDEPTH survey to the HDSS data. This will provide important new information on the feasibility of the use of these questions in household surveys. However, the frequent HDSS household visits might increase women's awareness of pregnancy duration and improve the reporting of gestational age.

Comparable data on abortion are limited [39]. In countries where abortion is illegal, data are underreported for fear of prosecution or stigma [18]. In contexts where abortion is legal, data may also be problematic. This study will add to the literature by testing the feasibility to asking a small set of abortion questions.

Fertility intentions are subject to substantial variability over time [40]. As part of a multi-country research protocol developed by the "STEP-UP" consortium that the LSHTM is co-leading with the Population Council [33], a set of new questions were developed to improve the measurement of ambivalence. We will test these questions, and because the study is nested in the HDSS sites, we will be able to prospectively assess the link between un-intendedness and pregnancy outcomes. The information collected will support a rigorous assessment of reasons for unmet need for family planning, as well as to assess whether unwanted childbearing is linked to negative pregnancy outcomes.

Registering a child's birth is a critical first step to protect the rights of every child, and non-registration might prevent the child from accessing health and education services. UNICEF estimates suggest that more than 230 million children under the age of 5 have not had their birth registered [41]. Household surveys represent the largest source of data on birth registration in low- and middle-income countries, [41]. Yet, registration and notification procedures vary, so more research into context specific survey questions is required [42]. In consultation with experts in the Child Protection team in UNICEF HQ, we selected birth registration questions to be evaluated in this study.

Whilst this study has strengths in terms of being randomised for the primary objective, as well as being multi-site and large-scale, pregnancies resulting in a stillbirth are less likely to be captured than those resulting in a live birth, especially if there is no frequent surveillance to capture new pregnancies and live births, even within relatively robust pregnancy surveillance systems. Hence, one limitation of this method is that women with only a stillbirth in the last five years and no live birth would not be surveyed, potentially underestimating the true SBR. In addition, the sites selected for this study have slightly different surveillance systems. Since we are collecting the data in the context of the demographic surveillance system, respondents might already be familiar with these survey questions and may be more likely than women in other settings to report pregnancy losses. If this is the case, we might have a higher reporting of events than in other settings. However, if respondents in the community are indeed more likely to report such events, this should affect women in the HDSS site equally and should not affect the randomised experiment.

The choice of Survey Solutions as our data collection tool might affect comparability with other studies using PAPI or CAPI using the CSPro Windows tablet interface. The main difference between these methods of data collection is that both PAPI and CAPI using the CSPro Windows tablet interface have a roster for the data collection of reproductive histories. In order to minimise such effect, we developed a summary of the reproductive history to mimic the reproductive history roster used in the original PAPI or CAPI using the CSPro Windows tablet application. In addition, another strength of this study is that our customised survey questionnaire developed with Survey Solutions Designer allows the inclusion of interviewer's instructions and these are visible to the interview for each question as the interviewer progresses during the interviewer visit. This addition might improve data quality.

CONCLUSIONS

Most of the 5.5 million deaths around the time of birth [1] occur in countries with the least data. Whilst improvement in CRVS and routine facility data systems is crucial, in the meantime the poorest countries rely on household surveys, and equity considerations should drive investment to improve the quality of data capture, especially for the large burden of pregnancy outcomes. We anticipate that the results of this study will inform improved tools and how these tools are applied and enable better measurement of the often-hidden outcomes associated with stigma and suffering of women in many countries. Better data alone will not change these outcomes, but counting and visibility is a crucial first step to change.

Acknowledgements: We would like to thank the Expert Advisory Group members for their inputs (alphabetical order): Fred Arnold; Peter Byass; Trevor Croft; Attila Hancio-glu; Stéphane Helleringer; Kobus Herbst; Shane M Khan; Sunita Kishor; Florina Serba-nescu; Turgay Unalan. We also acknowledge Michael Wild and the World Bank Survey Solutions Development Team for their technical support with the survey setup. We also would like to acknowledge the technical input provided by Claudia Cappa from UNICEF for the design of the birth registration questions. Appreciation to Claudia DaSilva, Fion Hay, Jacob Saah and Samuelina Arthur for their administrative support. We thank the women in the survey and the data collection staff from the HDSS sites at Bandim, Dabat, IgangaMayuge, Kintampo, and Matlab.

Ethics and consent to participate: *This study was granted ethical approval by the institutional review boards in all operating countries as well as from Institutional Ethical Review Committee of the London School of Hygiene & Tropical Medicine (Appendix S2 in* **Online Supplementary Document***).*

Availability of data and material: *Data sharing and transfer agreements have been made and signed by all collaborating partners.*

Disclaimer: *The information and views set out in this publication are those of the author(s) and do not necessarily reflect the views or the official opinion of the associated employer(s). The latter may not be held responsible for the use that may be made of the information contained therein.*

Funding: *This work is funded by the Children's Investment Fund Foundation (CIFF) by means of a grant to LSHTM (PI JEL), and a sub-award to the INDEPTH MNCH working group managed in Accra and with technical leadership by MakSPH (PI PW). A competitive RFA was issued to all 53 INDEPTH HDSS sites and the top five applicants were selected (as described above). SK is employed by ICF working on DHS programme, which is funded by USAID.*

Authorship contributions: *The study was conceptualised by JEL in 2014, and the initial protocol was developed with JEL, PW and HB and discussed in workshops in Kampala in 2015 and then refined in June 2016 with the five selected INDEPTH sites. AB joined in April 2016 and led the development of the data collection system, coordinated the research implementation activities and led the multi-country research implementation workshop that was held in Bangladesh in April 2017. AB with HB and JA and DK led the development of the questionnaire. VSG joined in mid-2016, coded the questionnaire into the software application and led the setup of multi-country data collection, data management, and monitoring systems. The data collection system was initially piloted in Bandim site with particular insights from ABF and SMT. All the site teams attended the design and implementation workshops and input to the concepts, data collection tools and training materials. DK led the development of the training materials and with HB is leading the work on barriers and enablers to data collection. The manuscript was drafted by AB and JEL, with inputs from VSG, HB, JA, and DK. All the authors reviewed and helped to revise the manuscript.*

Competing interests: *The authors completed the Unified Competing Interest form at www.icjme.org/coi_disclosure.pdf (available upon request from the corresponding author), and declare no conflicts of interest.*

References

1   United Nations Inter-agency Group for Child Mortality Estimation (UN IGME). Levels & Trends in Child Mortality: Report 2017, Estimates Developed by the UN Inter-agency Group for Child Mortality Estimation. New York: United Nations Children's Fund; 2017.

2   Blencowe H, Cousens S, Jassir FB, Say L, Chou D, Mathers C, et al. National, regional, and worldwide estimates of stillbirth rates in 2015, with trends from 2000: a systematic analysis. Lancet Glob Health. 2016;4:e98-108. Medline:26795602 doi:10.1016/S2214-109X(15)00275-2

3   World Health Organization. Trends in maternal mortality: 1990 to 2015: estimates by WHO, UNICEF, UNFPA, World Bank Group and the United Nations Population Division. Geneva: World Health Organization; 2015.

4   Lawn JE, Blencowe H, Waiswa P, Amouzou A, Mathers C, Hogan D, et al. Stillbirths: rates, risk factors, and acceleration towards 2030. Lancet. 2016;387:587-603. Medline:26794078 doi:10.1016/S0140-6736(15)00837-5

5   World Health Organization, United Nations Children's Fund. Every Newborn: an action plan to end preventable deaths. Geneva: World Health Organization; 2014.

6   United Nations. Transforming Our World: The 2030 Agenda for Sustainable Development. New York: UN Publishing; 2015.

7   United Nations. The Global Strategy for Women's, Children's and Adolescents' Health (2016-2030). New York: United Nations; 2015.

8   Day TL, Ruysen H, Gordeev VS, Gore-Langton GR, Boggs D, Cousens S, et al. "Every Newborn Birth Indicator Research Tracking in Hospitals" (EN-BIRTH) Observational Study Protocol in Tanzania, Bangkadesh and Nepal: Validating indicators for coverage and quality of maternal and newborn health care. J Glob Health. 2019;9:010902. doi:10.7189/jogh.09.010901

9   Moxon SG, Ruysen H, Kerber KJ, Amouzou A, Fournier S, Grove J, et al. Count every newborn; a measurement improvement roadmap for coverage data. BMC Pregnancy Childbirth. 2015;15 Suppl 2:S8. Medline:26391444 doi:10.1186/1471-2393-15-S2-S8

10 World Health Organization. WHO technical consultation on newborn health indicators: every newborn action plan metrics. Ferney Voltaire, France: 3-5 December 2014. Geneva: World Health Organization; 2015.

11 Lawn JE, Blencowe H, Pattinson R, Cousens S, Kumar R, Ibiebele I, et al. Stillbirths: Where? When? Why? How to make the data count? Lancet. 2011;377:1448-63. Medline:21496911 doi:10.1016/S0140-6736(10)62187-3

12 Lawn JE, Blencowe H, Oza S, You D, Lee AC, Waiswa P, et al. Every Newborn: progress, priorities, and potential beyond survival. Lancet. 2014;384:189-205. Medline:24853593 doi:10.1016/S0140-6736(14)60496-7

13 United Nations Children's Fund. Statistics and Monitoring: Multiple Indicator Cluster Surveys. Available: https://www.unicef.org/statistics/index_24302.html. Accessed: 1/2/2018.

14 International ICF. Demographic and Health Survey. Demographic and Health Surveys. Available: http://www.dhsprogram.com/. Accessed: 1 February 2018.

15 Blanc AK, Wardlaw T. Monitoring low birth weight: an evaluation of international estimates and an updated estimation procedure. Bull World Health Organ. 2005;83:178-85. Medline:15798841

16 Boerma JT, Weinstein KI, Rutstein SO, Sommerfelt AE. Data on birth weight in developing countries: can surveys help? Bull World Health Organ. 1996;74:209-16. Medline:8706237

17 Robles A, Goldman N. Can accurate data on birthweight be obtained from health interview surveys? Int J Epidemiol. 1999;28:925-31. Medline:10597993 doi:10.1093/ije/28.5.925

18 Sedgh G, Filippi V, Owolabi O, Singh SD, Ashew I, Bankole A, et al. Insights from an expert group meeting on the definition and measurement of unsafe abortion. Int J Gynaecol Obstet. 2016;134:104-6. Medline:27062249 doi:10.1016/j.ijgo.2015.11.017

19 Ghana Statistical Service (GSS), Ghana Health Service (GHS), and Macro International. Ghana Maternal Health Survey 2007. Calverton, Maryland, USA: GSS, GHS, and Macro International; 2009.

20 Ghana Statistical Service (GSS), Ghana Health Service (GHS), and ICF Macro. Ghana Demographic and Health Survey 2008. Accra, Ghana: GSS, GHS, and ICF Macro; 2009.

21 Stanton C. Perinatal Mortality in the Philippine: An investigation into the Use of Demographic Survey Data for the Study of Perinatal Mortality and its Determinants. PhD Thesis. Baltimore, Maryland: School of Hygiene and Public Health; 1996.

22 Espeut D, Becker S. The validity of birth and pregnancy histories in rural Bangladesh. J Health Popul Nutr. 2015;33:17. Medline:26825676 doi:10.1186/s41043-015-0027-8

23 Haws RA, Mashasi I, Mrisho M, Schellenberg J, Darmstadt GL, Winch PJ. "These are not good things for other people to know": How rural Tanzanian women's experiences of pregnancy loss and early neonatal death may impact survey data quality. Soc Sci Med. 2010;71:1764-72. Medline:20541305 doi:10.1016/j.socscimed.2010.03.051

24 Johnson K, Grant M, Khan S, Moore Z, Armstrong A, Sa Z. Fieldwork-related factors and data quality in the Demographic and Health Surveys program. DHS Analytical Studies No. 19. Calverton, Maryland, USA: ICF Macro; 2009.

25 Biswas A, Rahman F, Eriksson C, Halim A, Dalal K. Social Autopsy of maternal neonatal deaths and stillbirths in rural Bangladesh: qualitative exploration of its effect and community acceptance. BMJ Open. 2016;6:e010490. Medline:27554100 doi:10.1136/bmjopen-2015-010490

26 Boyden JY, Kavanaugh K, Issel M, Eldeirawi K, Meert K. Experiences of African American parents follwoing perinatal or pediatric death: a litterature review. Death Stud. 2014;38:374-80. Medline:24666143 doi:10.1080/07481187.2013.766656

27 Ellis A, Chebsey C, Storey C, Bradley S, Jackson S, Flenady V, et al. Systematic review to understand and improve care after stillbirth: a review of parents' and healthcare professional experinces. BMC Pregnancy Childbirth. 2016;16:16. Medline:26810220 doi:10.1186/s12884-016-0806-2

28 EN-INDEPTH Technical Secretariat. ENAP & INDEPTH Research Protocol Design Workshop. Kampala, Uganda. 15-17 June2016.

29 Kadobera D, Waiswa P, Peterson S, Blencowe H, Lawn J, Kerber K, et al. Comparing performance of methods used to identify pregnant women in the Iganga-Mayuge Health and Demographic Suirveillance Site, Uganda. Glob Health Action. 2017;10:1356641. Medline:28799450 doi:10.1080/16549716.2017.1356641

30 INDEPTH; Maternal Newborn Health Working Group. 2010. Available: http://www.indepth-network.org/groups/working-groups/maternal-and-newborn-health. Accessed: 1/2/2018.

31 INDEPTH. INDEPTH Network. 2016. Available: http://www.indepth-network.org/about-us. Accessed: 1/2/2018.

32 The World Bank. Survey Solutions CAPI/CAWI platform: Release 5.26. Accessed: 1 February 2018.

33   Machiyama K, Casterline J, Mumah J, Huda F, Obare F, Kabiru C, et al. Reasons for unmet need for family planning, with attention to the measurement of fertility preferences: protocol for a multi-site cohort study. Reprod Health. 2017;14:23. Medline:28183308 doi:10.1186/s12978-016-0268-z

34   ICF. Demographic and Health SurveyInterviewer's Manual. Rockville, Maryland: ICF; 2017.

35   The World Bank. Survey Solutions Manuals. 2018. Available: http://support.mysurvey. solutions. Accessed: 1/2/2018.

36   Liu L, Kalter H, Chu Y, Kazmi N, Koffi A, Amouzou A, et al. Understanding Misclassification between Neonatal Deaths and Stillbirths: Empirical Evidence from Malawi. PLoS One. 2016;11:e0168743. Medline:28030594 doi:10.1371/journal.pone.0168743

37   Hill K, Choi Y. Neonatal mortality in the developing world. Demogr Res. 2006;14:429-52. doi:10.4054/DemRes.2006.14.18

38   Channon AA, Padmadas SS, McDonald JW. Measuring birth weight in developing countries: does the method of reporting in retrospective surveys matter? Matern Child Health J. 2011;15:12-8. Medline:20063179 doi:10.1007/s10995-009-0553-3

39   Johnson BR, Mishra V, Lavelanet F, Khosla R, Ganatra B. A global database of abortion laws, policies, health standards and guidelines. Bull World Health Organ. 2017;95:542-4. Medline:28670021 doi:10.2471/BLT.17.197442

40   Machiyama K, Baschieri A, Dube A, Crampin M, Glynn J, French N, et al. An assessment of Childbearing Preferences in Northen Malawi. Stud Fam Plann. 2015;46:161-76. Medline:26059988 doi:10.1111/j.1728-4465.2015.00022.x

41   United Nations Children's Fund. Every Child's Birth Right: Inequities and trends in birth registration. New York: UNICEF; 2013.

42   United Nations Children's Fund. A Passport to Protection. A guide to birth registration programming. New York: UNICEF; 2013.

Measuring postnatal care contacts for mothers and newborns: An analysis of data from the MICS and DHS surveys

Agbessi Amouzou[1,2], Vrinda Mehra[2], Liliana Carvajal–Aguirre[2], Shane M. Khan[2], Deborah Sitrin[3], Lara ME Vaz[4]

[1] Johns Hopkins Bloomberg School of Public Health, Baltimore, Maryland, USA
[2] Data and Analytics Section, Division of Data, Research and Policy, UNICEF, New York, USA
[3] JHPIEGO, Baltimore, Maryland, USA
[4] Department of Global Health, Save the Children, Washington DC, USA

Background The postnatal period represents a vulnerable phase for mothers and newborns where both face increased risk of morbidity and death. WHO recommends postnatal care (PNC) for mothers and newborns to include a first contact within 24 hours following the birth of the child. However, measuring coverage of PNC in household surveys has been variable over time. The two largest household survey programs in low and middle–income countries, the UNICEF–supported Multiple Indicator Cluster Surveys (MICS) and USAID–funded Demographic and Health Surveys (DHS), now include modules that capture these measures. However, the measurement approach is slightly different between the two programs. We attempt to assess the possible measurement differences that might affect comparability of coverage measures.

Methods We first review the standard questionnaires of the two survey programs to compare approaches to collecting data on postnatal contacts for mothers and newborns. We then illustrate how the approaches used can affect PNC coverage estimates by analysing data from four countries; Bangladesh, Ghana, Kygyz Republic, and Nepal, with both MICS and DHS between 2010–2015.

Results We found that tools implemented todate by MICS and DHS (up to MICS round 5 and up to DHS phase 6) have collected PNC information in different ways. While MICS dedicated a full module to PNC and distinguishes immediate vs later PNC, DHS implemented a more blended module of pregnancy and postnatal and did not systematically distinguish those phases. The two survey programs differed in the way questions on postnatal care for mothers and newbors were framed. Subsequently, MICS and DHS surveys followed different methodological approach to compute the global indicator of postnatal contacts for mothers and newborns within two days following delivery. Regardless of the place of delivery, MICS estimates for postnatal contacts for mothers and newbors appeared consistently higher than those reported in DHS. The difference was however, far more pronounced in case of newborns.

Conclusions: Difference in questionnaires and the methodology adopted to measure PNC have created comparability issues in the coverage levels. Harmonization of survey instruments on postnatal contacts will allow comparable and better assessment of coverage levels and trends.

The postnatal period, days and weeks following childbirth, is a vulnerable phase in the lives of mothers and newborns. Deaths within the first month of life represent 45% of all under–five deaths [1] and of these, far too many occur within the first week of birth. In 2015, nearly one million neonatal deaths occurred on the day of birth and close to two million newborns died in the first week of life [2]. Women too face an increased risk of morbidity and death after delivery. Maternal complications such as bleeding and sepsis following childbirth are responsible for over one–third of the maternal deaths worldwide [3]. To support mothers and newborns during this critical phase, postnatal care (PNC) was identified as a critical need by the World Health Organization (WHO) in 1997 [4]. In 2004, this recommendation was again highlighted in WHO's guidelines for pregnancy, childbirth, postnatal and newborn care [5]. Postnatal care guidelines were recently reviewed to recommend the number, timing and content of postnatal care contacts. WHO recommends the first postnatal contact within 24 hours of birth, followed by three additional contacts on day 3, between days 7–14 and six weeks after birth. In case of facility based deliveries, newborns should receive an immediate check at birth, full clinical assessment around one hour after birth and before discharge [6].

Recent research estimates that increased coverage of postnatal interventions, along with quality interventions from preconception to birth can save 1.9 million neonatal deaths annually. [7]. Postnatal care home visit from a trained provider within two days of delivery can lead to 30–40% reduction in neonatal mortality [8,9]. Given the significance of postnatal period and the effectiveness of postnatal care, it was essential that its coverage is measured and monitored at global and country level. In 2010, the countdown to 2015 called on the importance of developing and expanding the measurement and availability of data on PNC [10]. More recently with the launch of the United Nations Global Strategy for Women's, Children's and Adolescent's Health [11] and the Lancet Every Newborn Series in 2014 [12] the international community has agreed on new frameworks for global monitoring of MNCH targets. These recent frameworks which include Every Newborn Action Plan (ENAP) and Ending Preventable Maternal Mortality (EPMM) have included and prioritized postnatal care as a core coverage monitoring indicator.[11,13,14].

Although there is consensus on the importance of care during this period, the definition and measurement of PNC contacts with the mother and newborn have been a challenge. With regard to definition, an important issue described by the Newborn Technical Working Group deals with timing of postnatal care [15]. There is a lack of consensus among experts as to when the intrapartum period ends and the postnatal period begins. Other studies have analyzed the validity and reliability of respondents' answers regarding the timing of postnatal health check [16–18]. Timing of postnatal health check has typically ranged from minutes to days. Thus, many of these contacts may be part of the routine intrapartum care rather than distinct postnatal care contacts [15,16]. The confusion in the timing and content of PNC also led to further challenges in the measurement from household surveys. To measure, PNC, it is essential to convey appropriately a clear understanding to the respondent of what interventions are considered PNC, the timing, location (facility or outside facility) and provider of the interventions.

Large–scale, nationally representative household surveys such as the UNICEF–supported Multiple Indicator Cluster Surveys (MICS) [19] and the USAID–funded Demographic and Health Surveys (DHS) [20] now systematically collect data on PNC in their standard tools. Both survey programs report on the global postnatal care indicator for mothers and newborns which is defined as the "postnatal health check for the mother (or newborn) within two days of delivery". However, there are differences in the survey tools with MICS round four introducing a detailed module on PNC, tested in consultation with the Newborn Technical Working Group [15,21]. A couple of studies have raised the difference in MICS and DHS protocols along with their potential implications on MNCH coverage indicators, and called for greater attention to harmonizing the indicators [15,22]. With regards to PNC, there has not been a systematic assessment comparing the measurement approaches implemented by MICS and DHS, the two largest source of population–based MNCH coverage data in low and middle–income countries, so it has not been clear how questionnaire differences may affect the level and interpretation of PNC coverage.

The aim of the present study is to assess the data on postnatal care of mothers and newborns collected by MICS and DHS and compare PNC measures. In the first part of this paper, we compare the standard questionnaires of MICS and DHS. To illustrate and further study how differences in questionnaires may affect coverage levels, we then review the computation approach of the PNC coverage indicators in four countries with available data from both surveys.

DATA AND METHODS

Data

The data for this study come from standard individual women's questionnaires used in MICS and DHS. The questionnaires were obtained from the website of these survey progams [23,24]. The MICS survey program works in rounds and is currently in its round six. DHS is implemented in phases and is currently in its seventh phase. PNC questions are asked to women age 15–49 years with a last live birth in the recent past, generally the past two to five years. Questions are asked regardless of whether the child is still alive or not.

For the quantitative assessment of data on postnatal care, we first used estimates on postnatal care coverage within two days of delivery for women and children from all available DHS and MICS reports during the period 2010–2015. We then identified six countries that had a MICS and a DHS survey of the 60 countries with DHS and/or MICS during this period. The selection of six countries namely, Bangladesh, Ghana, Kyrgyz Republic, Malawi, Nepal and Zimbabwe was intended to be illustrative rather than representative of countries across the two survey programs. Out of these, we retained four countries because the DHS survey in Malawi and Zimbabwe in 2010 and 2011 respectively, did not collect all the required information on postnatal contacts of mothers and newborns. Survey sample sizes in the four countries examined are included in **Table 1**.

Table 1. *Countries included in the analysis, data sources and sample sizes*

Country	MICS			DHS		
	Year	Number of households	Number of women (15–49 years)	Year	Number of households	Number of women (15–49 years)
Bangladesh	2012–2013	55 120	29 599	2014	17 989	18 245*
Ghana	2011	12 150	10 963	2014	12 841	10 963
Kyrgyzstan	2014	7 190	6 995	2011	8 208	8 286
Nepal	2014	13 000	14 936	2011	11 353	12 918

DHS – Demographic and Health Surveys, MICS – Multiple Indicator Cluster Surveys
*Data was collected only on ever married women.

Statistical analysis

We first described the coverage of postnatal care within two days of delivery for mothers and newborn using all available and consistent data from MICS and DHS reports during the period 2010–2015. Then for each survey program, we reviewed the model questionnaires starting from four 4 for DHS and round three for MICS, when questions on PNC were first introduced in each programme. We examined the wording of the PNC questions asked to mothers and the reference populations used. We finally compared data collected on postnatal contacts using questionnaires from MICS round five and DHS phase 6 as these survey rounds had quantitative data available at the time of analysis and mapped the algorithm of measurement of postnatal contacts across the 2 survey programs. We could not include data from the latest MICS round six and DHS phase 7 surveys as no databases on these revised tools were available at the time of completion of this analysis. The observed difference in questionnaires was then used to investigate any difference in the PNC indicator values across the two survey programs.

Focusing on the four countries listed above, we then carried out a quantitative description of variables on postnatal contact and timing of health check from MICS and DHS data sets. To investigate sources of differences between surveys, we calculated coverage of any PNC separately for mothers and newborns and for facility and non–facility births, then distinguished "immediate checks" and "postnatal care visits". Immediate checks refer to women who gave birth in a health facility and who received a check before discharge or to women who gave birth outside a health facility in presence of a birth attendant (health professional or trained birth attendant) and who had a check before the attendant left. A "postnatal care visit" is considered occurring after discharge or after the birth attendant has left or any check for women who gave birth without an attendant. A postnatal health check refers to either of those checks and is accounted for in the measurement of the PNC indicator [25]. We then calculated the global indicator of postnatal care within two days after birth. The global indicator as reported in survey reports was calculated separately for institutional and non–institutional births by consistently excluding postnatal health checks by a relative, family or friends. Our estimates for postnatal care of mothers and newborn differ from the survey report in case of Bangladesh DHS 2014 as the latter reports on postnatal health checks by only medically trained providers among live births in last three years while we follow a standardized approach of assessing postnatal care among live births in two years preceding the survey.

We then used the data collected in these 4 surveys to investigate the distribution of timing of health checks for mothers and newborns. Both survey programs report time of postnatal health checks in units of hours, days or weeks. However, for the purposes of this analysis, timing of postnatal health check was computed and assessed in terms of days, going from to 42 days.

Ethical review

Data used in this study come from publicly available data which are anonymized and therefore no ethical approval was sought. The Institutions that collected the data are responsible for securing the appropriate ethical approval prior to data collection.

RESULTS

PNC Coverage patterns

Figure 1 shows the coverage of postnatal care within two days for mothers and newborns, using all available consistent data from MICS and DHS surveys between 2010–2015. The figure compares PNC for mothers and newborns separately for DHS (A) and for MICS (B), and for different set of countries. The figure indicates variable levels of coverage across countries but highlights two important features. On the one hand, for DHS data, coverage levels of PNC appear higher for mothers than for newborns for all countries. On the other hand, for MICS, coverage of PNC appears fairly similar for mothers and for newborns, with newborns appearing to have a slight advantage over mothers in some countries (Tunisia, Saint Lucia, Zimbabwe and Malawi and Guinea–Bissau). The differential patterns between MICS and DHS persist in countries, such as Ghana and Kyrgyz Republic that had both types of surveys within the period examined.

Measuring PNC in DHS

Table 2 provides the evolution of introduction of PNC questions in DHS questionnaires by phase, and specific questions introduced. PNC questions were first introduced in phase 4 questionnaire in 1997. These questions were asked only to women who delivered outside a health facility. No attempts were made to measure PNC of newborns. In 2003, a new phase questionnaires were introduced (phase 5) which extended the PNC questions to all women regardless of place of delivery. In addition, questions on PNC for newborn were collected for the first time . However, they were asked only about facility births. From 2008, the phase 6 questionnaires extended PNC questions to all women and newborns, regardless of place of delivery. In addition, effort was made to ensure correct understanding of women's health check by the respondent by stating during the interview examples of actions that would be considered a health check.

A

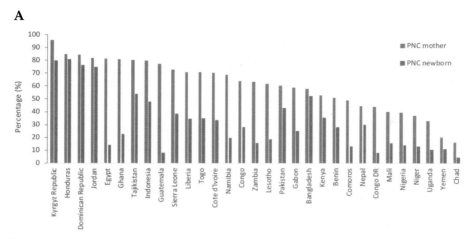

B

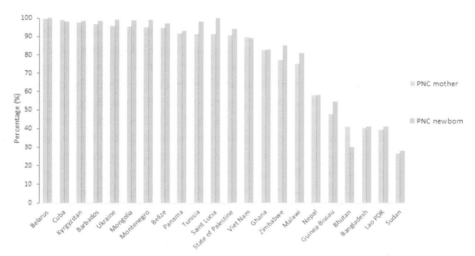

Figure 1. *Coverage of postnatal care within two days of delivery for mothers and newborns, Demographic and Health Surveys (DHS) and Multiple Indicator Cluster Surveys (MICS) (2010–2015).* **A.** *DHS data.* **B.** *MICS.*

The current phase 7 questionnaires introduced since 2013, continue to ask PNC questions of all women and newborns, but with additional questions to increase accuracy. Examples of what constitute a health check was provided for both women and newborns. Each category of respondents (ie, women with facility delivery who were checked before discharge, those who were not checked while in facility, and those who delivered outside a facility) has a separate set of questions investigating postnatal care for mothers and new-

Table 2. *Overview of PNC data collected in Demographic and Health Surveys (DHS)*

	Phase 4 (1997–2003)		Phase 5 (2003–2008)		Phase 6 (2008–2013)		Phase 7 (2013–2018)	
	Facility births	All home births	Facility births	All home births	Facility births	All home births	Facility births	All home births
Postnatal care: Women								
Timing of 1st check	X	Yes	Yes	Yes	Yes	Yes	Yes	Yes
Provider of 1st check	X	Yes	Yes	Yes	Yes	Yes	Yes	Yes
Place of 1st check	X	Yes	Yes	Yes	No	No	Yes	Yes
Postnatal care: Newborn								
Timing of 1st check	X	X	X	Yes	Yes	Yes	Yes	Yes
Provider of 1st check	X	X	X	Yes	Yes	Yes	Yes	Yes
Place of 1st check	X	X	X	Yes	Yes	Yes	Yes	Yes
Content of check	X	X	X	X	X	X	Yes	Yes

X – Information not collected in the survey

borns. For the first time in this round, women who delivered and were checked in a health facility before discharge are once again asked questions about any check on health, time, provider and location of health checks following discharge to capture a subsequent postnatal health check. Similarly, questions about any postnatal health check of the newborn after discharge are asked of women with a facility delivery. As a result, the current phase of DHS may provide data on an additional postnatal health check for facility births. Another substantial addition in this round of survey is questions on content of PNC for mother and newborn. All women, whether they delivered in or outside a health facility are asked if a health care provider examined the cord, measured temperature, counseled on danger signs, and observed breastfeeding within two days of birth of the baby.

Measuring PNC in MICS

Table 3 describes measurement of PNC in MICS questionnaires. MICS introduced standard PNC questions in a module referred to as "Postnatal Health Checks" during the fourth round of the survey starting from 2009, although there were few prior surveys that had included limited PNC questions based on countries' specific initiatives. The MICS4 module collected detailed information on postnatal health contacts after delivery and distinguished an immediate health check from a postnatal visit for all mothers and births regardless of place of delivery. The module was developed following consultation with the Newborn Indicators Technical Working Group, coordinated by Save the

Table 3. *Overview of postnatal care (PNC) data collected in Multiple Indicator Cluster Surveys (MICS)*

Postnatal care: Women & Newborn	MICS 1–3 (1993–2009)	MICS 4 (2009–2013)			MICS 5 (2013–2016)			MICS 6 (2017–ongoing)		
		Facility births	Assisted home births	Unassisted home births	Facility births	Assisted home births	Unassisted home births	Facility births	Assisted home births	Unassisted home births
Immediate check:										
Time of check	X	No	No	X	No	No	X	No	No	X
Provider of check	X	No	No	X	No	No	X	No	No	X
Place of check	X	Yes	Yes	X	Yes	Yes	X	Yes	Yes	X
Postnatal visit:										
Time of 1st visit	X	Yes	Yes	Yes	Yes	Yes	Yes	Yes	Yes	Yes
Place of 1st visit	X	Yes	Yes	Yes	Yes	Yes	Yes	Yes	Yes	Yes
Provider of 1st visit	X	Yes	Yes	Yes	Yes	Yes	Yes	Yes	Yes	Yes
Content of PNC visit	X	X	X	X	X	X	X	Yes	Yes	Yes

X – Information not collected in the survey

Children. Since MICS4, the PNC modules have been fairly consistent for both women and newborn. The latest round (MICS 7), initiated from 2017, introduced questions on PNC content, similar to the DHS questionnaires.

Implications for calculation of the global PNC indicator

Differences in the PNC questions between the two surveys programs have led to differences in the methodological approach used to compute the coverage of the PNC within two days after delivery, a potential source of incomparability (**Table 4**). To calculate this indicator, MICS distinguishes immediate check from PNC visits (post discharge or after attendant left in case of non–institutional deliveries) for mothers and newborns up to two days after delivery. A woman or newborn is then considered as having received PNC within two days after birth if an immediate check or a PNC visit occurred within these two days. DHS on the other hand, does not make this distinction and includes only the first health check after delivery that may occur anytime between birth

Table 4. *Comparison of postnatal care (PNC) indicator measured in Demographic and Health Surveys (DHS) phase 6 and Multiple Indicator Cluster Surveys (MICS) round 4–6 questionnaires*

DATA COLLECTED	DHS	MICS
Respondents:		
	Institutional births	Institutional births
	Non–institutional births	Non–institutional births with attendants
		Non–institutional births without attendants
Global indicator for postnatal care for mothers:		
Numerator	Number of women aged 15–49 years who received a health check within 2 days after delivery	Number of women aged 15–49 years who received a health check while in facility or at home following delivery, or a post–natal care visit within 2 days after delivery
Denominator	Total number of women aged 15–49 years with a live birth in the 2 years preceding the survey **(DHS changed reference period from five to two years)**	Total number of women aged 15–49 years with a live birth in the 2 years preceding the survey
Global indicator for postnatal care for newborns:		
Numerator	Number of last live births in the last 2 years who received a health check within 2 days after birth	Number of last live births in the last 2 years who received a health check while in facility or at home following delivery, or a post–natal care visit within 2 days after birth
Denominator	Total number of last live births in the last 2 years **(DHS changed reference period from five to two years)**	Total number of last live births in the last 2 years
First PNC contact	Unable to differentiate immediate health check from later postnatal visit	Able to distinctly assess and measure immediate health check from postnatal visit
Provider of first check	Yes	No, implied for institutional deliveries
Place of first check	Yes	Yes
Timing of first check	Yes	No
Duration of stay in facility	Yes	Yes
Postnatal visit	No	Yes, including timing, location and provider of first PNC visit
Content of PNC	Yes (starting in Phase 7)	Yes, starting in round 6

and two days following delivery, regardless of whether it was the immediate check or the later PNC visit (see Figure S1 and S2 in **Online Supplementary Document**). However, from phase 7 onwards DHS, questions separating out immediate check (pre–discharge check) from a later postnatal visit (post–discharge check) were introduced.

Assessment of the questionnaires from MICS 4 or 5 and DHS phase 6 further reveals that though the wording of questions about postnatal care of women are fairly similar across the two survey programs such as providing examples of a health check, a fundamental difference exists in the way questions are framed for postnatal care of newborns. While MICS asks about immediate health check and postnatal visits for the newborn without a specific reference period, DHS' questions on PNC for newborns considers checks within two months following the birth of the baby. However, in the most recent versions of the DHS (DHS phase 7) and MICS questionnaires, questions about postnatal care for women and newborns are closely aligned for institutional births but remain inconsistent for non–institutional births.

Comparing PNC coverage and timing between surveys

Table 5 and **Table 6** show measures of PNC respectively for women and newborns, comparing MICS and DHS results in the four countries. The pattern explained above, of broadly similar coverage of PNC for women between the two types of surveys and largely different coverage of PNC for newborns is seen in these four countries. Using MICS data, which allows us to distinguish

Table 5. *Postnatal care for women across Demographic and Health Surveys (DHS) and Multiple Indicator Cluster Surveys (MICS)*

	BANGLADESH		GHANA		KYRGYZSTAN		NEPAL	
Women with non–institutional births:								
	DHS 2014	MICS 2012–13	DHS 2014	MICS 2011	DHS 2012	MICS 2014	DHS 2011	MICS 2014
n	1932	5391	572	825	5	11	1143	894
Any postnatal care	46.9	26.2	53.7	57.1	NR		13.7	20.6
Immediate health check	NA	22.1	NA	47.2	NA		NA	16.3
Postnatal visit	NA	8.7	NA	21.9	NA		NA	7.2
Postnatal health check within 2 d of delivery	42.4	24.5	44.9	50.9	NR		11.3	18.4
Women with institutional births:								
n	1272	2461	1691	1703	1686	1648	888	1130
Any postnatal care	92.7	78.4	95.9	97.7	98.5	99.2	88.5	90.6
Immediate health check	92.2	76.5	95.2	97.5	98.3	99.1	87.8	90.5
Postnatal visit	NA	17.8	NA	26.6	NA	55.6	NA	17.0
Postnatal health check within 2 days of delivery	86.8	76.9	93.4	97.5	96.3	99.1	87.3	90.6
All women (check within 2 days)	60.1	40.4	81.2	82.3	95.9	97.8	44.5	57.9

NA – question not asked, NR – analysis not reported due to small sample size

Table 6. *Postnatal care for newborn across Demographic and Health Surveys (DHS) and Multiple Indicator Cluster Surveys (MICS)*

	BANGLADESH		GHANA		KYRGYZSTAN		NEPAL	
Non–institutional births:								
	DHS 2014	MICS 2012–13	DHS 2014	MICS 2011	DHS 2012	MICS 2014	DHS 2011	MICS 2014
n	1932	5391	572	825	5	11	1143	894
Any postnatal care	51.7	25.9	66.6	62.3	48.8	59.6	30.0	22.1
Immediate health check	NA	20.9	NA	47.4	NA	29.8	NA	15.0
Postnatal visit	NA	11.3	NA	35.9	NA	54.6	NA	11.7
Postnatal health check within 2 days of delivery	41.5	23.8	16.5	54.0	48.8	59.6	9.6	17.6
Institutional births:								
n	1272	2461	1691	1703	1686	1648	888	1130
Any postnatal care	81.7	83.3	73.4	97.9	89.5	99.9	68.5	91.2
Immediate health check	NA	80.5	NA	97.1	NA	99.7	NA	90.6
Postnatal visit	NA	26.6	NA	44.3	NA	94.9	NA	22.3
Postnatal health check within 2 days of delivery	74.3	80.9	24.9	97.1	80.0	99.7	56.5	90.6
All births (check within 2 days)	54.5	41.2	22.8	83.1	79.8	98.5	30.1	57.7

NA – question not asked, NR – analysis not reported due to small sample size

between immediate (pre–discharge) checks and (post–discharge) postnatal visits, we see a higher proportion of newborns receiving a postnatal visit compared to women, while coverage of the immediate check is not very dissimilar for women and newborns.

In **Figure 2** and **Figure 3**, we assess the distribution of timing of health check for women and newborn in Ghana, respectively for DHS and MICS. From the

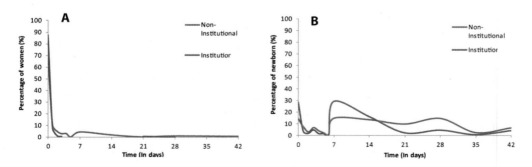

Figure 2. *Timing of health check, Ghana Demographic and Health Surveys (DHS) 2014.* **A.** *Women.* **B.** *Newborn.*

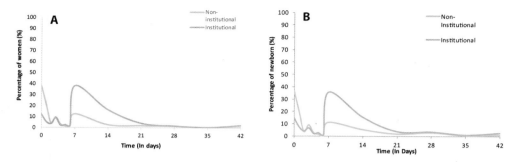

Figure 3. *Timing of postnatal visit, Ghana Multiple Indicator Cluster Surveys (MICS) 2011.* **A.** *Women.* **B.** *Newborn.*

DHS, most women appear to report a health check for themselves within the first days following delivery, most of the first day for institutional deliveries. However for their newborn, the reported coverage is much lower overall and the bimodal distribution (at day 0 and day 7) indicates that a substantial number of women report PNC on day 7 rather than within the first two days. For MICS, the figures include only the distribution of timing of the post–discharge or postnatal visit for women and newborn as the survey does not collect information on timing of immediate health check. The distribution of timing of postnatal visit is nearly identical for the mother and the newborn regardless of place of delivery.

DISCUSSION

Postnatal care is one of the essential strategies recommended for scale–up in many countries to improve health outcomes for women and newborn. The proportion of women receiving postnatal care within two days of delivery and the proportion of newborns receiving postnatal care within two days of delivery are the global consensus indicators for monitoring the coverage of this practice by countries. While enormous progress has been made in the past decade to accurately measure these indicators through household surveys, monitoring of levels and trend require consistent measurement across survey programs, time and geographies. We reviewed the way data on PNC indicators have been collected and the methodology used for their computation focusing on the two largest household survey programs, MICS and DHS. Results showed that the two survey programs have not measured the PNC indicator consistently, both in the way the questions are framed and the approach used for computation of this indicator. MICS dedicated a detailed standalone module to collect information on PNC for mother and newborn and included details that try to capture immediate checks following delivery from subsequent postnatal visit following discharge from health facility (in case of facility delivery) or when the attendant has left (in case of out–of facility deliveries with health professional or trained birth attendant). Their approach and questions used are similar for mothers and newborns. The calculation approach of the PNC indicators for either mothers or newborns thus captures occurrence of an immediate and/or a later postnatal visit occurring within the two–days window. By segmenting the postnatal period, this approach aims to better trigger the memory of the respondent toward a more accurate response. Consequently, coverage levels based on this approach tend to be higher than that of the DHS, and similar for both women and newborns.

DHS, on the other hand, implements a blended pregnancy and PNC module and measures the indicator differently for mothers and newborns. It does not systematically distinguish the immediate vs postnatal visit. Furthermore, for newborns, PNC questions in DHS refer to a check in the two month period following birth. The resulting coverage measures show a much lower PNC rate for newborns compared to women. We suspect that when mothers are asked during interviews about PNC of their newborn within the two months follow-ing the delivery, they are more likely to recall the most recent visit, which is likely to fall outside the first two days, resulting in an under–estimation of the coverage indicator. We indeed found a divergence in the distribution of timing of postnatal checks in DHS, with women reporting most immediate care for themselves (thus resulting in high coverage of PNC) while for their newborn, a substantial number of women tend to report the check at day 7, resulting in lower coverage of PNC within two–day of delivery for newborns. Because such two–month reference window is not applied to women themselves, they are likely to report more accurately a check that occurred within two days of delivery, especially given pre–discharge questions were specified. However, the confusion between when the intrapartum period ends and the postnatal period begins means that the immediate health check may also be capturing immediate intrapartum checks not necessarily considered as postnatal health check. A qualitative study in Malawi and Bangladesh suggested that women may potentially be reporting on a routine intrapartum check rather than a distinct postnatal contact [15,16]. This may result in overestimation of PNC measures in women for DHS and in both women and newborns for MICS.

While our analysis does not constitute a validation of one approach vs the other, a clear and most actionable implication is for MICS and DHS to coordi-nate and align the measurement of such critical indicators to improve comparability between measures coming from the two survey programs. Until such alignment occurs, measures produced will not be comparable. There are also increasing calls for going beyond measures of contact such as PNC to incorporate measure of content interventions received by mothers and newborns during these contacts [26,27]. A simple measure of contact does not provide any indication of the quality of care received, the duration and contents of such contacts. The most recent MICS round 6 and DHS phase 7 have both included a number of questions on the content of the first check within the first 2 days following birth, including cord examination, weight and temperature assessment, breastfeeding counseling and observation and counseling on symtpoms that cause a mother to take a newborn to health care. These efforts must also be guided by clear recommendation from the maternal and newborn community on content of PNC and its quality. The recent revisions to the DHS and MICS tools to improve alignment in the measurement of PNC indicators and incorporate information on PNC content is a welcome step toward filling these data gaps. However, the currents tools are still not fully aligned on PNC measurement, especially for out–of–facility deliveries.

Furthermore, more studies must to be carried out to validate reports from mothers on intrapartum and postpartum care during household survey to help fine tune the measurement tools.

Disclaimer: *The findings and conclusions in this report are those of the authors and do not necessarily represent the official position of the respective organization.*

Funding: *The analysis in this paper was partly supported by the Bill & Melinda Gates Foundation through the Countdown to 2015.*

Authorship contributions: *AA conceived and designed the analysis plan, VM carried out data analysis and wrote initial draft, LC, SMK, JF, DS, LV reviewed plan of analysis and early drafts; all authors reviewed and approved final draft.*

Competing interests: *The authors completed the Unified Competing Interest form at www.icmje.org/coi_disclosure.pdf (available upon request from the corresponding author), and have no competing interest to disclose.*

References

1 UNICEF. Committing to Child Survival: A promise renewed - Progress report 2015. New York: UNICEF; 2015.

2 United Nations Inter-agency Group for Child Mortality Estimation (IGME). Levels and Trends in Child Mortality: Report 2015. New York: UNICEF; 2015.

3 Say L, Chou D, Gemmill A, Tuncalp O, Moller AB, Daniels J, et al. Global causes of maternal death: a WHO systematic analysis. Lancet. 2014;2:e323-33. Medline:25103301

4 World Health Organization. Postpartum Care of the Mother and Newborn: a practical guide. Geneva: World Health Organization; 1998.

5   World Health Organization. Pregnancy, childbirth, postpartum and newborn care: a guide for essential practice. Geneva: World Health Organization; 2004.

6   World Health Organization. WHO recommendations on postnatal care of mother and newborn 2013. Geneva: World Health Organization; 2014.

7   Bhutta ZA, Das JK, Bahl R, Lawn JE, Salam RA, Paul VK, et al. Can available interventions end preventable deaths in mothers, newborn babies, and stillbirths, and at what cost? Lancet. 2014;384:347-70. Medline:24853604 doi:10.1016/S0140-6736(14)60792-3

8   Baqui AH, Ahmed S, El Arifeen S, Darmstadt GL, Rosecrans AM, Mannan I, et al. Effect of timing of first postnatal care home visit on neonatal mortality in Bangladesh: A observational cohort study. BMJ. 2009;339:b2826. Medline:19684100 doi:10.1136/bmj.b2826

9 Baqui AH, Arifeen SE, Williams EK, Ahmed S, Mannan I, Rahman SM, et al. Effectiveness of home-based management of newborn infections by community health workers in rural Bangladesh. Pediatr Infect Dis J. 2009;28:304-10. Medline:19289979 doi:10.1097/INF.0b013e31819069e8

10 World Health Organization and UNICEF. Countdown to 2015 decade report (2000–2010): taking stock of maternal, newborn and child survival. Geneva: World Health Organization; 2010.

11 Commission on Information and Accountability. Keeping Promises, Measuring Results: Commission on Information and Accountability for Women's and Children's Health. Geneva: World Health Organization; 2011.

12 Lawn JE, Blencowe H, Oza S, You D, Lee AC, Waiswa P, et al. Every Newborn: progress, priorties and potential beyond survival. Lancet. 2014;384:189-205. Medline:24853593 doi:10.1016/S0140-6736(14)60496-7

13 World Health Organization. Every Newborn Action Plan Metrics: WHO technical consultation on Newborn health indicators. Geneva: World Health Organization; 2015.

14 USAID. Ending Preventable Maternal Mortality: USAID Maternal Health Vision for Action Evidence for Strategic Approaches. 2015 Available: https://www.usaid.gov/sites/default/files/documents/1864/MH%20Strategy_web_red.pdf. Accessed: 30 October 2017.

15 Moran AC, Kerber K, Sitrin D, Guenther T, Morrissey CS, Newby H, et al. Measuring Coverage in MNCH: Indicators for Global Tracking of Newborn Care. PLoS Med. 2013;10:e1001415. Medline:23667335 doi:10.1371/journal.pmed.1001415

16 Yoder P, Rosato M, Mahmud R, Fort A, Rahman F, Armstrong A, et al. Women's recall of delivery and neonatal care in Bangladesh and Malawi: a study of terms, concepts, and survey questions. Calverton (Maryland): ICF Macro. 2010. Available http://www.measuredhs.com/pubs/pdf/QRS17/QRS17.pdf. Accessed: 30 October 2017.

17 Requejo JH, Newby H, Bryce J. Measuring Coverage in MNCH: Challenges and Opportunities in the Selection of Coverage Indicators for Global Monitoring. PLoS Med. 2013;10:e1001416. Medline:23667336 doi:10.1371/journal.pmed.1001416

18 Liu L, Li M, Yang L, Ju L, Tan B, Walker N, et al. Measuring coverage in MNCH: a validation study linking population survey derived coverage to maternal, newborn, and child health care records in rural China. PLoS One. 2013;8:e60762. Medline:23667429 doi:10.1371/journal.pone.0060762

19 UNICEF. Statistics and monitoring: Multiple Indicator Cluster Surveys. Available: http://mics.unicef.org/surveys. Accessed: 30 October 2017.

20 The DHS Program. Demographic and Health Surveys. Available: https://dhsprogram.com/. Accessed: 30 October 2017.

21 UNICEF. Multiple Indicator Cluster Surveys: Indicators for Global Reporting. Available: http://mics.unicef.org/tools?round=mics4. Accessed: 30 October 2017.

22 Hancioglu A, Arnold F. Measuring Coverage in MNCH: Tracking Progress in Health for Women and Children Using DHS and MICS Household Surveys. PLoS Med. 2013;10:e1001391. Medline:23667333 doi:10.1371/journal.pmed.1001391

23 UNICEF. Statistics and monitoring: Multiple Indicator Cluster Surveys. Available: http://mics.unicef.org/tools. Accessed: 30 October 2017.

24 The DHS Program. Demographic and Health Surveys. Available: https://dhsprogram. com/What-We-Do/Survey-Types/DHS-Questionnaires.cfm. Accessed: 30 October 2017.

25 Warren C, Daly P, Toure L, Mong P. Postnatal care. In: The Partnership for Maternal Newborn and Child Health. Opportunites for Africa's newborns. Practical data, policy and programmatic support for newborn care in Africa. Chap 4. Pp 79-90. Available: http://www.who.int/pmnch/media/publications/aonsectionIII_4.pdf. Accessed: 30 October 2017.

26 Marchant T, Tilley-Gyado RD, Tessema T, Singh K, Gautham M, Umar N, et al. Adding Content to Contacts: Measurement of High Quality Contacts for Maternal and Newborn Health in Ethiopia, North East Nigeria, and Uttar Pradesh, India. PLoS One. 2015;10:e0126840. Medline:26000829 doi:10.1371/journal.pone.0126840

27 Hodgins S, D'Agostino A. The quality–coverage gap in antenatal care: toward better measurement of effective coverage. Glob Health Sci Pract. 2014;2:173-81. Medline:25276575 doi:10.9745/GHSP-D-13-00176

Evidence from household surveys for measuring coverage of newborn care practices

Deborah Sitrin[1], Jamie Perin[2], Lara ME Vaz[1], Liliana Carvajal–Aguirre[3], Shane M Khan[3], Joy Fishel[4], Agbessi Amouzou[2,3]

[1] Department of Global Health, Save the Children, Washington DC, USA
[2] Institute for International Programs, Johns Hopkins School of Public Health, Baltimore, Maryland, USA
[3] Data and Analytics, Division of Data, Research and Policy, UNICEF, New York, New York, USA
[4] ICF, Rockville, Maryland, USA

Background Aside from breastfeeding, there are little data on use of essential newborn care practices, such as thermal protection and hygienic cord care, in high mortality countries. These practices have not typically been measured in national household surveys, often the main source for coverage data in these settings. The *Every Newborn* Action Plan proposed early breastfeeding as a tracer for essential newborn care due to data availability and evidence for the benefits of breastfeeding. In the past decade, a few national surveys have added questions on other practices, presenting an opportunity to assess the performance of early breastfeeding initiation as a tracer indicator.

Methods We identified twelve national surveys between 2005–2014 that included at least one indicator for immediate newborn care in addition to breastfeeding. Because question wording and reference populations varied, we standardized data to the extent possible to estimate coverage of newborn care practices, accounting for strata and multistage survey design. We assessed early breastfeeding as a tracer by: 1) examining associations with other indicators using Pearson correlations; and 2) stratifying by early breastfeeding to determine differences in coverage of other practices for initiators vs non–initiators in each survey, then pooling across surveys for a meta–analysis, using the inverse standard error as the weight for each observation.

Findings Associations between pairs of coverage indicators are generally weak, including those with breastfeeding. The exception is drying and wrapping, which have the strongest association of any two interventions in all five surveys where measured; estimated correlations for this range from 0.47 in Bangladesh's 2007 DHS to 0.83 in Nepal's 2006 DHS. The contrast in coverage for other practices by early breastfeeding is generally small; the greatest absolute difference was 6.7%, between coverage of immediate drying for newborns breastfed early compared to those who were not.

Conclusions Early initiation of breastfeeding is not a high performing tracer indicator for essential newborn care practices measured in previous national surveys. To have informative data on whether newborns are getting life–saving services, standardized questions about specific practices, in addition to breastfeeding initiation, need to be added to surveys.

Every year, 2.7 million babies die during the first month of life, largely from preventable causes [1]. The World Health Organization has prioritized several newborn care practices that could be used at home or facility to prevent many of these unnecessary deaths – thermal care to prevent hypothermia, hygienic cord and skin care to prevent infections, and early and exclusive breastfeeding [2]. Strong evidence on the mortality impact of specific practices is mostly unavailable, but the benefits are likely substantial. Delphi–based expert panels suggested clean postnatal practices could reduce deaths due to infections by 40% [3] and thermal care could reduce deaths due to preterm complications by 20% [4]. More robust evidence exists for the impact of early and exclusive breastfeeding, with a recent cohort trial finding late breastfeeding initiators had higher neonatal mortality (41% if initiated 2–24 hours after birth, 79% if more than 24 hours after birth) and infant mortality, which persisted even in exclusively breastfed babies, suggesting both early and exclusive breastfeeding independently reduce mortality [5].

Despite the importance of these behaviors, most countries do not have coverage data to know if they are practiced. Very few national health information systems collect data on these practices [6] and national surveys, such as the Demographic and Health Survey (DHS) and the Multiple Indicator Cluster Survey (MICS), usually only include questions on breastfeeding, but not other newborn care practices [7]. The *Every Newborn* Action Plan's (ENAP) Measurement Improvement Roadmap [8] was an important step forward in building momentum for improving measurement on newborn care, though mainly focused on coverage indicators for interventions to manage small or sick newborns, such as Kangaroo Mother Care and infection management. ENAP proposed early breastfeeding as a tracer for essential newborn care — preventive and supportive care all newborns need — due to the strong evidence for breastfeeding and its availability from DHS and MICS. However, the correlation between breastfeeding and use of other newborn care practices has not been examined, so it is not known if breastfeeding coverage corresponds with coverage of other practices. In the absence of data, it is generally assumed coverage of these practices is low in settings with high neonatal mortality. For example, a recent effort to model the impact of improving coverage of various interventions in high–burden countries assumed baseline coverage of clean postnatal practices and simple thermal were each just 11%, while coverage of exclusive breastfeeding at one month was estimated to be 62% (early initiation was not included) [4]. The lack of coverage data for other practices makes it difficult to monitor the effectiveness of strategies to promote them or identify unreached populations [9].

Population–based household surveys, particularly DHS and MICS, are often the main source for intervention coverage data in low– and middle–income countries. In many of these countries, a large proportion of deliveries occur outside health facilities and routine data systems are often weak [10]. Surveys are also used to collect sociodemographic data to identify inequities [11,12]. DHS and MICS measure contacts with the health system during the antenatal, birth, and postnatal periods, but contacts alone are poor indications of the content and quality of care and should not be used as a stand–in for effective coverage of high impact interventions [13,14]. Of the essential newborn care practices, only breastfeeding questions were included in standard DHS and MICS questionnaires until 2016. However, surveys are adapted to each country and a few national surveys prior to 2016 included additional questions on newborn care, presenting an opportunity to assess the performance of breastfeeding initiation as a tracer for essential newborn care practices.

This study first examines how DHS and MICS from 2005–2014 have asked about newborn care practices and standardizes the calculation of indicators, to the extent possible, to examine and compare coverage levels across countries. We then investigate the utility of early initiation of breastfeeding as a tracer indicator for essential newborn care. This analysis is especially important as countries weigh the need to include additional questions on newborn care into their next national survey. While both DHS and MICS recently included additional standardized newborn indicators in their model questionnaires based on global consensus around indicators that could be collected in household surveys (**Table 1**), most questions are optional and countries must choose to include them [15,16].

METHODS

We reviewed publicly available DHS and MICS reports from 2005–2014 to identify surveys capturing newborn care practices in addition to breastfeeding. Once surveys were identified, analysis proceeded with two primary components, the first descriptive and the second to examine relationships between indicators of coverage. Twelve national surveys in eight countries (four in South or Southeast Asia, three in sub–Saharan Africa, one in western Asia)

Table 1. *New questions in DHS (Phase 7) and MICS6 related to newborn care practices*

DHS Women's Model Questionnaire:
434 Immediately after the birth, was (NAME) put on your chest?
434A Was (NAME)'s bare skin touching your bare skin?
DHS Optional Newborn Module:
NB1 Was (NAME) wiped dry within a few minutes after birth?
NB2 How long after the birth was (NAME) bathed for the first time?
NB3 CHECK PLACE OF DELIVERY
NB4 What was used to cut the cord? (non–institutional births only)
NB5 Was it new or had it ever been used before? (non–institutional births only)
NB5A Was it boiled before it was used to cut the cord? (non–institutional births only)
NB6 Was anything applied to the stump of the cord at any time?
NB7 What was applied?
CH1 CHECK SUBSTANCES APPLIED TO CORD
CH2 Was chlorhexidine applied to the stump at any time?
CH3 How long after the cord was cut was chlorhexidine fist applied?
CH4 For how many days was chlorhexidine applied to the stump?
CH5 How many times per day was chlorhexidine applied to the stump: once a day, twice a day, three times a day, or four or more times a day?
MICS6 Questionnaire for Individual Women:
MN23 Immediately after the birth, was (*name*) put directly on the bare skin of your chest? [WITH PHOTO OF SKIN–TO–SKIN POSITION]
MN24 Before being placed on the bare skin of your chest, was the baby wrapped up?
MN25 Was (*name*) dried or wiped soon after birth?
MN26 How long after the birth was (*name*) bathed for the first time?
Recommended only for countries with high NMR, large programs on cord care, large proportion of non–facility births:
MN27 Check MN20: Was the child delivered in a health facility?
MN28 What was used to cut the cord? (non–institutional births only)
MN29 Was the instrument used to cut the cord boiled or sterilised prior to use? (non–institutional births only)
MN30 After the cord was cut and until it fell off, was anything applied to the cord?
MN31 What was applied to the cord?

were found that measured at least one indicator for immediate newborn care in addition to initiation of breastfeeding. Three countries (Bangladesh, Nepal, and Armenia) had more than one survey and therefore the potential to compare coverage over time. **Table 2** briefly describes all twelve surveys by the number of births recorded in the two years prior to each survey, the proportion of births occurring in non–institutional settings, and the proportion of Caesarean births. We compared how questions were asked in different surveys based on the following criteria: 1) wording of questionnaire items, 2) how responses were quantified, 3) target population of interest (eg, facility or home births), 4) reference period (eg, in the two or three years preceding survey), and 5) birth subset (all births in reference period or only most recent birth).

Table 2. *Twelve nationally representative household surveys that included measures of essential newborn care beyond breastfeeding*

Country	Year	Type	Number of House-holds Surveyed	Number of Births in Past Two Years	Number (%) of Non–Institu-tional Births in Past Two Years	Number (%) of Cesarean Births in the Past Two Years
Armenia	2005	DHS	4022	621	8 (1%)	59(10%)
Armenia	2010	DHS	3535	675	1 (0%)	90(13%)
Bangladesh	2007	DHS	8583	2469	1949 (79%)	262(11%)
Bangladesh	2011	DHS	14068	3483	2337 (67%)	648(19%)
Bangladesh	2014	DHS	14228	3283	1932 (59%)	805(25%)
Ghana	2014	DHS	6062	2517	698 (28%)	282(11%)
India	2005	DHS	76010	20837	9585 (46%)	2438(12%)
Malawi	2014	MICS	20772	7576	563 (7%)	412(5%)
Nepal	2006	DHS	6672	2270	1817(80%)	58(3%)
Nepal	2011	DHS	7874	2103	1156(55%)	127(6%)
Nigeria	2013	DHS	23364	13570	8345(61%)	326(2%)
Timor–Leste	2009	DHS	7516	4006	3107(78%)	74(2%)

DHS – Demographic and Health Survey, MICS – Multiple Indicator Cluster Survey

We estimated coverage of newborn care practices as defined by each survey, and then, to the extent possible, standardized indicators across surveys. Our standardized indicators are defined in **Table 3**, which also shows the comparability of these definitions to data that will be collected with the new DHS and MICS questionnaires. Given differences in wording and answer options, indicator numerators could not be perfectly harmonized across surveys. For example, the timing of interventions was recorded as an exact amount in some surveys, and as timing relative to other events in other surveys.

We standardized indicator denominators by recall period and population, using the shortest reference period across surveys (last birth in the two years preceding survey), and the smallest common reference population (births that were delivered at home). We used these standard populations and definitions to estimate coverage, accounting for strata and the multistage survey design in each case [17,18]. Once we standardized these coverage estimates, we examined their levels across countries and across time for multiple surveys in a single country.

We then examined the associations between various coverage indicators among those surveyed to determine how well early breastfeeding functions as a tracer for other indicators of newborn care. We used Pearson correlations to describe associations between each pair of estimated coverages [19]. We expected *a priori* that some types of coverage would be positively correlated: that is, an

Table 3. *Standardized definitions of newborn coverage indicators used for this analysis and comparability to DHS (Phase 7) module and MICS6*

INDICATOR GROUP	STANDARDIZED DEFINITION	COMPARABILITY TO DHS (PHASE 7)	COMPARABILITY TO MICS6
Breastfeeding initiation	Put to breast within one hour of birth	Comparable	Comparable
Thermal care	Dried within five minutes of birth OR before delivery of the placenta	Somewhat comparable DHS does not reference exact time or delivery of placenta' to 'DHS does not use five minutes or delivery of placenta for time reference	Somewhat comparable (MICS6 does not reference exact time or delivery of placenta' to 'MICS6 does not use five minutes or delivery of placenta for time reference)
	Wrapped within five minutes of birth OR before delivery of the placenta	Not comparable (not collected in DHS)	Not comparable (MICS6 asks if baby wrapped up before placed on mother's bare chest.)
	Neonate put on the belly or breast before delivery of the placenta OR directly on the bare skin of your chest	Somewhat comparable (DHS specifies bare skin must be touching in 2 questions)	Somewhat comparable (MICS specifies bare skin must be touching in 2 questions and a photo)
	Not given a bath in the first 24 h after birth	Comparable	Comparable
Hygienic cord care	A new or sterilized (boiled) instrument was used to cut the umbilical cord, or a clean delivery kit was used	Somewhat comparable (DHS does not ask about clean delivery kit)	Somewhat comparable (MICS6 does not ask about clean delivery kit)
	No substance was applied to the umbilical cord after it was cut	Comparable	Comparable

DHS – Demographic and Health Survey, MICS – Multiple Indicator Cluster Survey

infant receiving a specific intervention would be likely to receive a related intervention (for example, an infant who is dried may often be wrapped as well). We also hypothesized some coverages would be negatively correlated, indicating that an infant would be less likely to receive an intervention if another intervention had been received (for example, wrapping and placing skin–to–skin). We examined relationships with breastfeeding within one hour of delivery for each indicator at the individual level with these correlations.

We also aimed to describe the coverage of newborn care practices among newborns breastfed early and examine if it differed from coverage among newborns who did not breastfeed early. For each survey, we stratified by breastfeeding within one hour, and compared coverage estimates for each group. We statistically determined the difference between the coverage of newborn care practices for these groups. We then pooled observed differences across surveys in a meta–analysis. In order that different surveys contribute to the estimate overall, we used the inverse standard error as the weight for each observation. Using inverse standard errors as weights allows survey estimates with more uncertainty to contribute less information to overall estimates, per standard meta–analysis protocol. [20].

RESULTS

Two surveys (Nepal 2011 and Nigeria 2013) measured all seven indicators considered for the second part of our analysis (**Table 4**). Surveys in Armenia and Ghana each only collected one indicator of interest other than breastfeeding. The India 2005 survey included multiple newborn care practices, but asked as a composite question so it is not possible to tease out coverage of each practice. Except for early breastfeeding, coverage for other practices was often measured only for home births. However, in Armenia, Ghana, Malawi, and Bangladesh (2007 and 2014), some items were measured for all non–Caesarean

Table 4. *Immediate newborn care indicators included for each of twelve recent surveys*

	Armenia	Armenia	Ghana	India	Malawi	Bangladesh			Nepal		Nigeria	Timor–Leste
Indicator	2005	2010	2014	2005	2014	2007	2011	2014	2006	2011	2013	2014
Breastfed within first hour	A	A	A	A	A	A	A	A	A	A	A	A
Dried				H	H	H	A	H	H	H	H	H
Wrapped			A	H		H	A		H	H	H	
Bathed after 24 h				H	H	H	H	A	H	H	H	H
New or boiled blade				H	H	H	H	H	H	H	H	H
Nothing applied to cord					H	H	H	A	H	H	H	H
Skin to skin or baby put on mother's belly or chest	A	A						A		H	H	

A – Surveys that collected data for all non– Caesarean last births, H – Surveys that collected data only for home births

births. Questions and response categories for each survey can be found in Table S1 in **Online Supplementary Document** and respective coverage estimates from official survey reports in Figure S1 in **Online Supplementary Document**, though coverage is generally not comparable across surveys due to question wording, their reference populations, and time periods. We excluded four surveys from further analysis given the limited amount of comparable indicators – Armenia (2005 and 2010), Ghana, and India – leaving eight surveys for standardized coverage measurement.

We used the standardized definitions for most recent births which were also in non–institutional settings in the two years preceding the survey. Resulting coverage estimates are shown with 95% confidence intervals in **Figure 1** and Table S2 in **Online Supplementary Document**. Using a new or boiled instrument to cut the umbilical cord is generally the highest estimated coverage, except in Timor–Leste. Placing the baby skin–to–skin or on the mother's belly or chest was measured in only three of the eight surveys and generally had the

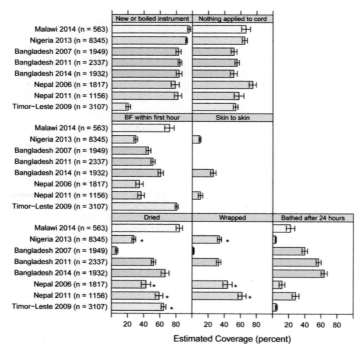

Figure 1. *Standardized coverage estimates for eight national surveys, with 95% confidence limits, for most recent births that were delivered in non–institutional settings in the two years preceding survey. Asterisk indicates that "before placenta delivery" was used for time reference, as opposed to "within five minutes" for drying or wrapping.*

lowest estimated coverage among the newborn care practices. Some measures had wide variation across surveys, such as drying, which ranges from 6.3% in Bangladesh (2007) to 84% in Malawi (2014). Trends in coverage over time can also be inferred from **Figure 1** for the two countries with more than one survey. Drying, wrapping, and delayed bathing increased in both Bangladesh and Nepal. There is no apparent change over time in using a new or boiled instrument in either country. Nepal had no change in early breastfeeding, but Bangladesh had a small increase between 2007 and 2014. For no application to the cord, there is a decline of 17 percentage points (95% confidence interval 6.8–28.0) in Nepal from 2006 to 2011. The 2011 survey added a follow–up question on what was applied to the cord with chlorhexidine as an answer option. Yet chlorhexidine use fails to explain this decrease in dry cord care: changing the 2011 coverage indicator to include nothing *or* chlorhexidine applied resulted in little change in the 2011 coverage estimate (only 1% respond regarding chlorhexidine, so coverage changes from 57.7% to 58.7%). Coverage for dry cord care was unchanged over time in Bangladesh.

We used these standardized coverage estimates in each survey to examine the associations between different newborn care practices at the individual level, to see whether neonates who receive a specific intervention are likely to receive another. We estimated the Pearson correlation between coverage indicators for each survey for all available measurements. The resulting associations are shown in **Figure 2** as a map, where interventions that tend to occur together are darker green the more they are positively correlated, and interventions that tend to occur separately are darker red the more they are negatively correlated. (See Table S3 in Online **Supplementary Document** for correlations.) Associations between pairs of newborn coverage indicators are generally weak, including those with breastfeeding. The exception is for drying and wrapping, which have the strongest association of any two interventions in all five surveys where they were measured, with an estimated correlation of 0.65 in Nigeria 2013; 0.83 and 0.73 in Nepal 2006 and 2001, respectively; and 0.47 and 0.58 in Bangladesh 2007 and 2011. Other correlations above 0.2 are between being placed "skin–to–skin" (includes babies placed mother's belly or chest in Nigeria and Nepal, babies placed on the mother's bare skin in Bangladesh) and both drying and wrapping in Nigeria 2013 and Nepal 2011. In Nigeria, infants placed "skin–to–skin" are somewhat more likely to have been dried (correlation 0.42) and wrapped (correlation 0.35). In Nepal 2011, infants placed "skin–to–skin" are also more likely to have been dried (correlation 0.24) and wrapped (correlation 0.23). Skin–to–skin and drying were not related in Bangladesh 2014 (correlation 0.013), while wrapping was not asked.

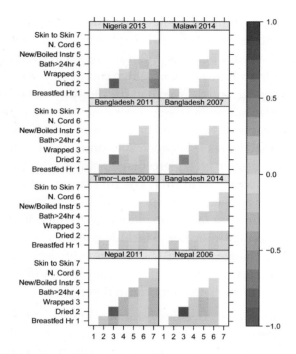

Figure 2. *Correlation matrices for eight national surveys and seven standardized coverage indicators, for most recent births in the two years preceding survey that were delivered in non–institutional settings. Strong correlations are indicated by dark green, negative correlations are indicated by red.*

In addition to these associations, we stratified surveys by early breastfeeding and examined the differences in coverage for those with early breastfeeding compared to those who did not breastfeed early. The estimated contrasts in coverage are shown for each survey and pooled across surveys in **Table 5**. The contrast in coverage between neonates by early breastfeeding is generally small, with pooled differences less than seven percentage points for each indicator. The absolute difference in coverage of essential practices between newborns breastfed early and those who were not ranged from less than one percent for having nothing applied to the cord to a difference of 6.7% for drying.

DISCUSSION

With little guidance on how to measure care for newborns and, until recently, little global attention on newborn health, few nationally representative household surveys have measured newborn care practices. In a ten year period,

Table 5. *Newborn coverage indicators, by survey and early breastfeeding status. The differences in coverage between those with early breastfeeding and those without was meta–analyzed for the pooled difference across surveys*

Description	Survey	Among those breastfed in first hour Estimate (%)	Among those not breastfed in first hour Estimate (%)	Differ-ence (BF – not BF) Estimate (%)	95% Confidence interval (%) Lower	Upper
Bathed after 24 h	Malawi 2014	21.6	23.1	–1.5	–12.8	9.9
	Nigeria 2013	4.9	3.2	1.6	0.3	2.9
	Bangladesh 2007	43.3	36.4	6.9	1.3	12.5
	Bangladesh 2011	61.5	52.0	9.5	4.7	14.3
	Bangladesh 2014	66.7	59.0	7.8	1.3	14.3
	Nepal 2006	12.2	10.6	1.6	–2.0	5.3
	Nepal 2011	36.2	24.8	11.3	3.9	18.8
	Timor–Leste 2009	4.6	6.3	–1.7	–4.0	0.6
	Pooled			4.0	1.1	6.9
Dried	Malawi 2014	85.9	79.2	6.7	–3.0	16.4
	Nigeria 2013*	30.3	26.7	3.6	0.1	7.1
	Bangladesh 2007	5.2	7.4	–2.2	–4.6	0.1
	Bangladesh 2011	55.0	48.9	6.2	1.3	11.1
	Bangladesh 2014	69.5	61.8	7.7	2.4	13.0
	Nepal 2006*	49.5	39.5	10.0	3.1	16.9
	Nepal 2011*	64.3	56.0	8.3	1.7	15.0
	Timor–Leste 2009*	67.6	51.5	16.1	10.0	22.1
	Pooled			6.7	2.2	11.2
New or boiled blade	Malawi 2014	96.0	95.4	0.6	–4.0	5.2
	Nigeria 2013	92.5	92.6	–0.1	–2.0	1.9
	Bangladesh 2007	82.5	82.7	–0.2	–4.2	3.8
	Bangladesh 2011	85.2	83.5	1.7	–2.0	5.5
	Bangladesh 2014	82.7	84.7	–1.9	–6.0	2.1
	Nepal 2006	82.0	76.9	5.1	–0.1	10.4
	Nepal 2011	85.7	80.2	5.5	0.1	11.0
	Timor–Leste	21.0	17.2	3.8	–0.4	8.1
	Pooled			1.3	–0.4	3.0
Nothing applied to cord	Malawi 2014	66.2	66.9	–0.7	–10.9	9.5
	Nigeria 2013	60.0	66.7	–6.7	–10.7	–2.8
	Bangladesh 2007	48.0	54.2	–6.1	–11.9	–0.4
	Bangladesh 2011	57.9	52.4	5.5	1.0	10.0
	Bangladesh 2014	49.6	52.7	–3.1	–9.9	3.6
	Nepal 2006	78.3	73.4	4.9	–0.1	9.8
	Nepal 2011	62.7	55.1	7.6	0.3	14.9
	Timor–Leste	52.3	60.2	–7.9	–13.7	–2.1
	Pooled			–0.1	–5.5	3.7

Table 5. *Continued*

		Among those breastfed in first hour	Among those not breastfed in first hour	Differ-ence (BF − not BF)	95% confi-dence interval (%)	
Skin to skin	Nigeria 2013	12.4	8.4	4.1	1.6	6.5
	Bangladesh 2014	25.9	25.8	0.1	−5.1	5.3
	Nepal 2011	13.1	8.7	4.4	0.5	8.4
	Pooled			3.6	1.7	5.5
Wrapped	Bangladesh 2007	1.7	2.1	−0.4	−1.6	0.8
	Bangladesh 2011	32.6	32.9	−0.3	−4.8	4.2
	Nepal 2006†	50.0	41.1	8.9	1.8	15.9
	Nepal 2011†	71.2	56.4	14.8	7.4	22.1
	Nigeria 201†	37.7	32.2	5.6	1.7	9.5
	Pooled			4.9	0.1	9.6

*Dried before delivery of placenta.
†Wrapped before delivery of placenta.

we identified only twelve surveys across eight countries, and several of these surveys asked about few practices. There was inconsistency across surveys in how and to whom newborn care questions were asked, which limits comparability. DHS and MICS have now offered standard questions to improve the consistency of data in coming years.

Early initiation of breastfeeding does not appear to be a high performing tracer indicator for essential newborn care, since it is poorly correlated with the all the other elements of newborn care in this analysis. Nor was there much difference in coverage of other practices when comparing babies who were breastfed within an hour and those who were not. In fact, no single practice was a good predictor of the coverage of other practices. In particular, there was very little correlation between coverage of any thermal care practices and coverage of cord care (and some had negative associations). Only drying and wrapping were highly correlated. Wrapping was not added to the DHS questionnaire because overlap between these two practices was previously seen in program surveys and thus it was deemed unnecessary to collect both [7]. Wrapping and "skin–to–skin" contact also appear to be weakly correlated in Nigeria 2013 and Nepal 2011. However, true skin–to–skin care and wrapping may be mutually exclusive events since a baby that is wrapped will not have exposed skin to place against the mother's bare skin. The correlation found in these two surveys may be explained by the fact that the question (Was the baby placed on the mother's belly/breast before delivery of the placenta?) did not specify skin–to–skin exposure, unlike how it was asked in Bangladesh 2014 or will be asked in future DHS and MICS (as shown in **Table 2**).

Indicator validation studies in Mozambique, Kenya, and Mexico have shown mothers have difficulty accurately reporting newborn care practices, though findings were inconsistent with drying, breastfeeding within an hour, and skin–to–skin contact meeting validation criteria in at least one study but not in other studies [21–24]. The weak correlations found in this study could be due to invalidity of indicators. On the other hand, newborn care practices may simply be inconsistently applied, which could also explain why correlations are weak with the exception of drying and wrapping. These past validation studies also had some design limitations. They could not include home birth observations, while this study was limited to only analyzing home births. Since validation for home births presents feasibility and ethical problems, triangulation of intervention coverage data with outcomes for babies born at home could be used to assess the plausibility of coverage levels. In addition, the validation studies did not ask all questions the same way they are asked in the new DHS and MICS questionnaires (including the question on initiation of breastfeeding) and did not examine the umbilical cord care practices now measured in DHS and MICS. While recall bias is a flaw of household surveys, most countries have no other means to assess coverage of these life–saving interventions. To have informative data on whether newborns are getting the services they need, questions about specific practices, aside from breastfeeding initiation, need to be added to surveys.

Nonetheless, surveys can mitigate bias due to mothers not witnessing certain practices, understanding terminology or what they saw being done for their baby, or remembering what was done, especially if a long time has passed since their last birth [25,26]. New DHS and MICS questions were developed and field tested to improve reporting. For example, validation research found a two–item question sequence improved mothers' reporting of skin–to–skin care, resulting in DHS and MICS adding two questions to their new questionnaires [22]. MICS6 also included a photo of a baby in the skin–to–skin position to help mothers understand the question. Mothers have also been shown to have difficulty reporting the exact timing of practices [16], so DHS and MICS limit the number of practices for which the mother is asked to give timing (breastfeeding initiation and first bathing) and simplified the need to recall precise timing by not requiring recall in minutes for practices within the first hour after birth. Instrument sterilization in facilities likely occurs outside the delivery room and many mothers who delivered in a facility report not knowing if the instrument was clean when asked [7], so DHS and MICS only ask questions on cutting the umbilical cord to mothers who delivered at home. Standard probes and follow–on questions could further improve recall and reduce use of leading questions [26,27], though not yet part of DHS or MICS interviewer manuals [28,29].

Many of the surveys reviewed in this paper only asked questions on newborn care for home births. The new DHS and MICS questionnaires are now designed to ask most questions for both facility and home births, because omitting facility births creates an information gap, especially as facility delivery rates rise; the exception is on questions on the instrument used to cut the cord [15,16]. In the future, therefore, correlations between newborn care practices for facility births can be examined. At the same time, routine data systems should be strengthened to capture newborn care practices delivered at facility and triangulate with survey data, as well as collect data on services to treat rare complications that cannot be reliably collected through national surveys.

After standardizing indicators to the extent possible, we found reported use of a clean instrument for cutting the cord among non–institutional births was high (around 80% or more) in all countries except Timor–Leste, and remained high over consecutive surveys in Bangladesh and Nepal. Coverage of dry cord care was more moderate, with a decline in Nepal from 75% in 2006 to 58% in 2011. Changing the indicator to include chlorhexidine application could not explain the decline; coverage of chlorhexidine application was low because Nepal only decided to proceed with national implementation of chlorhexidine in late 2011 [30]. As countries adopt the 2013 WHO guidelines recommending chlorhexidine application for newborns born at home in settings with high neonatal mortality [31], the appropriate indicator will be nothing *or* chlorhexidine only applied to the cord stump. Given the interest this new intervention, countries will need to know coverage. Increasing awareness of chlorhexidine may also help reporting accuracy.

Coverage levels for clean cutting and dry cord care practices in the surveys analyzed in this paper are much higher than Bhutta et al's modelled coverage estimate for the general category 'clean postnatal care practices', which was just 11% [4]. Bhutta's definition included handwashing and skin cleansing and did not include hygienic cord care, which likely explains why coverage is so different than what we found in these surveys. At the same time, countries that ask questions about hygienic cord care in national surveys may be more invested in changing these practices, so coverage may be higher than would be found others. The same may not be true for other hygienic postnatal care practices, which may be closer to Bhutta's estimate.

Early breastfeeding was generally moderate (ranging from 30% to 82%) with little change between surveys in Bangladesh and Nepal. These findings were in line with the average across all 75 countries tracked by *Countdown to 2015*, which was 50% [32]. Use of thermal care practices varied across countries, with drying, wrapping, and delayed bathing improving over time in Bangladesh and Nepal. Placing the neonate on the mother's belly or breast or on the mother's bare skin was low (10–25%). Overall, coverage estimates for thermal care practices in these surveys are substantially higher than Bhutta et al's modelled coverage estimate for 'simple thermal care' (11%). Though again, Bhutta's definition was not the same as used in this paper.

As the global community makes new commitments to the health and survival of newborns through the Sustainable Development Goals [33], countries need to know how newborns are cared for, beyond whether they are breastfed early. This study found coverage can vary greatly for different practices as well as differences across countries. There may not be a single way forward to improve the care of newborns, so country level data on multiple newborn care practices are critical. Essential newborn care may have even greater benefit for preterm babies, so having data to guide efforts to improve coverage of all practices will be important to reducing child mortality, now that prematurity is the leading cause of death for children under 5 [1]. New standards in household surveys will increase the availability of coverage estimates for these life–saving interventions for a key vulnerable population.

Acknowledgements: *The authors acknowledge the contribution of Vrinda Mehra And Liliana Carvajal in leading the supplement in which this paper is appearing.*

Disclaimers: *The findings and conclusions in this report are those of the authors and do not necessarily represent the official position of the respective organizations.*

Funding: *Save the Children's Saving Newborn Lives program funded this work.*

Authorship contributions: *DS, JF, AA conceptualized the study. DS reviewed DHS reports for the descriptive analysis. JP conducted quantitative data analysis. DS, JP, LV, LC, SK, AA participated in a workshop to review and interpret preliminary results. DS and JP prepared a first draft of the paper. All authors contributed to subsequent drafts and approved the final version.*

Competing interests: *The authors have completed the Unified Competing Interest form at www.icmje.org/coi_disclosure.pdf (available on request from the corresponding author) and declare no competing interests.*

References

1 Liu L, Oza S, Hogan D, Perin J, Rudan I, Lawn JE, et al. Global, regional, and national causes of child mortality in 2000-13, with projections to inform post-2015 priorities: an updated systematic analysis. Lancet. 2015;385:430-40. Medline:25280870 doi:10.1016/S0140-6736(14)61698-6

2   The Partnership for Maternal. Newborn & Child Health. A global review of the key interventions related to reproductive, maternal, newborn and child health (RMNCH). Geneva: PMNCH; 2011.

3   Blencowe H, Cousens S, Mullany LC, Lee AC, Kerber K, Wall S, et al. Clean birth and postnatal care practices to reduce neonatal deaths from sepsis and tetanus: a systematic review and Delphi estimation of mortality effect. BMC Public Health. 2011;11 Suppl 3:S11. Medline:21501428 doi:10.1186/1471-2458-11-S3-S11

4   Bhutta ZA, Das JK, Bahl R, Lawn JE, Salam RA, Paul VK, et al. Can available interventions end preventable deaths in mothers, newborn babies, and stillbirths, and at what cost? Lancet. 2014;384:347-70. Medline:24853604 doi:10.1016/S0140-6736(14)60792-3

5   NEOVITA study group. Timing of initiation, patterns of breastfeeding, and infant survival: prospective analysis of pooled data from three randomised trials. Lancet Glob Health. 2016;4:e266-75. Medline:27013313 doi:10.1016/S2214-109X(16)00040-1

6   Dwivedi V, Drake M, Rawlins B, Strachan M, Monga T, Unfried K. A review of the maternal and newborn health content of national health management information systems in 13 countires in sub-Saharan Africa and South Asia. Washington, DC: The Maternal and Child Health Ingrated Program. Available: http://www.mchip.net/sites/default/files/13%20country%20review%20of%20ANC%20and%20LandD.pdf. Accessed: 9 April 2017.

7   Moran AC, Kerber K, Sitrin D, Guenther T, Morrissey C, Newby H, et al. Measuring coverage in MNCH: indicators for global tracking of newborn care. PLoS Med. 2013;10:e1001415. Medline:23667335 doi:10.1371/journal.pmed.1001415

8   Moxon SG, Ruysen H, Kerber KJ, Amouzou A, Fournier S, Grove J, et al. Count every newborn; a measurement improvement roadmap for coverage data. BMC Pregnancy Childbirth. 2015;15 Suppl 2:S8. Medline:26391444 doi:10.1186/1471-2393-15-S2-S8

9   Bryce J, Arnold F, Blanc A, Hancioglu A, Newby H, Requejo R, et al. Measuring coverage in MNCH: new findings, new strategies, and recommendations for action. PLoS Med. 2013;10:e1001423. Medline:23667340 doi:10.1371/journal.pmed.1001423

10 Hancioglu A, Arnold F. Measuring coverage in MNCH: tracking progress in health for women and children using DHS and MICS household surveys. PLoS Med. 2013;10:e1001391. Medline:23667333 doi:10.1371/journal.pmed.1001391

11 Barros AJ, Victora CG. Measuring coverage in MNCH: determining and interpreting inequalities in coverage of maternal, newborn, and child health interventions. PLoS Med. 2013;10:e1001390. Medline:23667332 doi:10.1371/journal.pmed.1001390

12 Countdown to. 2015, Health Metrics Network, Unicef, Work Health Organization. Monitoring maternal, newborn and child health: understanding key progress indicators. Geneva: World Health Organization, 2011.

13 Marchant T, Tilley-Gyado RD, Tessema T, Singh K, Gautham M, Umar N, et al. Adding content to contacts: measurement of high quality contacts for maternal and newborn health in Ethiopia, north east Nigeria, and Uttar Pradesh, India. PLoS One. 2015;10:e0126840. Medline:26000829 doi:10.1371/journal.pone.0126840

14 Hodgins S, D'Agostino A. The quality-coverage gap in antenatal care: toward better measurement of effective coverage. Glob Health Sci Pract. 2014;2:173-81. Medline:25276575 doi:10.9745/GHSP-D-13-00176

15 International ICF. Demographic and Health Surveys: Model Woman's Questionnaire. 2015. Available: http://dhsprogram.com/pubs/pdf/DHSQ7/DHS7-Womans-QRE-EN-17May2016-DHSQ7.pdf. Accessed: 26 July 2016.

16 UNICEF. Multiple Indicator Cluster Surveys: Questionnaire for Individual Women. 2017. Available: http://mics.unicef.org/tools. Accessed: 7 April 2017.

17 National Institute of Population Research and Training (NIPORT), Mitra and Associates, Macro International Inc. Bangladesh Demographic and Health Survey 2007. Dhaka and Calverton, 2009.

18 National Statistical Office. Malawi MDG Endline Survey 2014. Zomba, Malawi: National Statistical Office, 2015.

19 Seed P. Confidence intervals for correlations. Stata Tech Bull. 2001;59:27-8.

20 Higgins JP, Thompson SG, Deeks JJ, Altman DG. Measuring inconsistency in meta-analyses. BMJ. 2003;327:557-60. Medline:12958120 doi:10.1136/bmj.327.7414.557

21 Stanton CK, Rawlins B, Drake M, dos Anjos M, Cantor D, Chongo L, et al. Measuring coverage in MNCH: testing the validity of women's self-report of key maternal and newborn health interventions during the peripartum period in Mozambique. PLoS One. 2013;8:e60694. Medline:23667427 doi:10.1371/journal.pone.0060694

22 Blanc AK, Warren C, McCarthy KJ, Kimani J, Ndwiga C. RamaRao S. Assessing the validity of indicators of the quality of maternal and newborn health care in Kenya. J Glob Health. 2016;6:010405. Medline:27231541 doi:10.7189/jogh.06.010405

23 Blanc AK, Diaz C, McCarthy KJ, Berdichevsky K. Measuring progress in maternal and newborn heatlh care in Mexico: validating indicators of health system contact and quality of care. BMC Pregnancy Childbirth. 2016;16:255. Medline:27577266 doi:10.1186/s12884-016-1047-0

24 McCarthy KJ, Blanc AK, Warren CE, Kimani J, Mdawida B, Ndwidga C. Can surveys of women accurately track indicators of maternal and newborn care? A validity and reliability study in Kenya. J Glob Health. 2016;6:020502. Medline:27606061 doi:10.7189/jogh.06.020502

25 Yoder P, Rosato M, Mahmud R, Fort A, Rahman F, Armstrong A, et al. Women's Recall of Delivery and Neonatal Care in Bangladesh and Malawi: A Study of Terms, Concepts, and Survey Questions. Calverton, Maryland, USA: ICF Macro, 2010.

26 Hill Z, Okyere E, Wickenden M, Tawiah-Agyemang C. What can we learn about postnatal care in Ghana if we ask the right questions? A qualitative study. Glob Health Action. 2015;8:28515. Medline:26350434doi:10.3402/gha.v8.28515

27 Salasibew MM, Dinsa G, Berhanu D, Filteau S, Marchant T. Measurement of delayed bathing and early initiation of breastfeeding: a cross-sectional survey exploring experiences of data collectors in Ethiopia. BMC Pediatr. 2015;15:35. Medline:25884185 doi:10.1186/s12887-015-0350-7

28 International I. Demographic and Health Surveys: Interviewer's Manual 2015. Available: http://dhsprogram.com/pubs/pdf/DHSM1/DHS7_Interviewer's_Manual_EN_28Feb2015_DHSM1.pdf. Accessed: 26 July 2016.

29 Unicef. Multiple Indicator Cluster Surveys: Instructions for Interviewers. Available: http://mics.unicef.org/tools#data-collection. Accessed: 26 July 2016).

30 Hodgins S, Pradhan YV, Khanal L, Upreti S. Chlorhexidine for umbilical cord care: game-changer for newborn survival? Glob Health Sci Pract. 2013;1:5-10. Medline:25276511 doi:10.9745/GHSP-D-12-00014

31 World Health Organization. WHO recommendations on postnatal care for mother and newborn. Geneva: World Health Organization, 2013.

32 Requejo J, Victora C, Bryce J. Countdown to 2015: A decade of tracking progress for maternal, newborn and child survival: The 2015 report. Geneva: World Health Organization, 2015.

33 United Nations. Transforming our world: the 2030 Agenda for Sustainable Development. Available: https://sustainabledevelopment.un.org/post2015/transformingourworld Accessed: 26 July 2016.

Appendix 1.

Links to online supplementary materials.

Online supplementary materials to chapter: Gap between contact and content in maternal and newborn care: An analysis of data from 20 countries in sub–Saharan Africa
http://www.jogh.org/documents/issue201702/jogh-07-020501-s001.pdf

Online supplementary materials to chapter: Assessment of health facility capacity to provide newborn care in Bangladesh, Haiti, Malawi, Senegal, and Tanzania
http://www.jogh.org/documents/issue201702/jogh-07-020509-s001.pdf

Online supplementary materials to chapter: "Every Newborn-BIRTH" protocol: observational study validating indicators for coverage and quality of maternal and newborn health care in Bangladesh, Nepal and Tanzania
http://www.jogh.org/documents/issue201901/jogh-09-010902-s001.pdf

Online supplementary materials to chapter: "Every Newborn-BIRTH" protocol: observational study validating indicators for coverage and quality of maternal and newborn health care in Bangladesh, Nepal and Tanzania
http://www.jogh.org/documents/issue201901/jogh-09-010901-s001.zip

Online supplementary materials to chapter: Measuring postnatal care contacts for mothers and newborns: An analysis of data from the MICS and DHS surveys
http://www.jogh.org/documents/issue201702/jogh-07-020502-s001.pdf

Online supplementary materials to chapter: Evidence from household surveys for measuring coverage of newborn care practices
http://www.jogh.org/documents/issue201702/jogh-07-020503-s001.pdf